The Well–Being of Farm Animals

Challenges and Solutions

To the farmers and ranchers who,
through animal husbandry,
renew and preserve our ancient contract
with farm animals

The Well-Being of Farm Animals

Challenges and Solutions

Edited by
G. John Benson
Bernard E. Rollin

Issues in Animal Bioethics Series
Bernard E. Rollin, Series Editor

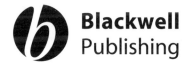

Blackwell
Publishing

G. John Benson received his DVM degree from the University of Illinois in 1971. Following three years of general practice in Petersburg, Illinois, involving primarily beef cattle and swine, he returned to the University of Illinois to pursue a Master's degree and residency in anesthesiology, becoming certified by the American College of Veterinary Anesthesiologists in 1979. He is a past president of the American College of Veterinary Anesthesiologists. Since then he has been a member of the Anesthesia Section in the Department of Veterinary Clinical Medicine and holds joint appointments in the Departments of Veterinary Pathobiology (Comparative Medicine Division) and Veterinary Biosciences (Pharmacology Division). Dr. Benson is presently Professor and Chief of the Anesthesia Section.

Bernard E. Rollin is University Distinguished Professor, Professor of Philosophy, Professor of Biomedical Sciences, and Professor of Animal Sciences at Colorado State University, where he is also University Bioethicist. He earned his BA, Magna cum Laude from the City College of New York, his PhD from Columbia, and was a Fulbright Fellow at the University of Edinburgh. Rollin is the author of 12 books and more than 200 papers dealing with animal ethics, animal consciousness, animal pain, and biotechnology. He has lectured over 800 times in 18 countries. He is the founder of the field of veterinary medical ethics and is a principal architect of 1985 laws protecting laboratory animals.

© 2004 Blackwell Publishing

Blackwell Publishing Professional
2121 State Avenue, Ames, Iowa 50014, USA

Orders:	1-800-862-6657	Fax:	1-515-292-3348
Office:	1-515-292-0140	Web site:	www.blackwellprofessional.com

Blackwell Publishing Ltd   Blackwell Publishing Asia
9600 Garsington Road, Oxford OX4 2DQ, UK   550 Swanston Street, Carlton, Victoria 3053, Australia
Tel.: +44 (0)1865 776868   Tel.: +61 (0)3 8359 1011

Printed on acid-free paper in the United States of America

First edition, 2004

Library of Congress Cataloging-in-Publication Data

The well-being of farm animals : challenges and solutions / edited by
G. John Benson, Bernard E. Rollin.—1st ed.
    p. cm.— (Issues in animal boiethics)
Includes bibliographical references (p.).
   ISBN-13: 978-0-8138-0473-6 (alk. paper)
   ISBN-10: 0-8138-0473-6 (alk. paper)
   1. Animal health. 2. Veterinary medicine. 3. Animal welfare. 4.
Livestock—Social aspects. 5. Animal industry—Moral and ethical
aspects. I. Benson, G. John. II. Rollin, Bernard E. III. Series.
   SF745.W45 2004
   636.089'3—dc22

                                                        2003020487

The last digit is the print number: 9 8 7 6 5 4 3 2

Contents

Contributors

Numbers in brackets following each name refer to chapters.

Michael C. Appleby [16], The Humane Society of the United States, Farm Animals and Sustainable Agriculture, 2100 L Street NW, Washington, DC 20037; mappleby @hsus.org, 301-258-3111, Fax: 301-258-3081

G. John Benson [4] University of Illinois, College of Veterinary Medicine, Dept of Veterinary Clinical Medicine, Urbana, IL 61802; gbenson@cvm.uiuc.edu

Timothy E. Blackwell [12], Veterinary Science, Ontario Ministry of Agriculture and Food, Wellington Place, RR#1, Fergus, Ontario N1M 2W3; tim.blackwell.omaf.gov.on.ca, 519-846-3413

Grahame Coleman [9], Monash University, Dept of Psychology, Room 08, Bldg F6, Caulfield, Victoria 3800, Australia; Grahame.coleman@med.monash.edu.au, +61-3-990-31524, Fax: +61-3-9903-2501

Ian J. H. Duncan [5, 14], University of Guelph, Dept of Animal and Poultry Science, Guelph, Ontario, Canada N1G 2W1; iduncan@uoguelph.ca, 519-824-4120 x53652, Fax: 519-836-9873

David Fraser [3, 15], University of British Columbia, Animal Welfare Program, Faculty of Agricultural Sciences, 2357 Mail Mall, Vancouver, B.C., Canada V6T 1Z4; fraserd @interchange.ubc.ca, 604-822-2040

Ted H. Friend [6], Texas A&M University, Dept of Animal Sciences, MS 2471, College Station, TX 77843; t-friend@tamu.edu, 979-845-5265

Franklyn B. Garry [11], Colorado State University, College of Veterinary Medicine, Dept of Clinical Sciences, Fort Collins, CO 80523; Franklyn.garry@colostate.edu, 970-297-0371

Temple Grandin [7, 8], Colorado State University, College of Veterinary Medicine, Dept of Animal Sciences, Fort Collins, CO 80523; grandin@lamar.colostate.edu

Paul H. Hemsworth [2], University of Melbourne, Animal Welfare Center, Institute of Land and Food Resources, Parkville VIC 3010, Australia; phh@unimelb.edu.au

Cleon V. Kimberling [13], Colorado State University, Dept of Clinical Sciences, Veterinary Teaching Hospital, Fort Collins, CO 80523; Ckimberl@lamar.colostate.edu, 970-491-1281

Robert E. Meyer [17], Mississippi State University, College of Veterinary Medicine, Mississippi State, MS 39762; meyer@cvm.msstate.edu, 662-325-1453

W. E. Morgan Morrow [17], Animal Science, Cooperative Extension Service, North Carolina State University, Raleigh, NC 27695; Morgan_Morrow@ncsu.edu, 919-515-4001

Gerilyn A. Parsons [13], Colorado State University, Veterinary Diagnostic Lab, Veterinary Teaching Hospital, Fort Collins, CO 80523; g.parsons@colostate.edu, 970-491-1248

Bernard E. Rollin [1], Colorado State University, Dept of Philosophy and College of Veterinary Medicine and Biomedical Sciences, Fort Collins, CO 80523; bernard.rollin @colostate.edu, 970-226-3355

Joseph M. Stookey [10], University of Saskatchewan, Western College of Veterinary Medicine, Large Animal Clinical Sciences, Saskatoon, Saskatchewan 57N 5B4; Joseph.stookey@usask.ca, 306-966-7154

Jon M. Watts [10], University of Saskatchewan, Western College of Veterinary Medicine, Large Animal Clinical Sciences, Saskatoon, Saskatchewan 57N 5B4; jon.watts@usask.ca, 306-966-7056

Daniel M. Weary [3, 15], University of British Columbia, Animal Welfare Program, Faculty of Agricultural Sciences, 2357 Main Mall, Vancouver, B.C., Canada V6T 1Z4; Danweary@interchange.ubc.ca, 604-822-3954, Fax: 604-822-4400

Preface

Over the last 30 years, animal treatment has emerged as a major social concern across the Western world. From the proliferation of legislation governing animal research in virtually every civilized society to recent laws raising the value of pets well beyond economic value, social ethics is changing to meet that concern.

While Europe has forged ahead in assuring the welfare of farm animals—witness the Swedish law of 1988, which the *New York Times* called "a bill of rights for farm animals," wherein the Swedish parliament abolished confinement agriculture as we know it in the United States, and European Union regulations—the United States has not yet experienced a major social effort in that direction. This is probably because the U.S. public still believes that farms are the Old McDonald's farms that are nostalgically depicted in children's books, and is ignorant of "factory farming." (How else can one explain one large confinement producer running advertisements for years showing the classic mixed animal barnyard scene, and intoning that he raises "happy chickens"?) Animal activists are working assiduously to raise public awareness; but despite the lessons of Europe, the industry has not instituted reforms except when forced to do so by pressure from PETA (People for the Ethical Treatment of Animals) on chain restaurants and grocers.

Part of the problem is the absence of sound literature on relieving farm animal suffering. A year ago one of us (BR), who had published one of the few extant U.S. books on the welfare of farm animals—*Farm Animal Welfare* (Iowa State University Press, 1995)—was shocked to learn how little research was available on farm animal analgesia despite the many painful procedures done on millions of farm animals, and sought to rectify this lacuna. Rather naively, Rollin looked for a veterinary anesthesiologist as a coeditor. He was again shocked to find that few anesthesiologists wished to risk the wrath of the industry by writing on analgesic regimens, and that there was far too little information for a book. Eventually, he found John Benson, who for 30 years had worked on relieving animal pain, including producing a major textbook of anesthesia and analgesia (Lumm and Jones, 1996, *Veterinary Anesthesia, Third Edition,* Pub. Williams and Wilkens). Benson, who fears no one, willingly agreed that a book on animal suffering was sorely needed and agreed to coedit this volume.

In order to create this volume, we recruited many of the world's finest scholars in the science of animal welfare. We are grateful that no one refused our offer, and all wrote original pieces for this volume. We believe we have thereby collected state-of-the-art, authoritative papers on many of the seminal and practical issues that need to be addressed to reduce farm animal suffering.

This book should be of interest to agriculturalists and animal welfare advocates alike, and particularly to those who actively work with animals. If we have created the groundwork for dialogue on these issues as well as some practical reforms, we will have succeeded in our goals.

We are grateful to our authors for the serious thought and effort that went into their contributions. We are especially appreciative of the efforts of David Rosenbaum, former acquisition editor *extraordinaire,* polymath, partner in dialogue, coach, and cheerleader at Iowa State Press (Blackwell Publishing), without whose enthusiasm and support this book would not have come to be.

I
Theoretical Framework

1

The Ethical Imperative to Control Pain and Suffering in Farm Animals

Bernard E. Rollin

I

It is easy to forget that the concept expressed in the term *profession* extends over many more instances than the usual array of law, medicine, veterinary medicine, and dentistry. If we think of a profession as comprising a group of individuals charged with doing a job deemed of paramount importance by society and given special privileges and autonomy to do that job, we realize that professional ethics is a far more important concept than it is usually considered to be.

Consider a standard example: Veterinarians are charged with ministering to the health of animals, be they companion animals, farm animals, or laboratory animals. To perform that function, they are given special privileges, for example, writing prescriptions and performing surgery. Though these are onerous responsibilities, society is loath to regulate them in detail, since laypeople (among whom are legislators) do not understand what is involved in surgery or prescribing medicine. So, society says to veterinarians, "you regulate yourselves the way we would regulate you if we understood in detail what you do—which we don't. But, we will know if you violate that trust, and if you do, you will pay for that breach of trust by loss of autonomy and having to endure regulations imposed on you by us." A classic example of this situation occurred in the 1980s when society became aware that some veterinarians were cavalierly prescribing antibiotics to animal agriculture for growth promotion. This practice was driving the evolution of bacterial resistance to antibiotics, and potentially endangering human and animal health. At that point, Congress was prepared to legislate an end to veterinarians' writing extra-label prescriptions, a restriction that would have destroyed veterinary medicine as we know it.

Unfortunately, throughout most of the twentieth century, professional ethics has not been seriously studied. It has instead devolved largely into intraprofessional etiquette, dealing with issues such as advertising, criticizing a colleague, fee splitting, and so on. Yet ignoring the true ethical dimensions of professions can lead to loss of the professional autonomy that comes from understanding the scope of professional activity better than legislators do. Despite the clarity of this point, it has been largely ignored. In 2002, in the wake of revelations of abuse of professional authority by accountants in the Enron case (specifically the accounting giant Arthur Andersen), accounting will be more strictly regulated by external authorities. Arthur Andersen abused the fact that no legislation or regulation existed curbing conflict of interest; instead, avoiding such conflict was left to the

3

profession. When it became known to the public that Arthur Andersen audited Enron's books while being highly paid as a local consultant to Enron, creating a patent conflict of interest between the two sides, society felt it could no longer trust the accounting profession to self-regulate. What regulatory rules will emerge is not yet clear, but we can be certain that accounting will lose some of the freedom it previously enjoyed.

The same sort of thing has happened in the last three decades to biomedical and social-scientific researchers using animal subjects and human subjects. In the wake of clear evidence emerging in the 1980s that the animal research profession was not providing the best care possible to research animals, despite protestations to the contrary, society imposed strong federal laws on researchers. More recently, revelations of cavalier treatment by researchers toward human subjects leading to unnecessary death and disease is moving the federal government toward restrictive regulations. For example, in the past, local review committees, chartered by the federal government, prospectively audited research protocols and assumed that researchers would keep their word. Now these rules demand a mechanism by which committees will need to inspect the actual conduct of research, a major erosion of researcher autonomy. Researchers are, we should recall, professionals as defined above. They can, for the sake of advancing scientific knowledge, risk the life, health, and suffering of research subjects, human and animal. Proven failure to meet the moral demands emerging from that privilege brought on draconian external regulation, which, most researchers agree, could have been even worse!

Plainly, agriculture is a profession as defined above—people in agriculture are entrusted with creating the U.S. food supply in a safe, environmentally sound way that also accords with demands regarding animal well-being, a task arguably as important as any of those entrusted to more standard occupations called professions. And perhaps the most overarching demand to all professionals—be they agriculturalists or physicians—is that they operate in accord with the extant and emerging social consensus ethic. We must recall that every society wishes to avoid chaos and anarchy in order to keep social life from being, in Thomas Hobbes's unparalleled phrasing, "nasty, miserable, brutish and short." As a result, those things that are deemed essential to harmonious social life and social justice are encoded in what we may aptly call the *social consensus ethic*. Such moral principles as the prohibition against murder, rape, robbery, theft, perjury, embezzlement, sexual harassment, and the like become, as Plato says, "written large" in laws and regulations, and adherence to them by all members of society, laypeople and professionals, is presupposed.

As societies evolve, moral principles may be added to, or dropped from, the social consensus ethic. For example, before the 1960s, the social ethic left the sale and rental of real property to individuals, or rather to their personal ethic regarding what they viewed as moral and immoral, right and proper. But when society perceives that leaving things up to individual morality leads to widespread unfairness and injustice, it will, as it does in professional ethics, remove the responsibilities in question from the realm of people's personal ethics, and instead encode them in law. For example, when society realized that leaving sale and rental of real estate to an individual's ethics resulted in failure to sell or rent such property to minorities, it removed that privilege from personal ethics and created strict rules, enforced by law, to stop such discriminatory practices. Society may, of course, also move in the other direction, relinquishing social control over choices it decides are best left to personal ethics. Such behaviors as homosexuality or abortion have pretty much been dropped from social control, and relinquished to individuals' personal ethics.

Thus, professionals and individuals wishing to preserve their autonomy must constantly monitor the social ethic to make sure that their behavior accords with changing social ethical concerns in an anticipatory way, lest they lose that autonomy.

It should be patent to anyone who even superficially examines ethical concerns across Western societies that moral concern for animals—how they are treated—and concern for their pain and suffering have been emerging as major issues during the past 30 years. According to both the National Cattlemen's Association and the National Institutes of Health, Congress received more letters, faxes, telephone calls, and so on dealing with animal welfare between 1980 and 1995 than any other issue. In 1991, a poll conducted by *Parents* magazine found that 85 percent of its readers affirmed that animals had rights (*Parents*, 1989).

Whereas, 25 years ago, the U.S. Congress saw no bills dealing with animal welfare, the last few years have witnessed legislative proposals numbering in the scores. According to an official of the American Quarter Horse Association, the largest equine association in the United States, the organization's largest expense in the late 1990s was hiring a research firm to monitor state and local legislation pertaining to equine welfare. In California, a law has been passed making shipping horses to slaughter a felony, as is knowingly selling a horse to someone who will so ship it. Animal cruelty has been made a felony in over 30 states, and some two dozen law schools now include courses in animal law, with numerous legal scholars working to raise the status of animals from property to quasi-personhood. Activist cities like San Francisco and Boulder, Colorado, have floated ordinances declaring that people who have pets are not owners of these animals, but guardians.

Europe has witnessed a steady increase in concern for farm animal welfare in recent years, largely due to careful scrutiny of intensive, industrialized confinement agriculture. Americans are generally surprised at the degree to which factory farming has captured public concern in Europe. Sweden passed a law in 1988 phasing out the high-confinement agriculture we take for granted in North America, which the *New York Times* called a "Bill of Rights for Farm Animals" (*New York Times*, 1988). Britain and the European Union have followed suit, with the latter announcing the elimination of sow stalls within a decade.

No area of animal use has failed to feel the effects of moral concern for animals. Animal circuses have lost the support of the public, with Cirque de Soleil, a show that does not use animals, the most popular in America. The American public's disaffection with wildlife authorities' management of wildlife populations for hunters, spring bear hunts that can lead to the death of a lactating mother bear and the consequent death by dehydration of her cubs, steel-jawed traps, lethal control of predators and pests, and mountain lion hunts have all resulted in what one authority called "management by referendum," with the public, by right of referendum, usurping the job of wildlife managers. Funds for "pest control" are ever-increasingly directed toward contraception and other nonlethal methods.

Somewhat surprisingly, PETA and other groups have found the public generally sympathetic when they target the welfare of aquatic animals, even fish. The fish importing industry was sufficiently concerned with this issue to invite me to lecture to two international meetings two years in a row. Sale of lobsters in Great Britain dropped precipitously until the industry developed a "lobster stunner" so that housewives did not have to drop a live, conscious animal into boiling water. The sale of live fish has precipitated major protests in San Francisco's Chinatown. Disavowal of animal testing for toxicity of cosmetics has propelled the Body Shop into a billion-dollar industry. As early as 1978, the readership of *Glamour Magazine*, when polled, affirmed that a new cosmetic does not justify the animal suffering required to develop it.

Most surprising, perhaps, was the virtually worldwide development of laws protecting laboratory animals, mostly rats and mice. In Switzerland, a law was promulgated by referendum banning animal research, which would have passed, according to polls, had the pharmaceutical industry not spent large sums of money at the last minute defending animal research. Laws in virtually all Western countries now mandate researcher control of animal distress. In many countries (e.g., Britain), an animal suffering intractable pain that cannot be controlled must be killed. (In the United States, the animals *may be* killed at the discretion of the Animal Care and Use Committee at a research institution.) In America, these laws address not only physical pain but also "distress," and they mandate exercise for dogs and environments for nonhuman primates that "enhance their psychological well-being." The National Institutes of Health *Guide to the Care and Use of Laboratory Animals* strongly urges enriching the captive environment for all laboratory animals, and trade journals regularly cover these issues. Zoos, also, have been forced by public concern into taking cognizance of animals' behavioral needs. In Germany, a constitutional amendment passed in the spring of 2002 protects animals from all but the most exigent reasons for inflicting pain.

One could list examples endlessly, but the point has been made. Society is concerned about the pain, suffering, and distress of all animals used for its benefit. The extent of such concern may be gleaned from the dramatic story of U.S. laboratory animal legislation. The research and medical communities were dead set against these laws, as were such ancillary groups as the American Associations of Medical Colleges, Veterinary Colleges, Land Grant Universities, and the pharmaceutical industry. In cleverly orchestrated campaigns, these powerful groups threatened the public with danger to human health if laws protecting research animals passed. Most extraordinary was a film entitled "Will I Be All Right, Doctor?" which said in essence that children's health was threatened by protection of laboratory animals. The public simply did not believe these preposterous claims, and in 1985 two laws were passed to that end.

Why, one may ask, have we not seen a similar furor regarding the protection of farm animals? The answer is simple—public ignorance. For reasons unclear to me, there seems to be a media blackout on issues of farm animal welfare. Even when the swine industry was being examined for environmental despoliations, no allusion was made to the related animal welfare issues. According to reporters I spoke to at the time, editors tend to see animal welfare as "fringe." Neither mass media nor the agricultural press cover these issues, and the ignorance of U.S. farmers and agricultural scientists as well as the general public on these issues in Europe is appalling.

The result is, as Paul Thompson has remarked, that the U.S. public still thinks that farms are Old McDonald's Farm—mixed, extensive, family-run small businesses (Thompson, 1991). For many years, high-confinement poultry producer Frank Perdue helped to perpetuate this misperception by running advertisements showing chickens pecking in a barnyard, complete with red barn and rising red sun, while a voiceover declared, "At Perdue, we raise happy chickens." In short, the public is largely clueless about how food animals are produced, though when the media did cover severe confinement of veal calves, the confinement veal industry was virtually destroyed.

The agriculture industry's response to all of this is curious. Rather than admitting that confinement agriculture raises welfare problems, spokesmen for the industry (but not farmers themselves) tend to fall back on the non sequitur that the public needs to know where its food comes from. "People think bacon and eggs come from the supermarket," I often hear. "We need to show them where it comes from." Needless to say, I have serious doubts about this claim. If people were to tour confinement egg production facilities and see the hens in small cages, debeaked, one sometimes walking and defecating on top of the other in an effort by the industry to get more production per cage; or if people could view confinement swine facilities, with a 600 pound sow forced into a "crate" that measures two and a half feet high by seven feet long by three feet wide (sometimes two feet wide in an effort to force more crates into a barn), where she can't lie down straight, much less turn around, they would not be happy. If they saw newborn baby pigs castrated and tattooed, with teeth clipped all without anesthesia, then saw them raised in pens that get more and more tight as they grow, never seeing daylight and breathing air that sometimes requires that employees wear respirators, they would be even less happy. If they saw pig and chicken shipping and slaughter, I doubt it would make them appreciate the industry more than they do now! What public ignorance entails is a grace period for the confinement industries to clean up their own acts, with Europe for a model. What the emerging ethic for animals demands for farm animals is pretty clear from the examples of Europe and Britain. Before exploring this in depth, however, it behooves us to examine why animal issues have suddenly come into focus internationally.

II

There are several reasons why animal issues have seized the public imagination during the last three decades. Most obvious, perhaps, is demographic change. Although a century ago over half the population made a living producing food, this has dramatically changed. Today, barely 1.7 percent of the population works in production agriculture, with perhaps half of that group or less in animal agriculture. Furthermore, few members of the population have relatives on farms either. As a result, concepts of animals have changed. A hundred years ago, if one ran a word association test on the rural or urban population asking what the word *animal* evokes, people would likely say *horse, cow, work, food*. As late as the 1960s, over 80 percent of veterinarians were employed by agriculture. Now, such veterinarians constitute less than 8 percent of veterinarians, most of whom work in the area of companion animals who are, in fact, the new paradigm for animals in society. (One rancher friend of mine was shocked when, upon bringing a range cow into our veterinary hospital, he was asked by the female and urban students, "What is her name?") Companion animals dominate the social mind, with almost 100 percent of the public claiming to view their pets as "members of the family." Such a paradigm is considerably jarred by farm animals in confinement.

Second, since we are largely removed from animals and animal life, we yearn for closer proximity, interaction, and knowledge. This is supplied by the mass media, who are quite cognizant, as one reporter told me, that "animals sell papers." My cable system has two 24-hour-a-day Animal Planet stations, and many other channels endlessly cover animal stories. (One large-city TV news producer told me that he routinely will begin the news with an animal story teaser and not finish the story until the end of the newscast, to hold viewers.) Recall that when two whales were trapped in an ice floe, they were freed by Soviet icebreakers! Was this an overflowing of Soviet compassion (surely an oxymoron for those who gave us pogroms, Stalin, and the Gulag)? It was rather that someone in the Kremlin was smart enough to realize that releasing the whales was a cheap way to win kudos from the U.S. public. If the U.S. public had been unaware of these whales, the Russians would probably have sent whaling boats, not icebreakers!

Third, the U.S. (and world) public has had 50 years of ethical sensitivity priming. The last 50 years have seen the rise of civil rights for minorities, women's rights, gay rights, children's rights, student rights, patients' rights, the rights of indigenous populations, environmentalism, and the rights of the disabled. Concern about the weakest and most disenfranchised part of human society, animals, was inevitable. Indeed, leaders of activist animal groups often come from other social movements such as civil rights, labor, the women's movement, the gay movement, and so on. These people take seriously the dictum that the morality of a society is best judged by how it treats its least enfranchised. Exploitation of animals is definitely politically incorrect.

Fourth, the nature of animal use changed quickly and dramatically at mid–twentieth century. Historically, the major use of animals in society was agriculture—food, fiber, locomotion, and power. The key to agricultural success was animal husbandry, from the old Norse word *hus/bond*—bonded to one's household. Animal husbandry betokened an ancient and symbiotic contract between humans and domestic animals, perhaps best expressed by western American cattle ranchers, the last large group of husbandmen in the United States, when they intone, "we take care of the animals and they take care of us." One of my colleagues, a rancher and beef specialist, has declared that the worst thing that ever happened to his department was betokened by the name change from Department of Animal Husbandry to Department of Animal Science. Animal husbandry was about putting square pegs into square holes, round pegs into round holes, and creating as little friction as possible while doing so. Animal science is about efficiency and productivity. The husbandman put the animal into optimal conditions of the sort the animal was evolved for, and then augmented the animal's natural ability to survive and thrive by providing the animal with food during famine, water during drought, medical attention, help in birthing, help during natural disasters, and so on. The animals gave us their products, their toil, and sometimes their lives; we gave them better, more comfortable lives. Not only was husbandry reinforced by practicality, it was also taught as an articulated ethic. So powerful was this ethic, that when the psalmist wished to create a metaphor for God's ideal relationship to people, he chose the image of the shepherd in the Twenty-third Psalm: "The lord is my shepherd; I shall not want. He maketh me to lie down in green pastures; he leadeth me beside the still waters. He restoreth my soul." We want no more from God than the shepherd gives his sheep!

This lovely ethic can still be seen among western ranchers, for whom husbandry is as much a way of life as it is a way of making a living. Cowboys routinely spend more on a sick calf than is economically justified; most ranchers and ranch wives will sit up all night with a sick or marginal calf in their kitchen. If this were a matter of economics alone, they would value their labor and sleep time at pennies an hour. Beyond economics, there is generally a strong love for the animals and a strong sense of duty. I know one cowboy who unhesitatingly plunged into a frozen pond to save a calf who had fallen through the ice, and who afterward incurred devastating lung problems. "And I would do it again," he wheezed.

Confinement agriculture sprang up in mid–twentieth century, when values of efficiency and productivity—business values—prevailed over values of husbandry and way of life. Intensification was born of fear that people were forsaking agriculture after the Dust Bowl and the depression. It was born of fear of loss of agricultural workers to better-paying urban jobs. It was born of fear that burgeoning population would encroach on agricultural land and make feeding that population by traditional means untenable. The issue of animal welfare, if considered at all, was erroneously thought to be assured by animal productivity. Alas! This was only true for husbandry agriculture, which, as we said earlier, was about putting square pegs into square holes and creating as little friction as possible. The producer did well if and only if the animal did well. This is not to say that there was no animal pain in husbandry agriculture—that claim is belied by knife castration, branding, and dehorning. But these were short-term insults seen as inevitable and as ones from which the animals recovered rapidly. Confinement agriculture was based on a brand new model, that of using technological sanders to help force square pegs into round holes. Whereas a nineteenth-century attempt to raise a hundred thousand chickens in one building would have ended abruptly with the deaths of the animals, technology gave us antibiotics, vaccines, bacterins, and air-handling systems, which allowed the animals to survive and produce, while still experiencing severely truncated welfare. Such compromised welfare was irrelevant to profitability and productivity of the operation as a whole.

Confinement swine producers do not jump into ponds to save animals. In fact, they don't even treat sick animals; rather they knock them in the head, since the value of each animal is too small to bother with. Although each animal may be miserable, the operation as a whole is economically solvent. No wonder that cowboys hate factory farms! As the president of the Colorado Cattlemen's Association once said at an agricultural meeting, "If I had to raise animals like the veal people do, I'd get the hell out of the business."

The Western world became aware that Old McDonald's Farm had become Old McDonald's Factory in the mid-1960s when journalist Ruth Harrison (Harrison, 1964) published her *Animal Machines* (significantly prefaced by Rachel Carson). Harrison's writings, buttressed by other journalists such as Elspeth Huxley, caused a furor among the British public, whose strong negative reaction led the British government to charter a commission of inquiry, the Brambell Committee (Brambell, 1965), headed by Sir Rogers Brambell. Though having no political authority, the Brambell Committee report immediately became a moral beacon for Britain and Europe when it stated that any agricultural system that failed to allow animals to perform the behaviors dictated by their biological natures was morally unacceptable, morally foreshadowing the Swedish law of 1988, and laying the basis for the conservative (rather than radical!) demand for husbandry we have called the emerging social ethic for animals.

III

The nature of the new ethic that would emerge in response to the new agriculture, as well as to the vastly increased mid-twentieth-century use of animals for research and toxicity testing (a use that violated the fair bargain found in husbandry agriculture, since we burned, poisoned, wounded, and inflicted disease upon animals for our benefit or for the benefit of other animals with no compensatory benefit to the research animals themselves) was quite rational and predictable. I did indeed foresee its development in my writings of the late 1970s and early 80s (Rollin, 1981). The traditional social ethic for animals—embodied in anticruelty laws—presupposed husbandry and thus could not replace it. The anticruelty ethic existed to deal with those (mainly sadists and psychopaths) who were not motivated by self-interest. These laws were directed against sadistic, deviant, intentional, and willful infliction of pain and suffering on an animal for fun or out of perverted desires, not normal social use or consumption of animals. For this reason, these laws could not be shaped to cover research or factory farming or steel-jawed traps. However, if one considers a pie chart representing all the suffering animals currently experience at human hands, one will quickly realize that only a tiny fraction of that chart—1 percent or less, my audiences typically estimate—is the result of deliberate, sadistic cruelty. Most comes, in fact, from the new approaches to agriculture and research enumerated above. It is estimated that U.S. confined broiler chickens go to slaughter with 80 percent of the eight billion produced bruised or fractured. If this is true, we have in that industry about 6.4 billion cases of suffering. Thank heavens, there is probably nothing like that number of acts of deliberate cruelty in the whole world. Thus, a new ethic is needed to replace the connected ethics of husbandry and anticruelty.

It was clear to me, as Plato taught, that new ethics doesn't come from nowhere, but builds on established ethics. It was thus also obvious to me that society would turn to our established ethic for humans to serve as the basis for our newly sought animal ethic. And our human ethic had indeed addressed the fundamental conflict of the good of the majority group of humans against the benefit of the minority. This is a perennial problem in human ethics that recurs in every society. If it benefits society as a whole (i.e., the majority) to tax the wealthy, is it morally acceptable? If the entire society is upset by my verbal message, may I ethically be silenced? If a disease needs to be studied and no one volunteers to be a research subject, is it ethically acceptable to force someone to serve? And so on. In absolutistic, totalitarian societies, there is no issue—sacrifice the minority. But in democratic societies like ours we endeavor to do minimum damage even to small minorities, a stance growing out of our making the individual the primary focus of moral concern. Pursuant to this goal, we build protective fences around key aspects of an individual human to protect his or her nature, or fundamental interests, from being submerged even for the general welfare. These fundamental protections for the individual from being submerged for the sake of the majority are called "rights." Those interests guarded by rights are the ones seen as fundamental to human life and human nature—not being tortured, being allowed to express oneself, holding on to one's property, being able to behave religiously (or not believe) as one chooses, being allowed to form associations by choice, and so on—and are fundamental human interests encoded in the Bill of Rights. This is, in essence, a theory of human nature. Other rights may be deduced from these and from more vague rights, such as "due process," as social conditions change.

Clearly, as the Brambell Committee noted, animals have natures, the thwarting of which matters to them as much as the thwarting of our interests matters to us. Under husbandry, protection of these interests was not an issue. Failure to nurture those interests led to diminished productivity. But now that husbandry has been replaced by industry, these "rights" are no longer naturally protected. Thus, the society would eventually demand that these rights be artificially imposed (i.e., protected in the legal system). This is why the *New York Times*, as we saw, designated the 1988 Swedish law as "a bill of rights for farm animals."

A nice example of what we are discussing can be found in a 1985 legal case brought by the Animal Legal Defense Fund (formerly Attorneys for Animals Rights) against the New York State Department of Environmental Conservation, which administers public land use in New York State. The lawyers attempted to argue that the department was guilty of violating the cruelty laws by failing to stipulate time requirements for those using the steel-jawed trap on public lands to check their traps. Lack of such a stipulation meant that an animal could be trapped with no food or water or medical attention if injured for an indefinite amount of time, which was alleged to count as neglect, given the anticruelty laws (Animal Legal Defense Fund, 1985). The judge's reason was fascinating. While condemning the traps, he affirmed that the society had not spoken against it, and thus it was a socially acceptable instrument. If people wished to ban the trap, he opined, they should go to the legislature, not the judiciary, to create new protections (i.e., rights) for animals to protect the needs flowing from their nature (or *telos*, as I have called it following Aristotle). This, as we saw earlier, is exactly what society has been doing! It is interesting support of our theory that the chief administrators from NIH and USDA responsible for enforcing the laboratory laws of 1985 asserted that these laws created new rights for animals, that is, their right to have the pain caused by research manipulations controlled!

IV

Thus agriculture must accord with the emerging social ethic for animals or risk losing its autonomy and being legislated as research was. As difficult as it was to legislate for science without destroying the creativity, freedom, and spontaneity essential to it, it would be considerably more difficult to legislate for agriculture in a manner that would be enforceable without being prohibitively expensive. Such legislation would need to cover the extensive management practices that cause pain to animals—castration, branding, and dehorning—as well as eliminate the aspects of confinement agriculture causing pain, suffering, and distress. It would be far wiser for producers to preempt legislation and to soften systems injurious to animal welfare. Much of the work necessary to effect such change has been done in Europe—for example, in Sweden and Britain. U.S. knowledge of such research is extremely limited. One thing the animal welfare movement could do that would help this situation is establish exchange programs between the United States and Europe so that American agriculture can learn how Europe has softened confinement systems. It is extremely unlikely that confinement can be fully reversed, but we can vector animals' welfare into the design of these systems and modify them to fit animals needs and natures.

Indeed, even if we were to return to fully extensive agriculture, we could not be sure that our managing of the animals was optimal for assuring their well-being. Although extensive systems require general satisfaction of the animals' needs and natures, no one to my knowledge had ascertained that the system in question was the best it could be vis-à-vis animal welfare and profitability. For example, although beef cattle production on western rangeland is the best of all current systems, from a welfare point of view, it could probably be better. Certainly, the management practices mentioned earlier—hot-iron branding, dehorning, and castration—could be improved or replaced. No one has done the research, but it may well be that the use of minimally expensive local anesthesia for castration not only decreases "shrink" (stress-induced weight loss) but also reduces disease susceptibility due to stress. And transportation of beef cattle has been known for a century to cause both welfare problems for the animals and losses for producers via shipping fever, bruising, and immunosuppression. As another example, it may be economically advantageous, as well as welfare advantageous, for ranchers using open range in hot climates to provide shade, cutting down on heat stress. In fact, in extensive systems, the more welfare is increased, the more likely is increased productivity.

One can argue that systems that are at the extreme end of extensive, such as turning cattle loose on enormous, harsh acreage like desert Australia where they cannot be at all under human surveillance, are deleterious to welfare because human husbandry assistance is rendered impossible, for example, in finding water. Similarly, the "survival of the fittest" approach, which has characterized sheep management in New Zealand, though extensive, clearly does not maximize animal welfare. For example, help is intentionally not given to animals in birthing, even under inclement conditions, since it is believed that one will thereby produce hardier animals. This may be the case, but it produces major welfare costs to individual animals. In short, we must recall that husbandry involves both putting the animals into conditions as close as possible to the ideal conditions they are evolved for *and* helping them when they need help.

The lesson is that merely managing animals extensively is no guarantee of welfare. Relationships with humans are also important, as papers in this volume point out. The problem is that in current confinement systems *neither* conditions for which they have evolved nor human "animal-smart" attention (cf. the good shepherd) are provided to them. Any "intelligence" is built into the system, making it inflexible and devoid of husbandry. Hence, we see the contrast between western cattle ranchers, who sometimes spend more in money or time than the animal is worth (e.g., on sick or marginal calves) as compared with confinement swine operations that treat disease by knocking the animals in the head!

One can, in fact, agree that the optimal production system, like the old small family dairy farm, is a balance between the extremes of extensive and intensive. In cold areas, barns were provided, which the animals voluntarily entered in inclement weather, even though pasture was available. At the same time, dairymen often gave each animal a name and knew their individual variations, with good and gentle treatment and herdsman personality assuring maximum milk production. In such operations, cows and owners bonded, and the animals lived for ten or more lactations. Today, with breeding cattle for maximal productivity *and,* in many cases, adding exogenous BST or BGH (bovine somatotropin or bovine growth hormone, which partitions nutrients into milk production), the animals last two lactations and "burn out," requiring replacement, which may not be economically sound and is certainly not welfare friendly.

Thus, contrary to industry caricature, welfare-friendly agriculture does not mean turning the animals loose on land we don't have. It does mean having husbandry-smart people to work with them. A friend of mine who grew morally sick of raising sows in total confinement moved to a system employing large sow pens and Quonset huts for the animals. His revenue remained the same and even grew some because his pork was more appealing to Japanese markets. One can find in agricultural magazines and newspapers ads requesting "pasture pork—top dollar paid." My friend was able to do this, and confinement factories could not, he said, because he employed three generations of Iowa "pig-smart" people—a grandfather, father, and son. Total confinement operations employ minimum-wage immigrants, ignorant labor that does not know—or care about—animal needs.

At a time when social concern for animal welfare is high, and people flee the cities, it might well behoove society to provide husbandry training to a new generation of young people. As Tim Blackwell and Dave Linton in Ontario have shown (Blackwell et al., 2002), pig-smart husbandmen can create and manage welfare-friendly barns, which are cheaper to capitalize and run and thus create more profit for the producer. In Colorado, for example, where corporate swine factories have been banished for environmental reasons, the lacuna created by their absence could help generate a renaissance in small husbandry-based swine operations, which could in turn revivify small communities turned into ghost towns by confinement operations, and restore the 80 percent of small producers displaced since the early 1970s by the large operators. (Small, partially extensive operations utilize manure as pasture fertilizer, turning what is an insoluble problem for huge confinement operations into an asset.)

V

In order to create welfare-compatible systems, we must overcome a number of barriers. Most formidable, perhaps, is the virtually universal acceptance among scientists, particularly in agricultural sciences, of what I have elsewhere called *scientific ideology*, the set of assumptions taught to nascent scientists along with the facts and theories relevant to their respective disciplines. All fields of human activity must begin with a set of assumptions because, as Aristotle pointed out, if we attempt to prove everything, we are led to an infinite regress, proving our assumptions on the basis of other assumptions, which are proven on the basis of other assumptions, and so on. Thus, as in the paradigm case of geometry, we just take certain assumptions for granted! That, however, does not mean that the assumptions cannot be challenged, examined, and discarded for good reasons, as Einstein ushered in contemporary physics by challenging Newton's assumptions about the existence of absolute space and time.

Sometimes, however, one's assumptions include the assumption that one's assumptions are not subject to questioning or criticism. Such a hardening creates an ideology where the assumptions are insulated from examination. Those raised in dogmatic Catholicism (including the belief that certain things cannot be rationally justified or explained—the Trinity, for example) can be fairly said to adhere to Catholic ideology. Ideology not only does not entertain criticism, it is very openly hostile to it. We most often use the term when talking about religious belief systems or political ones—Marxism, Nazism, Orthodox Judaism, Christian Biblical Fundamentalism are all views of the world that resist self-criticism. "God said it, I believe it, that's all there is to it," as one bumper sticker goes. Under the hold of ideology, one may do things that ordinary conscience finds unspeakable —burning infidels, torturing people to save their souls, or as Daniel Goldhagen (1996) has pointed out , exterminating Jews who one has been taught are "germs," infecting the body politic as bacteria invade the human body, and must be ruthlessly extirpated.

Two features of scientific ideology germane to our discussion must be noted. One is the claim that science is "value-free," that is, does not make value judgments in general nor ethical judgments in particular. One can find this view directly announced in science textbooks, and in pronouncements by leading scientists such as James Wyngaarden, then director of NIH, who announced in 1989 that though new areas of science such as genetic engineering are always controversial, science should "never be hindered by ethical considerations" (Michigan State *News*, 1989). When society questioned the morality of research animal use in the 1970s and 1980s, one often heard from researchers that animal use was not a moral issue but a "scientific necessity," as if that ended the issue. One heard similar defenses of research on humans that society found morally wrong, such as the Tuskegee syphilis experiments or the Willowbrook hepatitis studies. Such ideology was commonly used as a defense by researchers who worked on the atomic bomb and was also indirectly taught to science students by teachers, journals, and conferences failing to discuss or even raise ethical issues naturally growing out of science. Resistance by students to performing invasive experiments on animals was enough to cause a student to fail a class, or elicit threats to the effect that the student did not belong in science, or veterinary medicine, or human medicine. One associate dean of a medical school actually said in my presence in reference to a required hemorrhagic shock lab exercise on a dog that "our faculty does not believe you can be a good doctor unless you first kill a dog."

The second element of scientific ideology relevant to our discussion is the claim that one cannot know or study consciousness or states of awareness such as pain, fear, anxiety, boredom, or loneliness in animals or in people. This, in turn, led to a science that did not acknowledge felt pain in animals even in the study of anesthesia! The first textbook of veterinary anesthesia published in the United States in 1973 does not even *mention* control of felt pain as a reason for anesthesia (Lumb and Jones, 1973), and animal analgesia was essentially unknown until scientific attention was focused on it by federal legal mandate in 1985 to control pain in research animals.

The reason behind scientific ideology was laudable—to provide a clear criterion of demarcation between what is scientifically legitimate to talk about and what isn't. That criterion became observability, testability, and measurability in the early twentieth century. It was used to banish, as we saw, absolute space and time and aether from physics, and "life force" from biology. Since, as Wittgenstein once remarked, if we take an inventory of all the facts in the universe, we won't find it a fact that killing is wrong, science must also be value free. Since we cannot study states of consciousness or feelings objectively, they too must be banished from scientific discourse.

A moment's reflection reveals that scientific ideology must be wrong. Science makes value judgments such as, "double-blind studies are better sources of knowledge than are anecdotes," and ethical judgments when it affirms that the value of an invasive experiment on animals outweighs the pain and suffering or death of the animal. Further, not everything in science can be proven—neither the Big Bang nor the reality of an external world existing independently of our perceptions can be tested. Further, we cannot dismiss private experience from science, because our only approach to the "objective world" is by way of our subjective perceptions!

The ways in which these ideological components impact on farm animal welfare issues is clear. In the first place, the concept of welfare in animals cannot be evaluated without reference to value judgments. Consider: science can give us facts relevant to animal welfare—it can tell us whether the animal is or is not gaining weight, has or doesn't have a salmonella infection, has or doesn't have intestinal parasites, behaves in repetitive stereotypical ways or not, etc. However, to say the animal is "well-off" or "not well-off" requires a value judgment on what counts as well-off! (This is true of humans as well.) Historically, under confinement agriculture, agricultural scientists assumed that if an animal was well fed, free of infection, and gaining weight, it must be well-off. The Brambell Committee, on the other hand, affirmed that a social animal must be with others of its own kind to be well-off. The U.S. Congress, in framing the 1985 laboratory laws, affirmed that a dog could not be well-off without exercise, nor could a primate without an "enriched environment to enhance its psychological well-being"! So clearly, what constitutes welfare is going to be in part valuational; which values drive what facts are relevant to an animal's having positive welfare!

This, in turn, leads to the way in which denial of consciousness in science hindered research into—and even understanding of—animal welfare. For ordinary common sense, part of—indeed the main part of—a person's or animal's being in a state of positive welfare is whether it is happy (i.e., is in part defined by reference to the being in question's subjective state). We all know people with all the observable trappings of health, wealth, and success who are nonetheless miserable, and we would not say of such people that they enjoyed positive well-being. (For example, this state is depicted in *Richard Cory* by poet E. A. Robinson.) Similarly with an animal. Common sense says of the sow in confinement that exhibits compulsive, repetitive stereotypical behaviors such as bar-biting, that the animal cannot be well-off or happy, because it is "bored," or "driven crazy by the austere environment," or "has no one to play with." In my ethical writings, I have argued that in reference to animal welfare, how the animal feels subjectively, what it experiences, is the key feature of welfare or well-being. An irreducible component of being well-off is feeling well and not having enduring negative subjective experiences. But except for Marian Dawkins and Ian Duncan, most scientists working in this area have dismissed animal subjective experience in accord with the second component of scientific ideology articulated above.

This scientific ideology has in effect blocked agricultural scientists from viewing welfare as ordinary common sense (i.e., the general public) views it. Instead of thinking through the value judgments constituting welfare, the agricultural scientists have tended to assume that the productive animal is well-off or that having food and water and shelter suffices to guarantee animal welfare. Instead of looking at subjective states of happiness and unhappiness, the agricultural community has tended to lump all forms of subjective misery under the *psychological* rubric of "stress" as measured by cortisol, and to equate misery with levels of stress hormones. But it is plain that having certain levels of stress hormones such as cortisol is neither necessary nor sufficient to prove misery. Copulation and play, surely pleasant activities in animals and in humans, generate elevated stress hormones. Lack of such hormones does not prove that the animal is not miserable, as when animals achieve "learned helplessness."

Indeed, the traditional animal science/agriculture view of stress until about 1990 was that the psychological stress response was either on or off, like a light switch. This was dogma, despite the fact that scientists like Jay Weiss (1972) in psychology and John Mason (1971) in psychiatry had clearly shown that this allegedly nonspecific response view of stress—that it was all or nothing—was false. These researchers showed that animal psychological stress responses were variable given the same stressor, depending on the animal's *subjective cognitive state regarding the stressor.* Mason showed that if an animal could anticipate a stressor (elevated ambient temperature), it showed far less of a physiological stress response than when it was unable to anticipate the change. Similarly, Weiss showed that if an animal felt it could control a noxious stimulus (an electric shock), it showed far less of a physiological stress response to it than if it had no control over the stressor. Further augmenting the importance of an inherent psychological dimension of stress over its physical manifestations is the fact, long ago reported by Kilgour, that, for cattle, exposure to a new environment itself causes a greater stress response than does an electric shock (Kilgour, 1978)! This is again potentiated by research showing that how an animal is treated by caretakers can create a huge difference in an animal's reproductive success (Hemsworth, 1998), as well as in its response to disease agents (e.g., a 2 percent cholesterol diet in rabbits, who developed far less atherosclerosis when treated with TLC [Nerein et al., 1980]).

In short, whoever designs new systems with the intention of increasing animal welfare of farm animals must proceed in accordance with society's definition of animal welfare that can be reconstructed as something like this: Assuming that an animal has adequate welfare requires that it be in a position to actualize the needs and interests dictated by its biological and psychological nature or *telos*—the "cowness" of the cow, the "pigness" of the pig—and that, experientially, it does not experience prolonged noxious mental states, such as, fear, anxiety, boredom, loneliness, social isolation, and so on.

Though traditional scientific ideology scoffs at attributing such states to animals as at worst mystical and at least mindless anthropomorphism, those who live and work with animals cannot avoid such psychologistic locutions. In a classic study of zookeepers, psychologist David Hebb showed that they were unable to do their jobs if forbidden to use such mentalistic attributions (Hebb, 1946). My students who work with cattle have told me the same thing. The fact is that before the U.S. federal laboratory animal laws mandated the control of pain in laboratory animals, the scientific community complained that it could not even identify painful states in animals, much less control them (there were virtually no articles available on laboratory animal analgesia). Fifteen years later, articles on pain and treatment modalities for it have proliferated, as have useful pain classifications and the realization that, if we can study pain in animals as models for human pain, then what we know of human pain can be reciprocally employed to help understand animal pain!

Further, creative scientists have given us operational discussions and definitions of noxious mental states in animals. Wemelsfelder, for example, has discussed at great length the recognition, understanding and nature of boredom in farm animals and laboratory animals (Wemelsfelder, 1989). And the entire field of behavioral enrichment, as pioneered by ethologists like Hal Markowitz (1982), has pointed us in the direction of how to alleviate the noxious state of boredom. Others have studied play in animals, once thought to be a uniquely human phenomenon (Huizinga, 1950). Both NIH and USDA, in interpreting federal laws and regulations pertaining to the welfare of laboratory animals, are placing ever-increasing emphasis on the concepts of "distress" and "suffering," catchall phrases used at a time when essentially no one was recognizing subjective states as legitimately studiable in animals. We can be morally certain that, if someone were to offer 50 million dollars in research money to study loneliness or fear or anxiety in animals (or all of those), the money would not go "a-begging."

The U.S. public firmly believes in animal mental states and has a voracious appetite for knowing more about such states. Books like the *Horse Whisperer, The Secret Life of Dogs, When Elephants Weep*, Darwin's classic *The Expression of Emotion in Man and Animals,* and others eloquently attest to this belief, as do the endless television programs dealing with animal emotion and cognition. Thus, the U.S. public will simply not accept scientific agnosticism about the animal mind, particularly as far as the mental states pertaining to animal welfare are concerned. Those who believe that they understand the emotions of their pets, and that their own emotions are reciprocally understood—and empathized with—by these animals, will not accept a huge bifurcation between pets and farm animals. A society that believes, as polls show, that an animal's life matters to it as much as, and in the same way as, a human life matters to a human will not buy scientific agnosticism about morally relevant mental states.

VI

What all of this tells us is the direction that future agriculture must go. If animals are going to be raised for food, they must live, in balance, happy lives, or at least lives free from pain and suffering. New systems should combine the best of traditional extensive agriculture, particularly husbandry, with technological advances that allow us to satisfy an animal's basic interests, constitutive of its *telos*. Many models for this exist in the areas of "enhancing primate psychological well-being" or meeting animals' basic behavioral/psychological needs in the zoo. Hal Markowitz has described satisfying the serval's inborn interest in predating low-flying birds by shooting their rations across their enclosures at random with cannons (Markowitz and Line, 1989). Further long-term ethological studies should be conducted on farm species to determine their natural behavioral needs. Wood-Gush and Stolba's work with pigs in a small, naturalistic environment (a "pig park") over 25 years stands as a model (Wood-Gush and Stolba, 1981), as do the ethological studies done by Duncan, Hughes, Mench and others on behavior of great importance to laying hens. Housing should be designed in accordance with this knowledge. The handling of livestock should move beyond macho posturing to knowledge-based gentle science. People like Temple Grandin and Bud Williams have blazed trails in this area. Equipment for handling and transporting animals, be it squeeze chutes or trucks, should again be based on ethological knowledge—cattle defecating on other cattle in double-decker trucks is not morally acceptable, and probably never was. Again, Temple Grandin's work is an exemplar in this area. Systems of slaughter, too, should be accountable first to animal well-being and only second to efficiency. No animal should die in pain or terror. Kosher slaughter or halal slaughter should be held to the same high standards. Being a Jew who studied the Talmud, I believe it is clear that kosher slaughter as currently practiced is largely incompatible with the humane moral imperatives that inspired kosher slaughter in antiquity. Temple Grandin (1991) has again done an incomparable job in studying the Talmud and showing this incompatibility, even to the satisfaction of *Kashrut*, a magazine devoted to kosher living, whose editors endorsed her recommendations.

In summary, as the Bible indicated, if we are to use animals for our benefit, it is morally incumbent upon us to make sure that they benefit as well, by at least living decent lives, not lives of misery, fear, and pain. To expect any less is not only immoral, it is dishonorable. It is, as I hope we have shown, ethically timely to use our science and technology for the benefit of the animals we use, not merely for their exploitation.

REFERENCES

Animal Legal Defense Fund vs. The Department of Environment Conservation of the State of New York, 1985. Index a6670/85.

Blackwell, T., et al. 2002. *Alternative Housing for Gestating Sows* (a film). OMAFRA, Fergus, Ontario.

Brambell, F. W. R. 1965. Report of the Technical Committee to Enquire into the Welfare of Animals Kept Under Intensive Livestock Husbandry Systems. HMSO, London

Goldhagen, D. 1996. *Hitler's Willing Executioners.* Knopf, New York.

Grandin, T. 1991. Humane restraint equipment for kosher slaughter. *Kashrus* 11 (5): 18–21.

Harrison, R. 1964. *Animal Machines.* Vincent Stuart, London.

Hebb, D. O. 1946. Emotion in man and animals. *Psychology Review* 53: 88–106.

Hemsworth, P. 1998. *Human Livestock Interaction: The Stockperson and the Productivity and Welfare of Intensively Farmed Animals.* CAB International, New York.

Huizinga, J. 1950. *Homo Ludens: A Study of Play in Culture.* Beacon Press, Boston.

Kilgour, R. 1978. The application of animal behavior and the humane care of farm animals. *Journal of Animal Science* 46: 1478ff.

Lumb, W. V., and E. W. Jones. 1973. *Veterinary Anesthesia.* Lea and Febiger, Philadelphia.

Markowitz, H. 1982. *Behavioral Enrichment in the Zoo.* Van Nostrand Reinhold, New York.

Markowitz, H., and S. Line. 1989. The need for responsive environments. In: Rollin, B., and M. Kesel, The *Experimental Animal in Biomedical Research*, Volume 1. CRC Press, Boca-Raton, FL.

Mason, J. W. 1971. A re-evaluation of the concept of "non-specificity" in stress theory. *Journal of Psychiatry Research* 8:323–333.

Michigan State *News.* February 27, 1989, p. 8.

Nerein, R. M., et al. 1980. Social environment as a factor in diet-induced atherosclerosis. *Science* 208:1475–1476.

New York Times. October 25, 1988.

Parents. 1989. Parents poll on animals rights, attractiveness, television and abortion (survey by Kane and Parsons, New York).

Rollin, B. E. 1981. *Animals Rights and Human Morality.* Prometheus Books, Buffalo, NY.

Thompson, P. 1991. Unpublished paper read at USDA conference on animal welfare.

Weiss, J. 1972. Psychological factors in stress and disease. *Scientific American* 226 (March 1972): 101–113.

Wemelsfelder, F. 1989. Boredom and laboratory animal welfare. In Rollin, B., and M. Kesel. *The Experimental Animals in Biomedical Research*, Volume 1. CRC Press, Boca Raton, FL.

Wood-Gush, D., and A. Stolba. 1981. Behavior of pigs and the design of a new housing system. *Applied Animal Ethology* 8: 583–585.

2

Human-Livestock Interaction

Paul H. Hemsworth

INTRODUCTION

One of the first commentaries in the scientific literature on the influence of human-animal interactions on domestic animals was by Gross and Siegel (1979). In concluding on the results of three experiments examining the effects of human contact on domestic chickens, Gross and Siegel proposed that "providing only for their physical needs does not result in superior experimental animals. Also important factors in the outcome of experiments will be gentle care and familiarity of birds with the animal handlers and experimenters." Although the implications were obvious for experimental animals, the authors did not reflect on such implications for commercial livestock.

Reports first appeared in the scientific literature in the 1970s that implicated the influence of human-animal interactions on the productivity of livestock. In a study of dairy herds in the United Kingdom, Seabrook (1972) reported a significant relationship between the personality of the stockperson and the productivity of the herd: introverted and confident stockpeople were associated with higher milk yields. Seabrook also commented that herds in which cows appeared to readily approach the stockperson had higher productivity than herds in which cows appeared to less readily approach the stockperson. Hemsworth, Brand, and Willems (1981b) found a significant positive correlation, based on farm averages, between the approach behavior of commercial breeding pigs to an experimenter in a standard test and their reproductive performance indicating that productivity tended to be lower at farms in which breeding pigs showed less approach to humans.

One interpretation of these observations on dairy cattle, pigs, and poultry was that fear of humans, as a consequence of human-animal interactions, may reduce the productivity of intensively managed livestock. This interpretation has been supported by research in experimental and commercial situations over the last 20 years. This research has shown that interactions between stockpeople and their animals can indeed limit both the productivity and welfare of livestock. While stockpeople utilize a range of behaviors to inspect and handle their animals, the frequent use of some of these routine behaviors has been shown to result in farm animals becoming highly fearful of humans. It is these high fear levels, through stress, that will limit animal welfare and productivity.

Domestic animals such as farm animals are managed by humans. In situations in which this management is intense, as occurs in many forms of livestock production, it is not surprising that human-animal interactions may have implications for the animal. Nevertheless, the profound effects that human behavior can have on the behavior and physiology of animals are unexpected. The impact of interactions that are routinely but briefly used by stockpeople, many of which intuitively appear to be innocuous and innocent, is also surprising. Even after 20 years of research on this topic of human-animal interactions, I am still surprised at times by the effects of these interactions on the animal. This chapter will review some of the recent research on human-animal interactions in the dairy, pig, and poultry industries to demonstrate some of the important principles that may govern these interactions and their effects on the welfare of animals in intensive-managed livestock production systems.

HUMAN-ANIMAL INTERACTIONS IN LIVESTOCK PRODUCTION

Intensively managed livestock production involves several levels of interaction between stockpeople and their animals. Many interactions are associated with regular observation of the animals and their conditions, and thus this type of interaction often involves only visual contact between the stockperson and the animals. For example, stockpeople inspect meat chickens in indoor production systems by moving through the units several times a day. Animals in most production systems have to be moved and, in addition to visual and auditory contact, stockpeople often use tactile interactions to move their animals. Extensively grazed animals such as cattle and sheep are moved between pastures as part of optimal grass management, and extensively grazed dairy cows and indoor-housed dairy cows are moved several times a day during lactation to be milked. Growing pigs are generally moved from pen to pen, in order to provide accommodations suitable to their stage of growth, and breeding pigs may be regularly moved according to their stage of the breeding cycle. It is in situations in which animals are closely inspected or moved that human-animal interactions have considerable potential to influence animal welfare and animal performance.

Human-animal interactions also occur in situations in which animals must be restrained and subjected to management or health procedures. Some animals may never be restrained during their lives, while others are restrained on a regular basis. The association of fear and pain from these husbandry procedures with humans performing them will increase the fear of humans that animals subsequently exhibit in both similar situations involving humans and different situations involving humans, such as during routine inspections. The effects that these procedures have on the animal relate both to the aversiveness of the procedure and the association of people with that aversion. Rewarding experiences, such as provision of a preferred feed or even positive handling, around the time of the procedure may ameliorate the aversiveness of the procedure and reduce the chances that animals associate the punishment of the procedure with humans. For example, studies with pigs have shown that pigs will associate the rewarding elements of feeding with humans if handlers are present at feeding (Hemsworth, Verge, and Coleman, 1996b). Hutson (1985) found that although the effectiveness of food rewards diminished as the severity of the handling treatment increased, rewarding sheep with barley food improved subsequent ease of handling in the location in which the aversive treatment was previously imposed. Rushen and colleagues (Munksgaard et al., 1995; Rushen et al., 1995; de Passille et al., 1996) have shown that performing an aversive treatment at a specific location or by either an unfamiliar or familiar handler wearing different distinctive clothing may reduce the likelihood that dairy cows associate the procedure with the regular stockperson.

As Hemsworth and Gonyou (1997) have suggested, there are opportunities to reduce or even eliminate human involvement in some animal management procedures that are aversive to the animal. Examples include robotic shearing of sheep, robotic milking of cows, and automated handling facilities for sheep (Syme, Durham, and Elphick, 1981) and pigs (Barton Gade, Blaabjerg, and Christensen, 1992). The effect of eliminating humans from such handling procedures on the animals' responses is well illustrated by research on mechanical and manual harvesting of meat chickens (Duncan et al., 1986). While maximum heart rates of birds caught by either method were similar, the rates remained high for longer in manually caught birds than in birds caught by a specially designed machine. These results indicate that the stressfulness of some procedures may be reduced by eliminating humans from the procedure. In situations where the human contact component is highly aversive or even injurious to the animal, procedures that eliminate human involvement or changes in the behavior of the human should be sought. For instance, since the method of catching laying hens in cages affects the incidence of bird injuries (Gregory et al., 1993), catching techniques that minimize injury should be identified and adopted.

HUMAN-ANIMAL RELATIONSHIPS IN LIVESTOCK PRODUCTION

Human-animal relationships can be considered to be constructed from a series of interactions between humans and animals (Hemsworth, Barnett, and Coleman, 1992). These interactions between humans and animals may be tactile, visual, olfactory, gustatory, and auditory, and the nature of these interactions may be positive, neutral, or negative for the animal. For example, fear-provoking interactions such as the sudden unexpected appearance of a human or a human looming over an animal may be negative for the animal, while painful interactions such as being hit by a human are obviously negative to animals. It is the nature of these human interactions that will markedly determine the quality of the human-animal relationship for animals.

As reviewed by Rushen et al. (2001), the relationship between humans and domestic animals, particularly companion animals and to a lesser extent farm animals, is often considered a social relationship. If the definition of a social relationship between two individuals includes preference for interaction and proximity for each other (i.e., affiliative behavior) that is similar to that for conspecifics, it is questionable that human-animal relationships in commercial livestock systems are genuine social relationships. One could argue that such relationships exist between humans and their companion animals (Estep and Hetts, 1992). The extensive studies by John Paul Scott (1992) in which young dogs were shown to form long-lasting bonds or attachments to humans at an early age elegantly demonstrate the long-term effects of early human interaction. Human contact, as little as a few minutes of daily visual contact with humans or just two 20-minute periods of visual contact with humans, from the age of 3 to 8 weeks, will have profound effects on the subsequent behavioral responses of dogs to humans.

Nevertheless, the relationships that exist between humans and farm animals in livestock production are true relationships in that the interactions are frequent and often intense and, more important, the interactions have reciprocal effects on the partners. In intensive-management systems, livestock are dependent on the stockpeople for their welfare and survival. As will be considered in more detail in this chapter, the behavior of the stockperson is an influential determinant of the fear responses to humans and, in turn, the welfare and productivity of livestock. These fear responses to humans, by influencing aspects of the job such as ease of inspection and handling and the welfare and productivity of the animals, may affect a number of the job-related characteristics of the stockperson, such as job satisfaction, motivation, and commitment (Hemsworth and Coleman, 1998). These job-related characteristics, in turn, have obvious implications for the welfare and productivity of the animals under the care of the stockperson, because of their effects on the work performance of the stockperson. Interviews of stockpeople in the Australian pig and dairy industries indicate that, while many expressed a dislike for various aspects of the job, most stockpeople enjoyed working with their animals (Hemsworth and Coleman, 1998). Working with animals may provide stockpeople with benefits such as companionship and a commitment and interest that offers both responsibility and a sense of satisfaction for the health and welfare of lives other than their own or their families'. Therefore, the relationships that exist between humans and farm animals in livestock production appear to be genuine relationships because of their impact on both stockpeople and their livestock.

The quality of this relationship from the perspective of the animal can be assessed by measuring the behavioral and physiological responses of the animal to humans (Hemsworth and Coleman, 1998). Measurements of the behavioral response of the animal to humans as well as physiological responses such as heart rate and corticosteroid concentrations in the presence of humans will provide valuable information on the quality of the human-animal relationship for the animal. For instance, the approach behavior of individual pigs to a stationary experimenter in an arena in a standard test has been used to assess the animals' fear of humans. In these tests, although the degree of novelty of the test arena is reduced because of the similarity of the arena with the animals' home pen, pigs introduced into this new environment will be motivated to explore and familiarize themselves with the environment once the initial fear responses have waned. Therefore, although the pigs may be motivated to both avoid and explore the arena and the human stimulus, the pigs' fear of humans will have a major influence on the pigs' approach to the human stimulus. Because poultry show little locomotion in a novel arena in the short term, the avoidance responses of birds to an approaching human have often been used to assess fear levels. Studies with cattle have used both the approach behavior to a stationary experimenter and the distance at which an animal withdraws or escapes as a human approaches in a standard manner (flight distance to humans; Hediger, 1964) to measure the animal's fear of humans. Significant correlations between the behavioral and physiological responses of animals to humans in these tests support the validity of these measures (Hemsworth and Barnett, 1987; Lyons, Price, and Moberg, 1988; Breuer et al., 2000). Furthermore, the imposition of handling treatments designed to differentially affect the animal's fear of humans produced the expected variations in the behavioral responses of the animals to humans (Jones and Faure, 1981; Gonyou, Hemsworth, and Barnett, 1986; Hemsworth, Barnett, and Hansen, 1981a, 1986a, 1987; Hemsworth et al. 1994b, 1996a, 1996b; Hemsworth and Barnett, 1991; Barnett, Hemsworth, and Newman, 1992; Jones and Waddington, 1993).

DEVELOPMENT OF BEHAVIORAL RESPONSES
OF DOMESTIC ANIMALS TO HUMANS

Fear is considered a powerful emotional state that normally gives rise to defensive behavior or escape. In concert with these behavioral effects, fear normally activates the autonomic nervous system and the neuroendocrine system, which in turn through their effects on regulatory mechanisms such as energy availability and use, and cardiac and respiratory functions, assist the animal to meet physical or emotional challenges. Gray (1987) recognizes that fear may be triggered by environmental stimuli that are novel; have high intensity such as loud and large stimuli; have special evolutionary dangers such as heights, isolation, and darkness; arise from social interaction such as contagious learning; or have been paired with aversive experiences. In order to appreciate the influence of human-animal interactions on livestock, it is useful to consider the development of fear responses to humans.

There are marked between-species and within-species differences in fear of humans. For example, the behavioral response to humans varies markedly both between and within farm animal species. As reviewed by Hemsworth and Coleman (1998), considerable between-farm variation exists in the behavioral response of animals to humans in the dairy (Breuer et al., 2000; Hemsworth et al., 2000), egg (Barnett et al., 1992), meat chicken (Hemsworth et al., 1994b), and pig industries (Hemsworth, Brand, and Willems, 1981b; Hemsworth et al., 1989). Murphey, Moura Duarte, and Torres Penendo (1981) reported marked differences in the flight distance of *Bos indicus* and *Bos taurus* breeds of cattle to humans and Hearnshaw, Barlow, and Want (1979) reported marked differences in the behavior of crossbred Brahman cattle and British breeds to handling. Indeed, the latter authors reported that the behavioral response to restraint in a squeeze chute (or stall) in the close presence of humans, often referred to as temperament, is moderately heritable in *Bos indicus* cattle. Furthermore, the flight distance of extensively grazed farm animals is generally reported to be greater than that of intensively managed farm animals (Hemsworth and Coleman, 1998).

These differences in the behavioral responses of livestock to humans may, in part, reflect inherent species differences in their fear of unfamiliar stimuli (neophobia). Selection for neophobia will more likely affect the general fearfulness of naive animals rather than their responses to specific novel stimuli. Inherent species differences in neophobia will affect the initial responses of naive animals to novel stimuli such as humans. However, over time experience with humans should modify these responses to the extent that these responses become stimulus specific. There is some evidence that the behavioral response of relatively naive pigs to humans, which may be predominantly a result of general fearfulness, may be moderately heritable. However, subsequent experience with humans appears to dilute the genetic effects (Hemsworth et al., 1990): the behavioral response of relatively inexperienced pigs to humans only accounted for less than a quarter of the variance of their behavioral response to humans later in life. Murphy and Duncan (1977, 1978) studied two stocks of chickens, termed "flighty" and "docile" on the basis of their behavioral responses to humans, and found that early handling affected the behavioral responses of these two stocks of birds to humans, with the docile birds showing a more rapid reduction in their withdrawal responses to humans with regular exposure to humans than the flighty birds. These stock differences may be stimulus specific since observations indicated that the docile birds did not necessarily show less withdrawal responses to novel stimuli, such as a mechanical scraper and an inflating balloon, than the flighty birds (Murphy, 1976).

Further evidence that the handling effects on the behavioral response of animals to humans may be specific to humans and not generalized to a range of fear-provoking stimuli is provided by a series of studies by Jones and colleagues (Jones, Mills, and Faure, 1991; Jones and Waddington, 1992). These studies examined the effects of regular handling on the behavioral responses of quail and domestic chickens to novel stimuli (such as a blue light) and humans, and found that handling predominantly affected the responses of birds to humans, rather than to the novel stimuli. Handled birds showed less avoidance of humans but their responses to novel stimuli were unaffected. These data indicate that experience with humans results in stimulus-specific effects rather than effects on general fearfulness.

Over time, young domesticated animals that may have had limited experience with humans may habituate to the presence of humans and thus may perceive humans as part of the environment without any particular significance. Habituation will occur over time as the animals' fear of humans is gradually reduced by repeated exposure to humans in a neutral context; that is, the humans' presence has neither rewarding nor punishing elements. Even wild strains of rats and deer that are highly fearful of humans will habituate to humans over time (Galef, 1970; Matthews, 1993).

Some domestic animals such as farm and laboratory animals and, indeed, some pets such as aviary birds housed in groups, which may receive limited human contact, may perceive humans as predators. Selection for increased docility in the presence of humans has accompanied domestication; however, based on their withdrawal responses to humans, domestic animals may still find human contact aversive and thus perceive humans as predators rather than benevolent caretakers. *Bos indicus* cattle extensively grazed with infrequent human contact display extreme avoidance responses to restraint and human presence, including at times displaying tonic immobility or a catatonic-like state during restraint (Grandin, 1980), which are indicative of antipredator responses. Caine (1992) has challenged the widely held view that a captive animal's behavior can habituate to the presence of human observers. Her data suggest that the presence of observers, even for captive animals that have received considerable human contact, may result in antipredator behavior in these animals, often masking or confounding the behavior under study.

In situations in which they frequently interact with humans, domestic animals may, through conditioning, associate humans with rewarding and punishing events that occur at the time of these interactions, and thus conditioned responses to humans may develop. Studies examining the effects of a range of handling treatments on the behavior of pigs (Gonyou et al., 1986; Hemsworth et al., 1981a, 1986a; Hemsworth, Barnett, and Hansen, 1987; Hemsworth, Barnett, and Campbell, 1996a; Hemsworth and Barnett, 1991) indicate that conditioned approach-avoidance responses develop as a consequence of associations between the stockperson and aversive and rewarding elements of the handling bouts. Pigs that were slapped or shocked with a battery-operated prodder whenever they approached or failed to avoid the experimenter in daily handling bouts of 15 to 30 seconds learned to associate the presence of the handler with the punishment of the handling bouts. In contrast, pigs that received pats or strokes during brief daily handling bouts subsequently showed increased approach to humans. Furthermore, there is evidence that pigs may associate the rewarding experience of feeding with the handler and that this conditioning results in pigs being less fearful of humans (Hemsworth et al., 1996b). Although there is some controversy over the mechanism by which avoidance behavior becomes conditioned by punishment (Walker, 1987), it is well established that animals learn to avoid conditioned stimuli that are paired with aversive events. Thus, through conditioning, the behavioral responses of animals to humans may be regulated by the nature of the experiences occurring around the time of interactions with humans.

There is evidence in some farm animal species that the age of the animal at which handling occurs is influential, and this topic is well reviewed by Rushen et al. (2001). Human contact in early life has been shown to have persistent effects on fear of humans in cattle, horses, pigs, sheep, and silver foxes (for example Waring, 1983; Boissy and Bouissou, 1988; Lyons et al., 1988; Lyons, 1989; Pedersen and Jeppesen, 1990; Hemsworth and Barnett, 1992; Pedersen, 1993; Markowitz et al., 1998). Rearing young animals artificially or with their dams does not appear to affect the influence of early human contact on subsequent fear responses to humans (Rushen et al., 2001).

The literature on early handling of rodents is very extensive and is useful when considering the effects of early handling of livestock. There are basically two types of studies on rodents, those termed "handling studies," which involve brief removal of preweaned animals from their home cages, and those termed "gentling studies," which involve brief stroking of postweaned animals. Although the results have often been contradictory, these treatments at times have resulted in increased growth and accelerated development, reduced activity and defecation in an open-field test, improved performance in learning tasks, and physiological stress responses of lower magnitude to subsequent stressors (Dewsbury, 1992). These results have often been interpreted as a consequence of either direct stimulation or acute stress advancing the rate of development of some behavioral and physiological processes (Schaefer, 1968). Thus, early handling effects on fear, including fear of humans, may not necessarily be due to handling *per se* but may in part be a consequence of acute stress early in life associated with the separation and handling involved in the handling treatment and perhaps also early weaning in some studies.

Therefore, although handling at an early age may be highly influential (for a more detailed discussion of this, see Rushen et al., 2001), subsequent handling is also influential and has the potential to modify such early learning effects. Early human contact in comparison to subsequent human contact is often similar within most livestock production systems, and thus the considerable variation both within and between farms in the fear responses of cattle, pigs, and poultry to humans partly reflects the influence of human contact later in life. The two types of learning—conditioned fear responses and habituation to humans—occurring both early and subsequently in life are probably the most influential factors affecting the behavioral responses of livestock to humans.

EFFECTS OF HUMAN BEHAVIOR ON LIVESTOCK

Extensive research in the dairy, pig, and poultry industries over the last 20 years has shown that human-animal interactions, by affecting the animal's fear of humans, can markedly limit the welfare and productivity of livestock. Using the behavioral response of the animal to an experimenter to assess the animal's fear of humans, studies in commercial farms have found negative correlations between fear of humans and productivity in the dairy industry (Breuer et al., 2000; Hemsworth et al., 2000), egg industry (Barnett, Hemsworth, and Newman, 1992), meat chicken industry (Hemsworth et al., 1994b; Cransberg, Hemsworth, and Coleman, 2000), and pig industry (Hemsworth et al., 1981b; Hemsworth et al., 1989). These negative correlations, based on farm averages, indicate that high levels of fear of humans may be a major factor limiting the productivity of livestock in these industries.

There is evidence that these relationships observed in the livestock industries may have a causal basis. Handling studies have shown that handling treatments that result in high levels of fear may depress animal productivity and welfare. For example, studies in pigs indicate that high fear of humans can limit the growth and reproduction of pigs (for example, Gonyou et al., 1986; Hemsworth et al., 1981a, 1986a, 1987; Hemsworth, Barnett, and Campbell, 1996a; Hemsworth and Barnett, 1991). Studies of poultry have shown that chickens and laying hens are particularly sensitive to visual contact with humans (Jones, 1993; Barnett et al., 1994) and that handling treatments that increase fear of humans may depress growth (for example, Gross and Siegel, 1979, 1980, 1982; Collins and Siegel, 1987) and egg production (Barnett et al., 1994). Similarly, negative tactile handling by inducing high fear of humans may limit the productivity of commercial dairy cows (Breuer et al., 2000; Rushen, de Passille, and Munksgaard, 1999).

A number of these handling studies implicate stress in the deleterious effects of aversive handling on animal productivity. Negative tactile interaction, imposed daily for 15 to 30 seconds, consistently resulted in pigs showing increased fear of humans, increased basal cortisol concentrations, and reduced growth and reproductive performance (Hemsworth et al., 1981a, 1986a, 1987; Hemsworth and Barnett, 1991). Similarly, studies on dairy cattle by Rushen et al. (1999) and Breuer et al. (2000) suggest that aversive handling may depress the milk yield of cows through stress. The results of the former study implicate the secretion of catecholamines under the influence of the autonomic nervous system affecting milk letdown, while the latter study found evidence of chronic stress in negatively handled heifers.

Studies on stockpeople in the dairy and pig industries have shown significant sequential relationships between the stockperson's attitudes and behavior toward animals and the fear of humans by farm animals (Hemsworth et al., 1989, 2000; Coleman et al., 1998; Breuer et al., 2000). For instance, positive attitudes to the use of petting and the use of verbal and physical effort to handle cows and pigs were negatively correlated with the use of negative tactile interactions, such as slaps, pushes and hits, which in turn were positively associated with fear of humans by the animals. In studies on commercial meat chickens, Hemsworth et al. (1994b) and Cransberg et al. (2000) found a significant relationship between the behavior of the stockperson and the behavioral responses of birds to humans. For instance, these observations indicated that speed of movement by the stockperson is an important visual interaction influencing fear of humans at commercial meat chicken farms. In contrast to the results of studies in the dairy and pig industries, there was no evidence of a relationship between stockperson attitude and behavior. In retrospect, it appears that the wrong attitudinal variables may have been targeted in the questionnaire used to assess attitudes. The most pertinent attitudes in predicting behavior are those that are specifically directed toward relevant behaviors (Hemsworth and Coleman, 1998). The most important behavior exhibited by the stockperson that was found to be associated with fear responses by birds to humans was speed of movement, a behavior that was not specifically addressed in the attitude questionnaire in these studies.

Further evidence of a causal basis for these sequential human-animal relationships is the result of several recent studies aimed at improving behavior, productivity, and welfare of livestock by targeting for improvement the attitudes and behavior of stockpeople. Studies in the dairy and pig industries have shown that it is possible first to improve the attitudinal and behavioral profiles of stockpeople and second to reduce levels of fear and improve productivity of their farm animals (Coleman et al., 2000; Hemsworth, Coleman, and Barnett, 1994a; Hemsworth et al., 2002). This approach in improving the attitudes and behavior of stockpeople and its practical implications are discussed by G. J. Coleman in chapter 9. Basically, this process of inducing behavioral change not only involves imparting knowledge and skills, but also involves changing established habits; altering well-established attitudes and beliefs; addressing denial, offense, counterarguments, and counterexamples; and preparing the person to handle difficult situations such as stressful handling bouts and the reactions from others toward the individual following change. The training process is a comprehensive procedure in which all of the personal and external factors that are relevant to the behavioral situation are explicitly targeted.

Fear is an undesirable emotional state of suffering (Jones and Waddington, 1992), and the implications of fear of humans on the welfare of livestock are highlighted by the substantial between-farm variation in the avoidance response of commercial dairy cows, pigs, and poultry to humans (Hemsworth and Coleman, 1998). The risks to the welfare of these farm animals that are fearful of humans arise because of injuries that they may sustain in trying to avoid humans during routine inspections and handling, the evidence that these animals are likely to experience acute stress in the presence of humans and, in some situations, chronic stress, and, finally, the effects of this chronic stress response on immunosuppression (Hemsworth and Coleman, 1998), which may have serious consequences for the health of the animals. Furthermore, if the stockperson's attitude toward the animal is poor, the stockperson is likely to be less committed to inspecting and attending to welfare (and production) problems facing the animal.

Therefore, this extensive research indicates sequential relationships between the attitudes of stockpeople toward interacting with their animals, the behavior of the stockpeople toward their animals, the behavioral response of animals to humans (fear of humans), and the welfare and productivity of farm animals. These human-animal relationships, including the possible reciprocal relationships, are depicted in figure 2.1.

SENSITIVITY OF LIVESTOCK TO HUMANS

While it easy to appreciate that regular negative interactions with animals, particularly forceful negative interactions such as hits or shocks with a battery-operated prod, will produce high fear responses to humans, the sensitivity of livestock to brief human interactions or intuitively minor or moderate negative interactions is surprising. For instance, daily handling for 15 to 30 seconds consisting of a slap or brief shock with a commercial battery-operated prod when the animal approached or failed to avoid the experimenter, consistently resulted in pigs showing increased fear of humans and basal cortisol concentrations and reduced growth and reproductive performance (Hemsworth et al., 1981a, 1986a, 1987; Hemsworth and Barnett, 1991).

Animals also appear to be sensitive to brief nontactile human interactions. Handling studies on poultry clearly demonstrate the influence of brief visual contact with humans on fear. Jones (1993) found that regular treatments involving the experimenter placing his or her hand in the chicken's cage or allowing birds to observe other birds being handled resulted in reductions in the subsequent avoidance behavior of young chickens to humans. Barnett et al. (1994) found that regular visual contact, involving positive elements such as slow and deliberate movements, reduced the subsequent fear responses of mature laying hens to humans in comparison to minimal human contact that at times contained elements of sudden, unexpected human contact. The birds that had regular visual contact also had

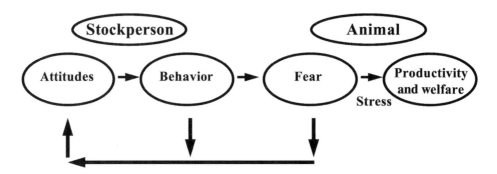

Figure 2.1.   A model of human-animal relationships in intensive livestock industries (From Hemsworth and Coleman, 1998).

higher egg production than those that received minimal human contact. Cransberg et al. (2000) found that the speed of movement of the stockperson in moving through meat chicken units to inspect birds was positively correlated with the level of fear of humans by birds.

There is also evidence that pigs and dairy cattle are sensitive to visual contact with humans. Gonyou et al. (1986) found that a regular handling treatment involving no tactile interactions but rapid and close approach by the experimenter resulted in pigs showing marked avoidance of humans, increased size of the adrenal glands, and reduced growth similar to those responses shown by pigs that received negative tactile interactions whenever they failed to avoid the approaching experimenter. Humans standing erect or approaching young pigs have been shown to be more threatening to pigs than humans squatting or avoiding pigs (Hemsworth, Gonyou, and Dzuik, 1986b). Breuer et al. (2000) found that frequency of waving by stockpeople was significantly and negatively correlated with the approach behavior of cows to an experimenter but not significantly correlated with restlessness of cows during milking. In contrast, speed of movement in moving cows from pasture to milking was positively and significantly correlated with restlessness during milking but not significantly correlated with the approach behavior of cows to an experimenter (Breuer et al., 2000).

Pajor, Rushen, and de Passille (2000), using aversion learning techniques in which animals learn to associate a location with a specific treatment, found that cattle showed a similar aversion, based on avoidance, to hitting and shouting by stockpeople. Breuer et al. (2000), in studying interfarm correlations in human and cow behavior, found a significant positive correlation between frequency of loud harsh vocalizations by stockpeople and restlessness by cows during milking and also a significant negative correlation between frequency of soft quiet vocalizations and cow restlessness. It is interesting that there was also a significant negative correlation between the use of loud, harsh vocalizations and milk yield. Waynert et al. (1999) studied the effects of noise on cattle and found that both heart rate and movement were greater when animals were exposed to a recording of humans shouting than a recording of the noise of metal-on-metal clanging.

While there were no differences in the approach behavior of young pigs to humans using a loud harsh voice or soft quiet voice, young pigs showed less approach to a human wearing gloves than to the ungloved human (Hemsworth et al., 1986b). It is possible that human odors particularly on the hands are used by pigs in recognition of humans and that masking these odors may create uncertainty or novelty for the animals.

Care is required in interpreting many of these studies in which individual cues have been studied since animals experienced with humans may learn through conditioning to associate insignificant cues from humans with those that have significance for the animals. For example, auditory cues from humans may be associated with negative tactile interactions by humans since many nontactile interactions may accompany negative interactions by humans. Another consideration is the identification of the nature of the interactions that stockpeople use and could use when interacting with their animals. For example, interactions such as pats, strokes, the hand of the stockperson resting on the animal, talking, and slow deliberate movement are often labeled as positive interactions in many studies. While

Pajor et al. (2000) found that similar effort and time were required to repeatedly move cattle to a location in which the animals were either provided with feed or petted (e.g., talking and stroking), it should be recognized that there is doubt about the nature of some of the interactions labeled as positive. Some may be positive in nature and through their increased use, conditioning should lead to reduced avoidance of humans by cows. Other interactions may be neutral in nature, but nevertheless their frequent use should lead to habituation by animals to the presence of the stockperson and thus fear of humans should decline. The identification of the nature of the range of behaviors used by stockpeople is an important area for future research because it is necessary in developing recommendations on the manner in which stockpeople should interact with their animals in order to minimize the elicitation of fear responses.

Identifying the nature of the interactions used by humans provides the prospect for stockpeople to use negative interactions only when necessary and conversely to utilize positive interactions when the opportunity arises so that the overall fear responses to humans can be minimized. There may also be valuable opportunities to use positive interactions to minimize the aversiveness of the husbandry procedures that humans impose on animals. Rewarding experiences, such as provision of a preferred feed or even positive handling around the time of the procedure, may ameliorate the aversiveness of the procedure and also reduce the chances that animals associate the punishment of the procedure with humans. Human contact, presumably of a positive nature, reduces the acute stress response of cows to rectal palpation, a moderately aversive husbandry procedure (Waiblinger et al., 1999). Furthermore, there is limited evidence that positive interactions by humans may reduce or ameliorate the chronic stress response shown by pigs to tether housing (Pederson et al., 1998).

Therefore, a number of studies indicate that farm animals are particularly sensitive to human contact. Even moderate slaps or hits regularly used will increase the fear responses of cattle and pigs to humans. Livestock not only are sensitive to brief tactile human contact but also are sensitive to nontactile interactions. For example, the regular use of shouting, fast speed of movement, and sudden, unexpected movement can be fear provoking to many livestock. The considerable impact of brief contact, moderate tactile contact, and nontactile contact by humans is surprising to many people both inside and outside of the livestock industries. Many of these interactions that stockpeople routinely use intuitively appear harmless and innocent, particularly when used to handle large animals such as pigs and cattle. Training stockpeople to handle farm animals is therefore a substantial challenge; however, as indicated previously, there are excellent opportunities to improve human-animal interactions in livestock production and thus reduce the substantial limitations that these interactions impose on both the animal and the handler.

DISCRIMINATION BETWEEN HUMANS BY LIVESTOCK

Evidence from handling studies and observations on human-animal interactions in the livestock industries indicate that the history of interactions between humans and the animal will determine the subsequent stimulus properties of humans for the animal. It has been proposed that, through the process of stimulus generalization, the behavioral response of a farm animal to an individual human will extend to all humans (Hemsworth and Coleman, 1998). Stimulus generalization can be defined as a tendency for stimuli similar to the original stimulus in a learning situation to produce the response originally acquired (Reber, 1988).

Evidence from a number of handling studies supports this view that the animal's response to a single human might extend to include all humans through this process of stimulus generalization. For example, pigs that previously were briefly but regularly handled by either a handler in a predominantly negative manner or two handlers who differed markedly in the nature of their behavior toward pigs, showed similar behavioral responses to familiar and unfamiliar handlers (Hemsworth et al., 1994c). Similar evidence is also available from studies with poultry and sheep (Barnett, Hemsworth, and Jones, 1993; Jones, 1993; Bouissou and Vandenheede, 1995).

However, it is possible that there are handling situations in which animals may not exhibit stimulus generalization. In situations in which there is intense handling, animals may learn to discriminate between this handler and other handlers to which the animals may be subsequently exposed. For example, several studies with rodents indicate that animals can discriminate between the caretaker, with whom the animals have had substantial contact presumably of a positive nature, and a stranger (see review by Dewsbury, 1992). Tanida et al. (1995) found that following an extensive period of intense human contact, young pigs showed greater approach to the familiar handler than to an unfamiliar handler, even though both handlers wore similar clothing. Furthermore, in situations in which the physical characteristics of the handlers may differ markedly, animals may learn to discriminate between the handlers. For example, in a series of experiments, de Passille et al. (1996) found that dairy calves exhibited clear avoidance of a handler that had previously handled them in a negative manner in comparison to handlers wearing clothing of a different color who were either unfamiliar to the calves or had previously handled them in a positive manner. Initially, there was a generalization of the aversive handling, with calves showing increasing avoidance of all handlers; but with repeated treatment, calves discriminated between handlers, and, in particular, between the "negative" and "positive" handlers. It is of interest that discrimination was greatest when tested in the area in which handling had previously occurred rather than in a novel location. These data on calves indicate that discrimination between people by animals will be easier if the animals have some distinct cues on which they can discriminate, such as color of clothing or location of handling.

CONCLUSION

It is clear that the behavior of stockpeople can result in the development by farm animals of stimulus-specific fear responses to humans, which can have large motivational and emotional effects on the animals. Even moderate negative interactions, such as sudden and unexpected appearance, if frequently used will result in animals becoming fearful of humans. It is these fear levels, through stress, that may adversely affect animal welfare and productivity. While most research examining the effects of human behavior on farm animals has focused on tactile interactions by humans, it should be appreciated that other types of human contact, such as visual and auditory contact, may also be influential.

In the last 20 years, scientists have explored the impact of the relationship between humans and farm animals on the animal. Farm animals are particularly sensitive to human contact, and the effects of brief contact, moderate tactile contact, or nontactile contact by humans is considerable and surprising. There is a clear need to reduce the substantial limitations that these interactions impose on the welfare of the animal. The risk to welfare arises as a consequence of the stress response in animals that are fearful of humans. The risk to animal welfare also exists in situations in which the attitude and behavior of the stockperson toward the animals are negative because the stockperson's commitment to the surveillance of and the attendance to welfare issues is most likely highly questionable. The existence of sequential relationships between these human and animal variables indicates opportunities to target stockperson attitudes and behavior in order to improve livestock welfare and productivity. Excellent opportunities exist and chapter 9 by G. J. Coleman explores these in more detail.

While our understanding of the regulation and impact of human-animal interactions has improved considerably over the last decade or so, recognition of the role of stockpeople in the welfare and productivity of livestock has only recently occurred. Much has been done to improve genetics, nutrition, health, and housing of livestock, but efforts to target the stockperson, who performs such a key function, has just begun. The role and impact of the stockperson should not be underestimated: to do so would seriously risk the welfare and productivity of livestock. Indeed, it is possible that the stockperson may be the most influential factor affecting animal welfare in intensively managed livestock production systems. It is therefore likely that in the near future both the livestock industries and the general community will place an increasing emphasis on ensuring the competency of stockpeople to manage the welfare of livestock.

REFERENCES

Barnett, J. L. Hemsworth, P. H. and Jones, R. B. 1993. Behavioural responses of commercial farmed laying hens to humans: Evidence of stimulus generalization. *Applied Animal Behaviour Science* 37: 139–146.

Barnett, J. L., Hemsworth, P. H. and Newman, E. A. 1992. Fear of humans and its relationships with productivity in laying hens at commercial farms. *British Poultry Science* 33: 699–710.

Barnett, J. L., Hemsworth, P. H., Hennessy, D. P., McCallum, T. M. and Newman, E. A. 1994. The effects of modifying the amount of human contact on the behavioural, physiological and production responses of laying hens. *Applied Animal Behaviour Science* 41: 87–100.

Barton Gade, P., Blaabjerg, L. and Christensen, L. 1992. New lairage system for slaughter pigs. Effects on behaviour and quality characteristics. *Proceedings 38th International Congress of Meat Science and Technology*, vol. 2, pp. 161–164. Clemont Ferrand, France.

Boissy, A. and Bouissou, M. F. 1988. Effects of early handling on heifers' subsequent reactivity to humans and to unfamiliar situations. *Applied Animal Behaviour Science* 20: 259–273.

Bouissou, M. F. and Vandenheede, M. 1995. Fear reactions of domestic sheep confronted with either a human or a human-like model. *Behavioural Processes* 43: 81–92.

Breuer, K., Hemsworth, P. H., Barnett, J. L., Matthews, L. R. and Coleman, G. J. 2000. Behavioural response to humans and the productivity of commercial dairy cows. *Applied Animal Behaviour Science* 66: 11–20.

Caine, N. G., 1992. Humans as predators: Observation studies and the risk of pseudohabituation. In Davis H. and Balfour A. D. (eds.), *Inevitable Bond: Examining Scientist-Animal Interactions*. Cambridge University Press, Cambridge, pp. 357–364.

Coleman, G. J., Hemsworth, P. H., Hay, M. and Cox, M. 1998. Predicting stockperson behaviour towards pigs from attitudinal and job-related variables and empathy. *Applied Animal Behaviour Science* 58: 63–75.

——. 2000. Modifying stockperson attitudes and behaviour towards pigs at a large commercial farm. *Applied Animal Behaviour Science* 66: 11–20.

Collins, J. W. and Siegel, P. B. 1987. Human handling, flock size and responses to an *E. coli* challenge in young chickens. *Applied Animal Behaviour Science* 19: 183–188.

Cransberg, P. H., Hemsworth, P. H. and Coleman, G. J. 2000. Human factors affecting the behaviour and productivity of commercial broiler chickens. *British Poultry Science* 41: 272–279.

de Passille, A. M., Rushen, J., Ladewig, J. and Petherick, C. 1996 Dairy calves' discrimination of people based on previous handling. *Journal of Animal Science* 74: 969–974.

Dewsbury, D. A. 1992. Studies of rodent-human interactions in animal psychology. In Davis, H. and Balfour, A. D. (eds.), *The Inevitable Bond—Examining Scientist-Animal Interactions*. Cambridge University Press, Cambridge, pp. 27–43.

Duncan, I. J. H., Slee, G. S., Kettlewell, P., Berry, P. and Carlisle, A. J. 1986. Comparison of the stressfulness of harvesting broiler chickens by machine and by hand. *British Poultry Science* 27: 109–114.

Estep, D. Q. and Hetts, S. 1992. Interactions, relationships, and bonds: The conceptual basis for scientist-animal relations. In Davis, H. and Balfour, A. D. (eds.), *The Inevitable Bond—Examining Scientist-Animal Interactions*. Cambridge University Press, Cambridge, pp. 6–26.

Galef, B. G., Jr. 1970. Aggression and timidity: Responses to novelty in feral Norway rats. *Journal of Comparative Physiology and Psychology* 70: 370–381.

Gonyou, H. W., Hemsworth, P. H. and Barnett, J. L. 1986. Effects of frequent interactions with humans on growing pigs. *Applied Animal Behaviour Science* 16: 269–278.

Grandin, T. 1980. Livestock behavior as related to handling facilities design. *International Journal for the Study of Animal Problems* 1: 33–52.

Gray, J. A. 1987. The psychology of fear and stress. 2d ed. Cambridge University Press, Cambridge.

Gregory, N. G., Wilkins, L. J., Alvey, D. M. and Tucker, S. A. 1993. Effect of catching method and lighting intensity on the prevalence of broken bones and on the ease of handling of end of lay hens. *Veterinary Record* 132: 127–129.

Gross, W. B. and Siegel, P. B. 1979. Adaptation of chickens to their handlers and experimental results. *Avian Diseases* 23: 708–714.

——. 1980. Effects of early environmental stresses on chicken body weight, antibody response to RBC antigens, feed efficiency and response to fasting. *Avian Diseases* 24: 549–579.

——. 1982. Influences of sequences of environmental factors on the responses of chickens to fasting and to *Staphylococcus aureus* infection. *American Journal of Veterinary Research* 43: 137–139.

Hearnshaw, H., Barlow, R. and Want, G. 1979. Development of a "temperament" or "handling difficulty" score for cattle. *Proceedings of the Inaugural Conference of Australian Animal Breed Genetics* 1: 164–166.

Hediger, H. 1964. The animals relationship with man. In *Wild Animals in Captivity*. Dover Publications, Inc., New York.

Hemsworth, P. H. and Barnett, J. L. 1987. Human-animal interactions. In Price, E. O. (ed.), *The Veterinary Clinics of North America, Food Animal Practice*. W. B. Saunders Co., Philadelphia. Vol. 3: 339–356.

——. 1991. The effects of aversively handling pigs either individually or in groups on their behaviour, growth and corticosteroids. *Applied Animal Behaviour Science* 30: 61–72.

——. 1992. The effects of early contact with humans on the subsequent level of fear of humans in pigs. *Applied Animal Behaviour Science* 35: 83–90.

Hemsworth, P. H. and Coleman, G. J. 1998. *Human-Livestock Interactions: The Stockperson and the Productivity and Welfare of Intensively-Farmed Animals*. CAB International, Oxon, UK.

Hemsworth P. H. and Gonyou, H. W. 1997. Human contact. In Appleby, M. C. and Hughes, B. O. (eds.), *Animal Welfare*. CAB International, Oxon, UK, pp. 205–305.

Hemsworth, P. H., Barnett, J. L. and Campbell, R. G. 1996a. A study of the relative aversiveness of a new daily injection procedure for pigs. *Applied Animal Behaviour Science* 49: 389–401.

Hemsworth, P. H., Barnett, J. L. and Coleman, G. J. 1992. Fear of humans and its consequences for the domestic pig. In Davis, H. and Balfour, A. D. (eds.), *The Inevitable Bond—Examining Scientist-Animal Interactions*. Cambridge University Press, Cambridge, pp. 264–284.

Hemsworth, P. H., Barnett, J. L. and Hansen, C. 1981a. The influence of handling by humans on the behaviour, growth and corticosteroids in the juvenile female pig. *Hormones and Behavior* 15: 396–403.

——. 1986a. The influence of handling by humans on the behaviour, reproduction and corticosteroids of male and female pigs. *Applied Animal Behaviour Science* 15: 303–314.

——. 1987. The influence of inconsistent handling on the behaviour, growth and corticosteroids of young pigs. *Applied Animal Behaviour Science* 17: 245–252.

Hemsworth, P. H., Barnett, J. L., Coleman, G. J. and Hansen, C. 1989. A study of the relationships between the attitudinal and behavioural profiles of stockpersons and the level of fear of humans and reproductive performance of commercial pigs. *Applied Animal Behaviour Science* 23: 301–314.

Hemsworth, P. H., Barnett, J. L., Treacy, D. and Madgwick, P. 1990. The heritability of the trait fear of humans and the association between this trait and the subsequent reproductive performance of gilts. *Applied Animal Behavioural Science* 25: 85–95.

Hemsworth, P. H., Brand, A. and Willems, P. J. 1981b. The behavioural response of sows to the presence of human beings and their productivity. *Livestock Production Science* 8: 67–74.

Hemsworth, P. H., Coleman, G. J. and Barnett, J. L. 1994a. Improving the attitude and behaviour of stockpersons towards pigs and the consequences on the behaviour and reproductive performance of commercial pigs. *Applied Animal Behaviour Science* 39: 349–362.

Hemsworth, P. H., Coleman, G. J., Barnett, J. L. and Borg, S. 2000. Relationships between human-animal interactions and productivity of commercial dairy cows. *Journal of Animal Science* 78: 2821–2831.

Hemsworth, P. H., Coleman, G. J., Barnett, J. L. and Jones, R. B. 1994b. Fear of humans and the productivity of commercial broiler chickens. *Applied Animal Behaviour Science* 41: 101–114.

Hemsworth, P. H., Coleman, G. J., Barnett, J. L., Borg, S. and Dowling, S. 2002. The effects of cognitive behavioral intervention on the attitude and behavior of stockpersons and the behavior and productivity of commercial dairy cows. *Journal of Animal Science* 80: 68–78.

Hemsworth, P. H., Coleman, G. J., Cox, M. and Barnett, J. L. 1994c. Stimulus generalisation: The inability of pigs to discriminate between humans on the basis of their previous handling experience. *Applied Animal Behaviour Science* 40: 129–142.

Hemsworth, P. H., Gonyou, H. W. and Dzuik, P. J. 1986b. Human communication with pigs: The behavioural response of pigs to specific human signals. *Applied Animal Behaviour Science* 15: 45–54.

Hemsworth, P. H., Verge, J. and Coleman, G. J. 1996b. Conditioned approach avoidance responses to humans: The ability of pigs to associate feeding and aversive social experiences in the presence of humans with humans. *Applied Animal Behaviour Science* 50: 71–82.

Hutson, G. D. 1985. The influence of barley food rewards on sheep movement through a handling system. *Applied Animal Behaviour Science* 14: 263–273.

Jones, R. B. 1993. Reduction of the domestic chick's fear of humans by regular handling and related treatments. *Animal Behaviour* 46: 991–998.

Jones, R. B. and Faure, J. M. 1981. The effects of regular handling on fear responses in the domestic chick. *Behavioural Processes* 6: 135–143.

Jones, R. B. and Waddington, D. 1992. Modification of fear in domestic chicks, *Gallus gallus domesticus,* via regular handling and early environmental enrichment. *Animal Behaviour* 43: 1021–1033.

——. 1993. Attenuation of the domestic chick's fear of human beings via regular handling: In search of a sensitive period. *Applied Animal Behaviour Science* 36: 185–195.

Jones, R. B., Mills, A. D. and Faure, J. M. 1991. Genetic and experimental manipulation of fear-related behaviour in Japanese Quail chicks *(Coturnix coturnix japonica). Journal of Comparative Psychology* 105: 15–24.

Lyons, D. M. 1989. Individual differences in temperament of dairy goats and the inhibition of milk ejection. *Applied Animal Behaviour Science* 22: 269–282.

Lyons, D. M., Price, E. D. and Moberg, G. P. 1988. Individual differences in temperament of domestic dairy goats: Constancy and change. *Animal Behaviour* 36: 1323–1333.

Markowitz, T. M., Dally, M. R., Gursky, K. and Price E. O. 1998. Early handling increases lamb affinity for humans. *Animal Behaviour* 55: 187–195.

Matthews, L. R. 1993. Deer handling and transport. In Grandin, T. (ed.), *Livestock Handling and Transport.* CAB International, Oxon, UK, pp. 253–272.

Munksgaard, L., de Passille, A. M., Rushen, J., Thodberg, K. and Jensen, M. B. 1995. The ability of dairy cows to distinguish between people. *Proceedings of the 29th International Congress of the International Society of Applied Ethology,* Exeter, 3–5 August, pp. 19–20 (Abstract).

Murphey, R. M., Moura Duarte, F. A. and Torres Penendo, M. C. 1981. Responses of cattle to humans in open spaces: Breed comparisons and approach-avoidance relationships. *Behaviour Genetics* 2(1): 37–47.

Murphy, L. B. 1976. *A Study of the Behavioural Expression of Fear and Exploration in Two Stocks of Domestic Fowl.* Ph.D. Dissertation, Edinburgh University, UK.

Murphy, L. B. and Duncan, L. J. H. 1977. Attempts to modify the responses of domestic fowl towards human beings. I. The association of human contact with a food reward. *Applied Animal Ethology* 3: 321–334.

——. 1978. Attempts to modify the responses of domestic fowl towards human beings. II. The effect of early experience. *Applied Animal Ethology* 4: 5–12.

Pajor, E. A., Rushen, J. and de Passille, A. M. B. 2000. Aversion learning techniques to evaluate dairy cattle handling practices. *Applied Animal Behaviour Science* 69: 89–102.

Pederson, V. 1993. Effects of difference post-weaning handling procedures on the later behaviour of silver foxes. *Applied Animal Behaviour Science* 37: 239–250.

Pedersen, V., and Jeppesen, L. L. 1990. Effects of early handling on better behaviour and stress responses in the silver fox (*Vulpes vulpes*). *Applied Animal Behaviour Science* 26: 383–393.

Pedersen, V., Barnett, J. L., Hemsworth, P. H., Newman, E. A. and Schirmer B. 1998. The effects of handling on behavioural and physiological responses to housing in tether-stalls in pregnant pigs. *Animal Welfare* 7: 137–150.

Reber, A. S. 1988. *Dictionary of Psychology*. Penguin Books, London.

Rushen, J., de Passille, A. M. B. and Munksgaard L., 1999. Fear of people by cows and effects on milk yield, behaviour and heart rate at milking. *J. Dairy Sci* 82: 720–727.

Rushen, J., de Passille, A. M. B., Munksgaard L. and Tanida, H., 2001. People as social actors in the world of animals. In Keeling, L. J. and Gonyou, H. W. (eds.), *Social Behaviour in Farm Animals*. CAB International, Oxon UK, pp. 353–372.

Rushen, J., Munksgaard L., de Passille, A. M. B., Jensen, M. B. and Thodberg K. 1995. Location of handling and dairy cows' ability to discrimate between gentle and aversive handlers. *Proceedings of the 29th International Congress of the International Society for Applied Ethology,* Exeter, UK.

Schaefer, T. 1968. Some methodological implications of the research on "early handling" in the rat. In Newton, G. and Levine, S. (eds.), *Early Experience and Behaviour: The Psychobiology of Development*. Charles C. Thomas Publisher, Florida.

Scott, J. P. 1992. The phenomenon of attachment in human-non human relationships. In Davis, H. and Balfour, A. D. (eds.), *The Inevitable Bond—Examining Scientist-Animal Interactions*. Cambridge University Press, Cambridge, pp. 72–92.

Seabrook, M. F. 1972. A study to determine the influence of the herdsman's personality on milk yield. *Journal of Agricultural Labour Science* 1: 45–59.

Syme, L. A., Durham, I. H. and Elphick, G. R. 1981. Microprocessor control of sheep movement. In *Proceedings 2nd Conference on Wool Harvesting Research and Development*. Australian Wool Corporation, pp. 237–245.

Tanida, H., Miura, A., Tanaka, T. and Yoshimoto, T. 1995. Behavioural response to humans in individually handled weanling pigs. *Applied Animal Behaviour Science* 42: 249–259.

Waiblinger, S., Menke, C., Korff, J., Palme, R., and Bucher, A. 1999. Effects of handling and the presence of different persons on the behaviour and heart rate of dairy cows during rectalisation. *Proceedings of the 33rd International Congress of the International Society for Applied Ethology, Lillehammer, Norway*, p. 49 (Abstract).

Walker, S. 1987. *Animal learning: An introduction*. Routledge and Kegan Ltd., London.

Waring, G. H. 1983. *Horse behaviour. The behavioural traits and adaptations of domestic and wild horses, including ponies*. Noyes Publications, Park Ridge, NJ.

Waynert, D. F., Stookey, J. M., Schwartzkopf-Genwein, K. S., Watts, J. M. and Waltz, C. S. 1999. Response of beef cattle to noise during handling. *Applied Animal Behaviour Science* 62: 27–42.

3

Quality of Life for Farm Animals: Linking Science, Ethics, and Animal Welfare

David Fraser and Daniel M. Weary

INTRODUCTION

Ethical concern about the proper treatment of animals has spanned many centuries and many cultures; expressing those concerns in terms of "animal welfare" is a more culture-specific development. For social reformers of nineteenth-century England, better treatment of animals was part of a drive to improve the moral tone of society by stamping out the vice of cruelty. For members of the Jain religion, proper treatment of animals flows from a broader concern to avoid causing harm to other living beings. For early pastoralists of the Middle East, the diligent care of animals was virtuous behavior modeled after God's treatment of the world. Presumably, each of these value systems helped to promote the welfare of animals, yet animal welfare was not the central, organizing principle.

In contemporary Western culture, however, where many people take for granted a reasonable level of nutrition, shelter, and safety, "well-being," or "quality of life," has become an important concept and focus of ethical concern. Philosophers analyze quality of life; psychologists devise research methods to assess it; medical and mental health workers see quality of life as a key goal of their professions. In this cultural context, quality-of-life concerns often play a central role in ethical debate about the proper treatment of animals. People express concern, for example, about the effects of over-crowding on the well-being of hens in cages, about frustration among sows that cannot build nests, about distress among calves removed from their mothers, about lameness among confined dairy cows, about acute stress among excitable pigs during transport, about pain from procedures such as branding and castration, and about abnormal behavior by horses confined in small paddocks. Here the focus is not mainly on eradicating cruelty (as with English reformers), or avoiding harm (as in Jainism), or providing diligent care (as with Middle Eastern pastoralists), but on the quality of life or well-being or welfare of the animals themselves.

By focusing on animal welfare in this way, our culture has opened the door for science to play a key role in operationalizing and addressing ethical concerns about the treatment of animals. For example, scientists have studied the effects of crowding on animals and have recommended space allowances on this basis; they have developed methods to recognize and mitigate pain and distress in animals; they have conducted surveys on the causes of lameness and recommended preventive measures; and they have analyzed physiological "stress" responses and identified ways to reduce these responses. These and other

39

lines of research constitute an emerging field of research and technical innovation that Dawkins (1980) termed the "science of animal welfare."

However, the application of science to animal welfare places research in a somewhat unusual role. Animal welfare science developed not out of human curiosity (like paleontology) nor as an attempt to develop new products (like applied electronics), but as a response to ethical concerns. In pursuing the science, therefore, we need to be clear on what the ethical concerns are, on how well these concerns are captured in scientists' conceptions of animal welfare, on the strengths and weaknesses of using science to address these concerns, and on the interplay between the scientific and ethical elements (Tannenbaum, 1991; Sandøe and Simonsen, 1992; Rollin, 1993, 1995; Stafleu, Grommers, and Vorstenbosch, 1996).

In this chapter, we will (1) briefly identify the ethical concerns that have arisen over the quality of life of animals, (2) review the scientific and technical approaches that are being used to address these concerns, and (3) discuss some of the confusions that have arisen in trying to apply science to issues that are fundamentally ethical in nature.

DIFFERENT CONCEPTIONS OF THE QUALITY OF LIFE OF ANIMALS

Three Issues

Social critics, ethicists, and others have expressed three different but overlapping types of concern about the quality of life of animals (Duncan and Fraser, 1997; Fraser et al., 1997).

A traditional set of concerns—often expressed by veterinarians, animal producers, and others with practical responsibilities for animal care—centers on the basic **biological functioning** of animals including normal health, growth, behavior, and development. For example, in the early years of intensive animal production systems, veterinarian George Taylor (1972) argued that animal welfare is generally better in these systems than in the older, extensive systems, because the animal "is certainly much freer from disease and attack by its mates; it receives much better attention from the attendants, is sure of shelter and bedding and a reasonable amount of good food and water."

Since Taylor's article, concerns about the biological functioning of animals have extended well beyond these basic elements. Issues today include abnormal and seemingly functionless types of behavior that some animals perform, especially in confinement; "production diseases," such as mastitis and laminitis among dairy cattle, which appear to be more common among animals bred and managed for very high productivity; and bodily damage resulting from environments to which the animals are not adapted.

A second major concern centers on the **affective states** of animals—emotions and feelings, especially unpleasant states such as fear, pain, hunger, and distress. Concern arises, for example, over pain caused by branding and castration, over fear caused by rough handling, and over separation distress caused by abrupt weaning or social isolation. In addition to these traditional issues, concerns have arisen over other unpleasant states, such as boredom, anxiety, and depression, which may occur in animals, and about depriving animals of pleasant affective states. For example, humane advocate Ruth Harrison (1964) asked, "Have we the right to rob [animals] of all pleasure in life simply to make more money more quickly out of their carcasses?"

However, biological functioning and affective states do not fully exhaust the range of ethical concerns that arise over animals' quality of life. Consider, for example, a chimpanzee kept isolated from birth in a small steel cage. Imagine that we have such sophisticated technology that we can keep the chimpanzee perfectly free from disease and injury, nourished so as to promote normal growth, drugged so as to prevent any pain, discomfort, or frustration, and infused with opioids from time to time to create feelings of pleasure. Would we have ethical concerns about the quality of life of such an animal? At least some people would object that good quality of life requires that animals be allowed to live **relatively natural lives**, in accordance with their basic nature. Astrid Lindgren, the Swedish novelist and critic of intensive animal production, objected to the unnaturalness of modern production facilities and urged that farm animals should have, "at least a temporary reprieve from the floors of barns and the crowded spaces where the poor animals are stored until they die. Let them see the sun just once, get away from the murderous roar of the fans. Let them get to breathe fresh air for once, instead of manure gas" (Anonymous, 1989).

A more analytic version of this concern was expressed by philosopher Bernard Rollin (1993, 1995) who proposed that animals have "natures—the pigness of the pig, the cowness of the cow . . . —which are as essential to their well-being as speech and assembly are to us." What Rollin perceived as the "new social ethic" for animals demands that "animals' basic natures will not be submerged in the course of their being used by humans" (Rollin, 1993, p. 11). Interpreted in the context of the biological sciences, the "nature" of an animal can be understood to mean the set of adaptations that is characteristic of the species, and the set of genetically encoded instructions that guides the animal's normal development (Fraser et al., 1997). Hence, to allow animals to live in accordance with their natures would mean allowing them to live in a manner to which they are adapted and to develop in a manner that is normal for the species.

Three Issues or One?

But do these three concerns not boil down to the same thing? In some cases they may well. A pig in hot weather will normally wallow in mud; if an overheated pig is confined in a pen where wallowing is impossible, its quality of life is arguably affected according to all three criteria: the natural behavior is prevented; the animal is likely to undergo a heat-stress reaction, which involves reduced growth and reproduction; and the animal is likely to feel uncomfortably hot. Such examples have led some commentators to claim that by addressing any one of the concerns, such as ensuring a high level of biological functioning, we will address the others as well.

The situation can be different, however, when animals are kept in environments very unlike those in which the species evolved. Figure 3.1 provides a visual representation. Circle A represents the set of adaptations possessed by the animal mainly as a result of its evolutionary ancestry and perhaps modified by genetic changes during domestication and the individual's own learning and experiences. Some adaptations involve affective states, such

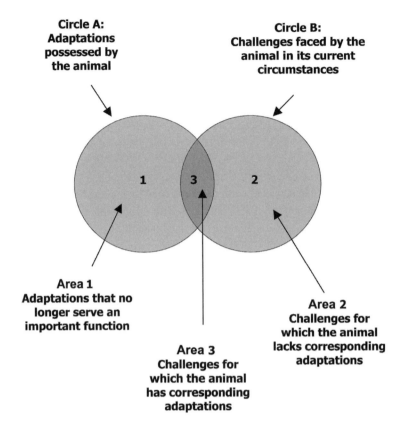

Figure 3.1.   Conceptual model illustrating three types of problems that may arise when the adaptations possessed by an animal (circle A) make an imperfect fit to the challenges it faces in the circumstances in which it is kept (circle B). The different types of problems, taken together, constitute the subject matter of much animal welfare research (From Fraser et al., 1997).

as hunger, cold, and pain, which motivate the animal to act in certain ways. Circle B represents the challenges faced by the animal in its current circumstances. These may include cold temperatures, exposure to pathogens, and aggression from other animals. If animals are kept in environments very similar to those in which the species evolved and the individual developed, then we may expect a close correspondence between the adaptations and the challenges. For many captive and domestic animals, however, we expect some discrepancy between the adaptations and the challenges, producing the three areas shown in figure 3.1.

In area 1 of circle A, we find adaptations possessed by the animal that no longer serve their original role in meeting challenges in the environment. Some such adaptations involve strong motivation to carry out a particular type of behavior. For example, in the days before they give birth, pregnant sows appear highly motivated to find and prepare a nest, presumably because this behavior was essential for the survival of their young in the environment in which the species evolved. Modern sows retain this motivation, and if confined in farrowing crates, they become intensely restless, make persistent attempts to escape, and root vigorously on the solid floor sometimes to the point of injuring themselves, even though the behavior is likely irrelevant to piglet survival in the animal's current environment. In such cases, the inability to carry out the behavior may be very unpleasant for the animal (a negative affective state), even though the survival of the young (the behavior's original contribution to biological functioning) is not affected.

In area 2 of circle B, we find challenges in the environment for which the animal lacks corresponding adaptations. For example, animals may be poorly equipped to avoid becoming obese if concentrated food is available, to avoid losing physical condition if exercise is not required, to avoid pathogens when kept close to diseased animals, and to avoid polluted air even at levels that damage their respiratory systems. These problems may seriously impair biological functioning, without the animal showing any evidence of suffering, at least until pathological changes are well advanced.

Area 3—the overlap of circles A and B—represents the situation where an adaptation the animal possesses corresponds to a challenge it faces. For example, the animal will be exposed to a range of temperatures, and it will possess certain thermoregulatory adaptations. This correspondence does not eliminate problems of animal welfare. The animal may, for example, still suffer when very hot or very cold. In these cases, however, we expect unpleasant affective states (feeling cold) to correspond more closely to biological functioning (actual or incipient cold stress). Hence, providing a "natural environment" for the species does not eliminate all welfare concerns, although it may eliminate the two classes of problems represented by areas 1 and 2, which have become prominent issues in the debate about the welfare of farm animals.

Thus, we see a set of ethical concerns—biological functioning, affective states, and natural living—that arises over the welfare of animals, and a conceptual framework (fig. 3.1) that shows that these concerns may arise singly as well as together.

SCIENTIFIC AND TECHNICAL APPROACHES

These concerns have stimulated a range of scientific and technical efforts to study, assess, and improve animal welfare.

Achieving High Levels of Agricultural Productivity

In certain circumstances, simple measures of agricultural productivity, such as rate of growth and reproduction, can identify problems in biological functioning. When laying hens are crowded beyond certain minimal space allowances, their rate of lay declines and death rate increases. When pigs are kept in hot summer conditions without any means of cooling, young animals grow more slowly and breeding animals conceive smaller litters. Such links between productivity and animal welfare tend to be clearest when, as in these examples, there is some depression of normal health, growth, reproduction, and survival, reflecting a clear problem with normal functioning. In such cases, improved survival, growth, and reproduction, as may be achieved through improved nutrition, health, and shelter, can indicate positive improvements in the quality of life of animals.

However, there are many confounding factors that weaken the link between productivity and other aspects of biological functioning, especially where productivity is already high. One confounding factor is intense genetic selection for specific production traits. For example, hens highly bred for egg production will draw calcium from their bones for shell deposition, to the point of becoming prone to leg bone fractures; and strong selection of pigs for lean growth has sometimes led to high-strung animals that are susceptible to sudden death when stressed. In these cases, high productivity is achieved at the expense of other aspects of biological functioning. Another confounding factor is the use of hormones, antibiotics, and other interventions to enhance productivity. For example, beef calves are sometimes removed abruptly from the cow before their normal weaning age, transported to auctions, mixed with unfamiliar calves, and then transported again to the feedlot. This can cause digestive problems and weight loss extending for several days, but such practices can still be commercially advantageous if the animals are given antibiotics. Similarly, injections of growth hormone may cause a high-producing cow to increase her milk yield even more, but also increase the risk of certain diseases if her feed intake and feed quality are not carefully managed. Moreover, productivity should not be confused with profitability. For example, the highest profit in egg production is often achieved when hens are crowded to the point that their individual rate of lay is reduced (Adams and Craig, 1985; Rousch, 1986).

In short, there are cases where improving productivity can play a real role in improving farm animal welfare, but the relationship between productivity, profit, and welfare is often too complex for any simple inferences to be drawn.

Preventing Disease and Injury

Preventing disease and injury is a more straightforward means of improving animal welfare through maintaining good biological functioning. Traditional examples include much of veterinary medicine, especially the treatment of sick and injured animals, vaccination programs, measures to eliminate pathogens from herds and flocks, and measures to prevent long-distance transfer of diseases. More recently scientists have used pathological and epidemiological data to improve animal housing and management. For example, Tauson (1984) used such simple indicators as foot abnormalities and feather damage to propose changes in cage design for laying hens, and these led to major improvements in bird welfare. Using epidemiological data, Martin (1983) showed that certain management practices —notably, mixing calves from different farms, large group size, and certain changes in diet —increase the likelihood that calves in feedlots will develop bovine respiratory disease. Numerous studies have shown that the incidence of mastitis in dairy cows is influenced by aspects of the physical environment including stall length and width, drafts, the type of bedding, and restriction of movement (International Dairy Federation, 1987).

In these examples, research that allows us to reduce disease and injury problems improves biological functioning and, hence, animal welfare. Where there is no such clear evidence of impaired functioning, scientists have often developed less direct indicators of altered animal welfare.

Avoiding "Stress"

Since the early twentieth century, theories have arisen over how the body responds to adverse conditions. The great physiologist Walter Cannon proposed that a wide range of emotional states, including pain, hunger, and fear, involve activation of the sympathetic nervous system and secretion of adrenaline from the medulla of the adrenal gland. This generalized response is sometimes termed the "fight or flight" response or the "SAM" response (for sympathetic-adrenal-medullary). A second major response system was described by physiologist Hans Selye who found that a variety of adverse conditions, including disease, physical restraint, and exposure to cold, produce a characteristic set of responses that Selye termed the "General Adaptation Syndrome." These involve release of corticotropin releasing hormone (CRH) from the hypothalamus, which stimulates release of adrenocorticotropic hormone (ACTH) from the anterior pituitary gland, which in turn stimulates secretion of glucocorticoid hormones (such as cortisol) from the adrenal cortex. Selye's bold hypothesis was that this "HPA" response (for hypothalamus-pituitary-adrenal cortex) serves as a generalized response, preparing the body to respond to all manner of challenges (Sapolsky, 1992).

The theories of Cannon and Selye led some scientists to use the HPA response, the SAM response, and many related endocrine, immunological, and hematological measures as a generalized means of studying how animal welfare is affected by all manner of factors including crowding, aggression, and physical restraint. For example, various studies have compared plasma cortisol levels and related measures in calves housed under different degrees of restriction. Cortisol levels are sometimes higher in certain of the more restrictive housing systems (Wilson et al., 1999), but other studies show the opposite result, perhaps because of the greater difficulty in catching loose-housed calves for blood sampling (Stull and McDonough, 1994). Similarly, studies have compared measures of HPA activity among sows in stalls, tethers, and group-housing systems. Cortisol levels are often found to be particularly high among tethered sows, but much of this may be due to specific features of the tethering system used, rather than to tethering itself (Barnett et al., 2000).

Other scientists have emphasized the limitations of using physiological stress responses in assessing animal welfare (e.g., Dantzer, 2001; Dantzer and Mormède, 1983; Rushen, 1991; Rushen and de Passillé, 1992). One limitation is that activation of these responses is not specific to unpleasant states. For example, cortisol secretion is increased simply by exposure to novel environments, by exercise, and by such presumably pleasurable activities as mating and nursing (Rushen and de Passillé, 1992). Hence, these generalized responses may really represent a form of activation when the body meets some kind of challenge, but not necessarily an unpleasant one. Furthermore, some forms of long-term discomfort, including hot conditions and uncomfortable housing, are not reflected by increased HPA activity once the animal's initial reaction to the conditions is past (Dantzer and Mormède, 1983; Ladewig and Smidt, 1989). Moreover, given that the SAM and HPA responses are natural and often adaptive adjustments of the body, there is much debate over how to distinguish between normal bodily responses and impaired welfare (Barnett and Hemsworth, 1990; Mendl, 1991).

In response to these and other problems, Moberg (1985) proposed an alternative approach to assessing animal welfare within the context of stress biology. Moberg noted that although the common stress responses are often natural and adaptive, if sufficiently intense or prolonged they can lead to pathological changes such as clinical disease, failure of reproduction, or outbreaks of harmful behavior. However, such breakdowns of normal biological functioning are often preceded by some "prepathological" condition; for example, sustained high levels of the HPA response can lead to reduced immune competence and to altered secretion of reproductive hormones, before any disease or reproductive dysfunction is observed. Moberg proposed that full-blown pathology is neither a humane nor an efficient measure of impaired well-being, and recommended the occurrence of prepathological states as better welfare indicators.

Although the HPA and SAM responses do not necessarily reflect adverse conditions, they may still be useful for quantifying and comparing an animal's reactions in cases where short-term adverse conditions are clearly present. In particular, some scientists have used cortisol responses as an index of the degree of pain experienced by animals as a result of surgical procedures. For example, lambs show a surge in plasma cortisol after castration and tail docking, but Sutherland et al. (1999) found that this response is reduced if the animals receive a local anesthetic to block the pain.

Ensuring High Levels of Fitness or Its Correlates

The theory of natural selection has also been used to provide a rationale for assessing animal welfare. Natural selection causes genetic traits to increase in frequency in a population if these traits provide individuals with an advantage in terms of their "fitness," that is, their ability to survive and reproduce. Many of the physiological and behavioral responses used in welfare assessment can be seen as genetically selected adaptations that promote fitness (Dawkins, 1998). Some authors have also suggested that the fitness consequences of such adaptations (i.e., differential reproduction and survival) can themselves be considered as welfare indicators (Broom, 1991a,b). For example, Hurnik (1993) emphasized longevity as an integrative measure that serves as an "indirect indicator of quality of life." Hurnik argued that an animal's quality of life is directly related to the satisfaction of the many needs that are important for survival, health, and comfort, and that the more adequately these needs are satisfied, the longer the animal may be expected to live. Hence, Hurnik argued that longevity integrates the various needs over the life of the animal, and that we can enhance animal welfare by keeping animals in circumstances that promote long life.

However, fitness requires animals not only to survive, but also to mate, give birth, and rear young, and sometimes they pursue these activities at considerable cost to their longevity (Sachser, 2002). In fact, Barnard and Hurst (1996) propose that although humans have been selected to achieve fitness by long life and relatively slow reproduction, some species (many rodents and fish, for example) achieve fitness by expending themselves through high rates of reproduction. Hence, Barnard and Hurst argue that the common reliance on health, long life, and low stress as measures of animal welfare reflects a human-centered bias. According to this logic, to achieve good welfare among animals we need to understand the "design rules" by which they achieve high fitness, and allow animals to exercise these "natural . . . strategies of self-expenditure" (p. 415). This could potentially give rise to different approaches to studying animal welfare, especially for short-lived, rapidly reproducing species.

Preventing Abnormal Behavior

When animals are kept in circumstances unlike those in which the species evolved, they sometimes show unexpected behavior that appears to serve no adaptive purpose. Caged tigers may trace and retrace the same route in their cages; sheep may denude their pen-mates by chewing their wool; horses may grip a rail with their teeth and suck air into the esophagus. These types of seemingly unadaptive behavior pose a welfare concern in that they appear to involve some breakdown of the normal functioning of the animal; they might also provide evidence of unpleasant affective states if the basis of the abnormal behavior could be properly understood.

A striking example is seen with pregnant sows. During pregnancy most sows have to be limited in their calorie intake in order to prevent excessive weight gain and later health problems, but the restricted diet can lead to serious aggression if the animals are fed in groups. A common solution is to house sows individually, usually in narrow stalls. Some such sows develop stereotyped movement patterns; for example, a sow may make three rooting movements to the left, swing her head to the right, and bite the bar of the stall, and then repeat that same sequence of movements for several hours every day. Observations suggest that the stereotyped actions result from food restriction, which causes a motivation to forage for food (Appleby and Lawrence, 1987). In a barren environment where normal foraging is impossible, elements of foraging behavior are performed in repetitive sequences, and perhaps because such behavior never leads to actual eating, it does not turn off in the normal manner (Hughes and Duncan, 1988). Hence, as well as representing a failure of normal functioning, the behavior may indicate that the sow is experiencing a state of chronic hunger.

Tail biting by pigs (that is, chewing the tail of other pigs to the point of causing injury) is one of many forms of abnormal behavior thought to result from a mismatch between the animal's natural behavior and restrictive environments. An explanatory hypothesis for tail biting (fig. 3.2) suggests that there are complex links between this behavior and animal welfare. According to the hypothesis, the animals direct their natural foraging and exploratory activities, including rooting and chewing, to their pen-mates if more suitable substrates are not available. Most of this behavior is harmless, but the amount or intensity of the behavior can be increased by many factors, such as crowding, hunger, or discomfort, which cause an increase in the animal's general activity. Once the behavior has led to a bleeding injury, any strong attraction to the taste of blood, which can result from diets deficient in salt or protein, may cause the tail biting to escalate. Thus, a high incidence of tail

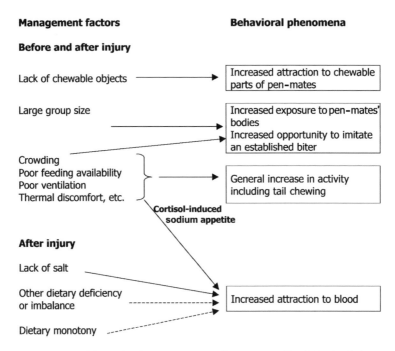

Management factors   **Behavioral phenomena**

Before and after injury

Lack of chewable objects ──────────▶ Increased attraction to chewable parts of pen-mates

Large group size
                        ──────────▶ Increased exposure to pen-mates' bodies
                        ──────────▶ Increased opportunity to imitate an established biter

Crowding
Poor feeding availability
Poor ventilation   ────────▶ General increase in activity including tail chewing
Thermal discomfort, etc.

Cortisol-induced
sodium appetite

After injury

Lack of salt

Other dietary deficiency
or imbalance   ------------▶ Increased attraction to blood

Dietary monotony ------

Figure 3.2.   Proposed model showing how management factors may affect behavioral phenomena leading to tail biting among pigs. The more speculative links are shown with broken lines (Adapted from Fraser, 1987).

biting can reflect many different problems in the animal's environment, diet, and management (Fraser, 1987). Like many other types of abnormal behavior, tail biting is also a cause of injury among recipient animals; hence, the behavior is linked to animal welfare in numerous ways.

Despite the importance of dealing with abnormal behavior, there are difficult definitional problems in distinguishing normal, adaptive behavior from the abnormal and maladaptive (Mason, 1991). For example, veal calves that perform a high level of stereotyped tongue rolling—a seemingly abnormal and nonadaptive behavior—have fewer ulcers of the abomasum (Wiepkema et al., 1987), suggesting that in some cases the performance of seemingly abnormal behavior may actually help animals to cope with an adverse situation.

Accommodating Natural Behavior

One common approach to improving animal welfare is to accommodate the "natural behavior" of animals. For example, dairy calves are normally removed from the mother within the first day after birth, and are often given a milk-based or milklike diet, which they drink in just a few minutes if it is provided in a bucket. At this age, calves are highly motivated to suck and will often suck avidly on the navel, ears, or prepuce of other calves, sometimes to the point of causing damage. However, if the calves obtain their milk by sucking from artificial teats, this appears to satisfy their motivation both for milk and for the act of sucking, and allows the animals to be raised in groups with fewer problems from mutual sucking. Even a dummy teat attached to the wall allows the animals to suck in a harmless way, and the behavior is followed by a release of digestive enzymes that is not seen with bucket feeding (de Passillé and Rushen, 1997). In this case, accommodating natural behavior helps prevent the damage caused by mutual sucking, allows calves to satisfy their motivation to suck, and may also improve the functioning of the digestive system.

Attempts to accommodate natural behavior have led to many refinements in animal housing and handling. For example, research on laying hens has identified four environmental features that birds need in order to perform normal behavior that is impossible in standard "battery" cages. The features are (1) a nest box where the hen can retreat to lay; (2) sand or other loose material that she can use for "dust bathing" and feather care; (3) a perch for resting; and (4) sufficient space to allow normal movement without feather damage (Appleby and Hughes, 1995). In 1999, when the 15 countries of the European Union agreed to phase out the standard battery cage, they drew on this research in approving an "enriched" cage containing these four features as an alternative.

Nonetheless, accommodating natural behavior is no panacea for solving animal welfare problems. The natural behavior of animals includes some activities that are adaptations to adverse circumstances. Pigs, for example, flee when chased by predators, huddle together in the cold, and wallow in mud when hot. Keeping pigs in environments where these behaviors are seen would presumably be detrimental to welfare, at least by some criteria. However, in the "higher" animals, at least, evolution has often favored not simply a repertoire of actions that are performed with a characteristic frequency, but a series of conditional rules whereby the animal is motivated to act in certain ways in response to certain circumstances. If we construe natural behavior to mean these conditional rules rather than a simple repertoire of actions, then the concept may be more relevant to quality of life. That pigs fail to wallow or huddle in a given type of housing may not indicate a problem, but if pigs are prevented from wallowing when hot and huddling when cold, then their welfare may well be compromised.

Providing Animals with Environments That They Prefer

One of the most widely discussed proposals for improving animal welfare is to provide animals with living conditions that they themselves prefer. In one of the earliest examples, Hughes and Black (1973) attempted to identify suitable flooring materials for hens by housing birds in cages where they could move freely between compartments with different types of flooring. Records of the time the birds spent on the different options indicated that the birds actually preferred a particular flooring product that had previously been criticized as unsuitable for hens. From such simple experiments, tests of environmental preference have evolved rapidly over the past 30 years (Fraser and Matthews, 1997), and have been used in the design of pens, perches, loading ramps, and many other aspects of animal housing.

By themselves, however, preferences do not indicate the degree of importance that animals attach to the preferred options. This weakness led to attempts to assess how strongly animals are motivated to obtain different rewards. For example, American mink (*Mustela vison*) are partially aquatic carnivores that are raised commercially for fur. In the wild, mink perform a wide range of behavior that is impossible in captivity, including swimming, resting in several nest sites, surveying the environment from raised perching places, and exploring the burrows of potential prey animals. In one study, mink in standard cages were trained to push against weighted doors for access to various rewards including a tunnel, a raised platform, an alternative nest box, and a small pool of water where they could swim. The experimenters then varied the amount of weight that the animals had to lift to open the different doors. The animals performed much more work for access to the pool of water than for the raised platform, the tunnel, and other options (Mason et al., 2001), and the authors concluded that an opportunity to swim is of substantial importance for the welfare of mink.

Despite the obvious strengths of the approach, accommodating animals' preferences is not a universal means of solving animal welfare problems. In some cases, animals may not have evolved the capacity to detect certain benefits and harms; pigs, for example, seem to have only a weak aversion to the smell of ammonia, even at harmful levels (Jones et al., 1996). Some preferences seem to reflect short-term comfort rather than long-term welfare; in the hen study mentioned above, for example, Hughes and Black (1973) found that the most preferred flooring, being less rigid than the others, was also most likely to break and cause leg injuries. Similarly, animals' preferences may not reliably reflect their welfare if choices are too complex. For example, we might wish to know whether a cow is better off in a crowded shed or on pasture with less abundant feed and occasional snow storms, but it is not realistic to assume that a preference experiment would give a definitive comparison of animal welfare over the long term in two such different environments.

Identifying and Mitigating Negative Affective States

One of the key concerns about the quality of life of animals centers on unpleasant affective states such as fear, pain, and distress. Animal welfare scientists have responded by trying to find ways to identify and reduce such states in animals.

Of the various affective states, fear is one of the most studied (Jones, 1997). A widely used behavioral test for fear in chickens involves flipping the bird suddenly onto its back, whereupon the bird will often stay totally immobile for many minutes in a reaction called "tonic immobility." It can be shown experimentally that chickens tend to remain in tonic immobility longer if they have been frightened before the test. Duncan et al. (1986) used this method to assess fear caused by the mechanical "harvesting" of chickens raised for meat. When these birds reach market weight, crews of people are traditionally employed to catch the birds, usually grabbing them by the legs and carrying them upside-down to the shipping crates. An alternative is a machine that moves through the pens, gathers the birds in rotating rubber fingers, and transfers them to the shipping crates by a conveyor belt. When mechanical harvesters first appeared, there was concern that they would cause unnecessary fear in the birds. However, Duncan et al. (1986) found that immediately after being caught, birds captured by machine maintained tonic immobility for significantly less time than birds that had been captured by hand. The evidence thus suggested that machine catching actually caused less fear than manual catching, probably because the mechanical device did not trigger any form of predator recognition.

Pain is another important subject of animal welfare research. Many routine procedures performed on animals—such as castration of piglets and dehorning of calves—are presumably painful, and a number of behavioral methods of pain assessment have been developed. For example, Schwartzkopf-Genswein et al. (1998) tested whether freeze branding is a less painful alternative to hot-iron branding for identifying beef cattle. In the study, steers were subjected to either hot-iron or freeze branding, and their movements were recorded by video-recording and subsequently digitized for analysis. Cattle branded with a hot iron showed more head movements, and more rapid head movements, than those that were freeze branded, suggesting that the freeze branding is a less painful method. However, steers branded using either method were much more likely to flick their tails, kick, fall, and vocalize than were animals that were simply restrained and not branded, indicating that both methods are painful.

Farm management practices often involve disrupting normal social bonds. For example, dairy calves are typically separated from their mothers soon after birth, and piglets are often weaned by sudden removal from their mothers at only two to four weeks of age. Measures have been used to assess separation distress in such situations. If an unweaned piglet is removed to an isolated pen, it gives a characteristic set of calls, beginning with quiet, closed-mouth grunts and progressing to loud, high-pitched squeaks and squeals (fig. 3.3). Experiments have shown that piglets give more calls, especially more of the loud, high-pitched calls, if they have not been fed recently or if they are in a cool environment—both conditions that presumably increase their need to be reunited with their mother. Moreover, sows respond more vigorously to calls given by piglets in conditions of greater need. The current thinking is that these calls form a communication system that helps to reunite isolated piglets with their mothers, and that the number and type of calls reflect the animals' level of distress at being separated (Weary and Fraser, 1995). Hence, the calls may be useful for testing ways to mitigate separation distress. For example, experiments show that piglets separated from the sow call much less if they are kept with several familiar littermates; hence, maintaining intact litters at weaning may help reduce the distress caused by the practice (Fraser, 1975).

"Avoidance learning"—testing whether animals will learn to avoid an event or situation—provides a more direct way of showing that animals perceive an event as unpleasant. An example arose over the "electro-immobilization" of sheep. Electro-immobilization involves passing a pulsed, low-voltage current through the body to immobilize animals temporarily for procedures such as shearing. Promoters of electro-immobilization claimed that it functions as an analgesic, making procedures such as shearing less unpleasant for the animals, but critics noted that it might merely make animals unable to move. To test these ideas, Rushen (1986) trained sheep to move along a runway to a pen where they received mildly aversive treatments, such as rough shearing, with and without electro-immobilization. The results showed that over repeated trials, sheep that received the electrical treatment became more difficult to move along the runway than those that received the mildly aversive treatments without electro-immobilization. Rushen concluded that electro-immobilization actually made unpleasant procedures more aversive, not less.

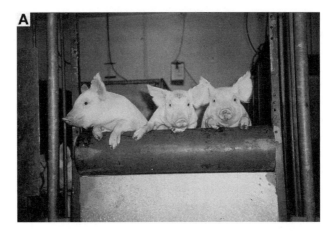

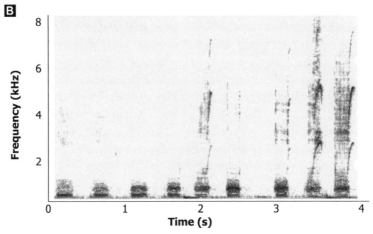

Figure 3.3.   (A) Piglets looking over a barrier after their mother has left, and (B) a sound spectrogram of a sequence of nine "separation calls" given by a piglet in this situation (From Fraser and Weary, 2003; photo by Dr. E. A. Pajor).

Pain, fear, and other unpleasant states are obviously relevant to the quality of life of animals, but they pose a challenge for science. Unlike overt behavioral and physiological responses that can be observed directly, the affective states experienced by animals have to be inferred from other evidence, but the theoretical basis for making these inferences remains relatively weak. The emergence of "affective neuroscience" (Panksepp, 1998)—or the scientific study of emotions in animals and humans—holds great promise for the study of animal welfare, but the field is still in an early stage of development.

Identifying and Enhancing Positive Affective States

In addition to identifying and preventing negative affective states, could we also detect and enhance positive affective states such as comfort, contentment, and pleasure? One promising example comes from the ultrasonic vocalizations produced by rats. Adolescent rats are known to produce "chirps" at about 50 kHz in frequency, during presumably pleasurable social interactions such as sex and play, as well as during tickling by human handlers. This has led to the speculation that these calls are analogous to human laughter. One recent study (Burgdorf and Panksepp, 2001) suggests that the calls are indeed associated with positive affect. In this study, rats that were tickled in a series of training sessions approached the handler's hand much more quickly than if they had been gently touched but not tickled during training. Rats that were tickled also approached the hand more and more quickly as training progressed, and produced more chirps during the tickling session; moreover, those rats that approached most quickly vocalized most often. Interestingly, rats that were individually housed were more likely to show these effects than those that were socially housed, indicating that tickling was more pleasurable for rats that could not engage in normal social interactions with other rats.

There is also a growing understanding of the neuroendocrine basis for certain positive affective states. Carter (2002) notes that oxytocin and other peptide hormones appear to be closely involved in positive social contact such as affiliative, sexual, and maternal behaviors. Oxytocin release is stimulated by seemingly pleasurable tactile stimulation and may also play an important role in social bonding, including the attachment of the mother to her newborn and the bonding of sexual partners in socially monogamous species. In many species, oxytocin also appears to reduce the reaction of the HPA system and the sympathetic nervous system to stressors. Hence, oxytocin and the neural processes leading to its release may play a key role both in pleasurable experiences and in modulating stress responses. However, the secretion and action of oxytocin within the central nervous system may be poorly correlated with levels in the blood; therefore, the action of oxytocin on emotions and social behavior may be difficult to study directly (Knierim et al., 2002).

In a hypothesis linking negative and positive affect to evolutionary biology, Fraser and Duncan (1998) distinguished between "need situations" where there is a potential fitness cost from not performing certain behavior (e.g., failing to drink when dehydrated, failing to escape from an approaching predator), and "opportunity situations" where there is a potential fitness benefit from performing certain behavior (e.g., playing, exploring) at times when the cost of performing the behavior is low. They proposed that unpleasant affective states (thirst, fear) evolved to stimulate behavior in need situations, whereas positive affective states (the pleasure of playing or exploring) evolved to motivate behavior in opportunity situations. The hypothesis suggests that positive effect is likely to accompany common behavioral activities that can plausibly be seen as contributing to fitness but that do not appear to meet any pressing threat to fitness. Depending on the species and life history, such pleasurable behavior is likely to include play, grooming, hoarding, exploring, renewing territorial markings, and certain types of social behavior. Hence, accommodating these types of behavior could make a positive contribution to an animal's welfare through promoting positive effect.

Drawing on neurobiological and behavioral evidence mainly from mammals, Panksepp (1998) identified evolutionarily ancient neural systems in subcortical regions of the brain that control behavior that appears to involve emotional states. Activation of some of these systems—especially those controlling fear, rage, and separation distress—appears to create unpleasant states that the animal will try to avoid. Activation of certain other systems appears to involve pleasant states and can serve as positive incentives. These include the systems that underlie vigorous social play, exploration and anticipation, maternal and related care of others, and sexual behavior.

The above lines of investigation, each embryonic in itself, tend to lead to the intuitively plausible conclusion that, at least in mammals, activities such as play, exploration, and certain forms of social behavior are pleasurable to perform and thus contribute to well-being. In the past, these commonsense ideas have proven difficult for science to address. By being brought into the realm of scientific enquiry, they may take on a respectability in animal welfare discourse that they have not previously enjoyed.

Nonetheless, our understanding of positive affective states in animals remains very limited and tentative. Some negative states, such as pain and fear, appear to have "downstream" physiological indicators, such as increased cortisol production, whereas positive states may not have such convenient peripheral indicators. It may require new tools, such as magnetic resonance imaging of the brain, to make significant headway in understanding positive affective states in other species.

THE INTERPLAY OF ETHICAL AND EMPIRICAL ELEMENTS

In summary, we see certain ethical concerns over the welfare of animals, and a wide range of scientific approaches that have been used to address those concerns. The science maps onto the ethical concerns in complex ways (fig. 3.4). For example, preventing disease and injury obviously addresses concerns over biological functioning and may help deal with related affective states such as pain and malaise. Accommodating natural behavior addresses concerns over natural living and, depending on the example, it may also improve certain aspects of biological functioning and allow animals to experience pleasure from behavior such as play. However, as figure 3.4 illustrates, no one scientific approach fully covers the range of concerns.

There are some obvious advantages to using scientific research in addressing ethical concerns about the quality of life of animals. By having a better understanding of animals' health, preferences, and aversions, and how these relate to elements in the environment, we are less likely to use naive or purely anthropomorphic ideas when assessing animal welfare. However, there are also potential problems and areas of confusion.

One problem is that certain aspects of animal welfare lend themselves more readily to scientific study than others, and there is a risk that scientists will focus on those aspects that they can study most easily and ignore the rest. For example, some scientists focus on easily quantifiable variables reflecting biological functioning (disease rates, stress responses) and ignore affective states. Duncan (1996) rightly argues that if we focus on measures of health and stress physiology while ignoring the animal's psychological response to these states, we will miss a major aspect—perhaps *the* major aspect—of ethical concern about animal welfare. Duncan argues that because the animal's affective states are a key part of its welfare, science must find ways to study these states and not simply focus

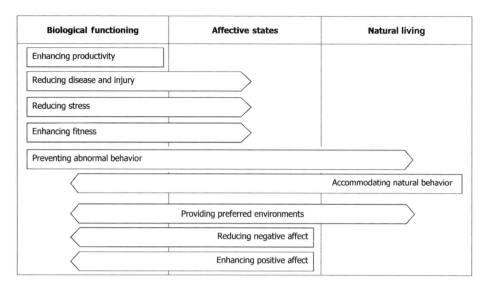

Figure 3.4.   A conceptual framework showing three ethical concerns that arise over the quality of life of animals (biological functioning, affective states, and natural living) and how different scientific approaches relate to these concerns. Scientific approaches are listed under the ethical concern to which they most closely correspond. Arrows indicate possible additional implications. *Brief explanation:* The first four measures are focused on biological functioning as defined especially by agriculturalists (productivity), veterinarians (disease and injury), physiologists (stress), and evolutionary biologists (fitness). Enhancing biological functioning in these ways may also influence animals' affective states, for example by reducing suffering resulting from injury, disease, and stress. Preventing abnormal behavior addresses concerns over biological functioning, and often has implications for affective states and natural living, as abnormal behavior may arise from negative affect and unnatural environments. Accommodating natural behavior tends to promote natural living, but also promotes biological functioning (as defined by ethologists) and may enhance affective states, for example by permitting animals to perform pleasurable types of behavior. Providing animals with preferred environments is often done to promote positive affective states and reduce negative affective states because animals presumably choose environments where they experience more comfort, less fear, and so on. Under some circumstances, animals may also select environments that permit more natural living and better biological functioning. The two final criteria are focused on affective states but may also enhance biological functioning; for example, negative affect (pain) may result from impaired functioning (injury).

on other measures that are more amenable to scientific research. Even among affective states, animal welfare science may tend to overemphasize pain, fear, and distress because these lead to easily measured responses, whereas positive states—pleasure, enjoyment, contentment—have perhaps been underemphasized because their physiological and behavioral correlates are more difficult to identify.

Another problem is the illusion that because there is now a science of animal welfare, scientists will be able to "measure" animal welfare in a purely objective, scientific manner, much as they might measure viscosity or atomic weight. However, animal welfare is a socially constructed concept with important ethical implications. Stafleu et al. (1996) noted that when scientists deal with such concepts, they are likely to narrow the concept so as to link it to a scientific theory (the theory of stress physiology, the theory of evolution) and then restrict it further to available methods of measurement within that theory (cortisol levels, fitness correlates). This makes the assessment of animal welfare seem like a purely empirical and objective matter; but when animal welfare is thus redefined, important elements of the concept are likely to be lost. Hence, a scientist relying on injury rates and cortisol levels might claim that sows have better welfare in stalls than on pasture, whereas a critic might argue that the science has not adequately reflected the animals' welfare.

In describing the interplay of science and animal welfare concerns, it helps to think of animal welfare as an "evaluative concept," roughly analogous to terms such as *product quality* and *building safety* (Fraser, 1999). In assessing the safety of a building, there are many relevant variables that can be studied and measured objectively—the strength of the fire escapes, the quality of the air—but the decisions about which variables to study and the relative weight to assign them involve value-related judgments about what is important for a building to be considered safe. Thus, an evaluative concept organizes relevant empirical information within a value-based framework. Animal welfare is an evaluative concept of this type, with the provision that the study of animal welfare attempts to incorporate, as much as is possible, the animal's own perceptions of its quality of life. Animal welfare thus encompasses many variables that can be studied scientifically and objectively. However, our decisions about which variables to study, and how to weight and interpret them in terms of an animal's welfare, involve value-dependent judgments about what we believe to be desirable and important for the quality of life of animals.

These constraints on the scientific study of animal welfare have implications for efforts to assess the "overall" welfare of animals. Dawkins (2002) notes that animals face many different challenges in their natural environment and have been shaped by natural selection to respond to them in different ways. Hence, it will likely prove fruitless to look for "overall" indicators of welfare. But could the various responses not be combined into an overall welfare score? Recent years have seen the creation of scoring systems, for example to identify animal products as coming from farms meeting certain animal welfare standards (e.g., Bartussek, 2001), where marks are awarded for certain variables and then combined into overall scores. Science can help in the development of these systems by shedding light on what animals prefer and what factors affect their health and reproduction. Ultimately, however, there is no logically or empirically correct way of deciding how to weight disparate factors. Thus, while scoring systems for "overall welfare" can be informed by science, they inevitably include value-dependent judgments about what is important for the quality of life of animals.

It also follows that science remains limited in its ability to deal with certain multivariable comparisons. We might want to know, for example, whether chickens have better welfare when kept in cramped cages in heated barns with balanced rations, or on pasture with fresh air, foxes, and occasional storms. Here again, there is no empirically or logically correct way to balance the different variables in such complex comparisons.

These issues force us to think clearly about the role of animal welfare science and how it can be applied to ethical concerns that arise over the quality of life of animals. With other evaluative concepts, such as the health of a person or the safety of a building, the key goal is rarely to perform overall measurement or comparison. Physicians, for example, rarely try to measure the "overall" health of a person or determine whether one patient is, on net, healthier than another. Rather, their role is to improve health, largely by identifying, solving, and preventing health problems. Similarly, although animal welfare science can help to inform multivariable scoring systems and comparisons of disparate management methods, it is on its firmest ground when it tries to identify, solve, and prevent animal welfare problems.

REFERENCES

Adams, A. W. and Craig, J. V. 1985. Effect of crowding and cage shape on productivity and profitability of caged layers: A survey. *Poultry Science* 64: 238–242.

Anonymous. 1989. *How Astrid Lindgren Achieved Enactment of the 1988 Law Protecting Farm Animals in Sweden.* Animal Welfare Institute, Washington, DC.

Appleby, M. C. and Hughes, B. O. 1995. The Edinburgh Modified Cage for laying hens. *British Poultry Science* 36: 707–718.

Appleby, M. C. and Lawrence, A. B. 1987. Food restriction as a cause of stereotypic behaviour in tethered gilts. *Animal Production* 45: 103–110.

Barnard, C. J. and Hurst, J. L. 1996 Welfare by design: The natural selection of welfare criteria. *Animal Welfare* 5: 405–433.

Barnett, J. L. and Hemsworth, P. H. 1990. The validity of physiological and behavioral measures of animal welfare. *Applied Animal Behaviour Science* 25: 177–187.

Barnett, J. L., Hemsworth, P. H., Cronin, G. M., Jongman, E. C. and Hutson, G. D. 2000. A review of the welfare issues for sows and piglets in relation to housing. *Australian Journal of Agricultural Research* 52: 1–28.

Bartussek, H. 2001. An historical account of the development of the Animal Needs Index ANI-35L as part of the attempt to promote and regulate farm animal welfare in Austria: An example of the interaction between animal welfare science and society. *Acta Agriculturae Scandanavica, Section A, Animal Science*, Supplement 30: 34–41.

Broom, D. M. 1991a. Animal welfare: Concepts and measurement. *Journal of Animal Science* 69: 4167–4175.

——. 1991b. Assessing welfare and suffering. *Behavioural Processes* 25: 117–123.

Burgdorf, J. and Panksepp, J. 2001. Tickling induces reward in adolescent rats. *Physiology and Behavior* 72: 25–38.

Carter, C. S. 2002. Is there a neurobiology of good welfare? Pages 11–30 in D. M. Broom (ed.), *Coping with Challenge: Welfare in Animals Including Humans.* Dahlem Workshop Report 87. Dahlem University Press, Berlin.

Dantzer R. 2001. Stress, emotions and health: Where do we stand? *Social Science Information* 40: 61–78.

Dantzer, R. and Mormède, P. 1983. Stress in farm animals: A need for reevaluation. *Journal of Animal Science* 57: 6–18.

Dawkins, M. S. 1980. *Animal Suffering: The Science of Animal Welfare.* Chapman and Hall, London.

——. 1998. Evolution and animal welfare. *Quarterly Review of Biology* 73: 305–328.

——. 2002. How can we recognize and assess good welfare? Pages 63–76 in D. M. Broom (ed.), *Coping with Challenge: Welfare in Animals Including Humans.* Dahlem Workshop Report 87. Dahlem University Press, Berlin.

de Passillé, A. M. B. and Rushen, J. 1997. Motivational and physiological analysis of the causes and consequences of non-nutritive sucking by calves. *Applied Animal Behaviour Science* 53: 15–31.

Duncan, I. J. H. 1996. Animal welfare defined in terms of feelings. *Acta Agriculturae Scandinavica, Section A, Animal Science*, Supplement 27: 29–35.

Duncan, I. J. H. and Fraser, D. 1997. Understanding animal welfare. Pages 19–31 in M. C. Appleby and B. O. Hughes (ed.), *Animal Welfare.* CAB International, Wallingford, UK.

Duncan, I. J. H., Slee, G., Kettlewell, P., Berry, P. and Carlisle, A. J. 1986. Comparison of the stressfulness of harvesting broiler chickens by machine and by hand. *British Poultry Science* 27: 109–114.

Fraser, D. 1975. Vocalizations of isolated piglets. II. Some environmental factors. *Applied Animal Ethology* 2: 19–24.

——. 1987. Mineral-deficient diets and the pig's attraction to blood: Implications for tail-biting. *Canadian Journal of Animal Science* 67: 909–918.

——. 1999. Animal ethics and animal welfare science: Bridging the two cultures (The D. G. M. Wood-Gush Memorial Lecture). *Applied Animal Behaviour Science* 65: 171–189.

Fraser, D. and Duncan, I. J. H. 1998. "Pleasures", "pains" and animal welfare: Toward a natural history of affect. *Animal Welfare* 7: 383–396.

Fraser, D. and Matthews, L. R. 1997. Preference and motivation testing. Pages 159–173 in M. C. Appleby and B. O. Hughes (eds.), *Animal Welfare.* CAB International, Wallingford, UK.

Fraser, D. and Weary, D. M. 2003. Applied animal behaviour and animal welfare. In press in L. A. Giraldeau and J. Bolhuis (eds.), *The Behavior of Animals: Mechanisms, Function and Evolution.* Blackwell Scientific, Oxford.

Fraser, D., Weary, D. M., Pajor, E. A. and Milligan, B. N. 1997. A scientific conception of animal welfare that reflects ethical concerns. *Animal Welfare* 6: 187–205.

Harrison, R. 1964. *Animal Machines.* Vincent Stuart, London.

Hughes, B. O. and Black, A. J. 1973. The preference of domestic hens for different types of battery cage floor. *British Poultry Science* 14: 615–619.

Hughes, B. O. and Duncan, I. J. H. 1988. The notion of ethological "need", models of motivation and animal welfare. *Animal Behaviour* 36: 1697–1707.

Hurnik, J. F. 1993. Ethics and animal agriculture. *Journal of Agricultural and Environmental Ethics* 6 (Supplement 1): 21–35.

International Dairy Federation. 1987. *Environmental influences on bovine mastitis.* Bulletin No. 217. International Dairy Federation, Brussels.

Jones, J. B., Burgess, L. R., Webster, A. J. F. and Wathes, C. M. 1996. Behavioural responses of pigs to atmospheric ammonia in a chronic choice test. *Animal Science* 63: 437–445.

Jones, R. B. 1997. Fear and distress. Pages 75–87 in M. C. Appleby and B. O. Hughes (eds.), *Animal Welfare.* CAB International, Wallingford, UK.

Knierim, U., Carter, C. S., Fraser, D., Gartner, K., Lutgendorf, S. K., Mineka, S., Panksepp, J. and Sachser, N. 2002. Good welfare: Improving quality of life. Pages 79–100 in D. M. Broom (ed.), *Coping with Challenge: Welfare in Animals including Humans.* Dahlem Workshop Report 87. Dahlem University Press, Berlin.

Ladewig, J. and Smidt, D. 1989. Behavior, episodic secretion of cortisol, and adrenocortical reactivity in bulls subjected to tethering. *Hormones and Behavior* 23: 344–360.

Martin, S. W. 1983. Factors influencing morbidity and mortality in feedlot calves in Ontario. *Veterinary Clinics of North America, Large Animal Practice* 5: 75–86.

Mason, G. J. 1991. Stereotypies: A critical review. *Animal Behaviour* 41: 1015–1037.

Mason, G. J., Cooper, J. and Clarebrough, C. 2001. Frustrations of fur-farmed mink. *Nature* 410: 35–36.

Mendl, M. 1991. Some problems with the concept of a cut-off point for determining when an animal's welfare is at risk. *Applied Animal Behaviour Science* 31: 139–146.

Moberg, G. P. 1985. Biological response to stress: Key to assessment of animal well-being? Pages 27–49 in G. P. Moberg (ed.), *Animal Stress*. American Physiological Society, Bethesda, MD.

Panksepp, J. 1998. *Affective Neuroscience: The Foundations of Human and Animal Emotions*. Oxford University Press, New York.

Rollin, B. E. 1993. Animal welfare, science and value. *Journal of Agricultural and Environmental Ethics* 6 (Supplement 2): 44–50.

——. 1995. *Farm Animal Welfare: Social, Bioethical, and Research Issues*. Iowa State University Press, Ames.

Rousch, W. B. 1986. A decision analysis approach to the determination of population density in laying cages. *World's Poultry Science Journal* 42: 26–31.

Rushen, J. 1986. Aversion of sheep to electro-immobilization and physical restraint. *Applied Animal Behaviour Science* 15: 315–324.

——. 1991. Problems associated with the interpretation of physiological data in the assessment of animal welfare. *Applied Animal Behaviour Science* 28: 381–386.

Rushen, J. and de Passillé, A. M. B. 1992. The scientific assessment of the impact of housing on animal welfare: A critical review. *Canadian Journal of Animal Science* 72: 721–743.

Sachser, N. 2002. What is important to achieve good welfare in animals? Pages 31–48 in D. M. Broom (ed.), *Coping with Challenge: Welfare in Animals Including Humans*. Dahlem Workshop Report 87. Dahlem University Press, Berlin.

Sandøe, P. and Simonsen, H. B. 1992. Assessing animal welfare: where does science end and philosophy begin? *Animal Welfare* 1: 257–267.

Sapolsky, R. M. 1992. Neuroendocrinology of the stress-response. Pages 287–324 in J. B. Becker, S. M. Breedlove, and D. Crews (eds.), *Behavioral Endocrinology*. MIT Press, Cambridge, MA.

Schwartzkopf-Genswein, K. S., Stookey, J. M., Crowe, T. G. and Genswein, B. M. A. 1998. Comparison of image analysis, exertion force, and behavior measurements for use in the assessment of beef cattle responses to hot-iron and freeze branding. *Journal of Animal Science* 76: 972–979.

Stafleu, F. R., Grommers, F. J. and Vorstenbosch, J. 1996. Animal welfare: Evolution and erosion of a moral concept. *Animal Welfare* 5: 225–234.

Stull, C. L. and McDonough, S. P. 1994. Multidisciplinary approach to evaluating welfare of veal calves in commercial facilities. *Journal of Animal Science* 72: 2518–2524.

Sutherland, M. A., Mellor, D. J., Stafford, K. J., Gregory, N. G., Bruce, R. A., Ward, R. N. and Todd, S. E. 1999. Acute cortisol responses of lambs to ring castration and docking after the injection of lignocaine into the scrotal neck or testes at the time of ring application. *Australian Veterinary Journal* 77: 738–741.

Tannenbaum, J. 1991. Ethics and animal welfare: The inextricable connection. *Journal of the American Veterinary Medical Association* 198: 1360–1376.

Tauson, R. 1984. Plumage condition in SCWL laying hens kept in conventional cages of different designs. *Acta Agriculturae Scandanavica* 34: 221–230.

Taylor, G. B. 1972. One man's philosophy of welfare. *Veterinary Record* 91: 426–428.

Weary, D. M. and Fraser, D. 1995. Calling by domestic piglets: Reliable signals of need? *Animal Behaviour* 50: 1046–1055.

Wiepkema, P. R., van Hellemond, K. K., Roessingh, P. and Romberg, H. 1987. Behaviour and abomasal damage in individual veal calves. *Applied Animal Behaviour Science* 18: 257–268.

Wilson, L. L., Terosky, T. L., Stull, C. L. and Stricklin, W. R. 1999. Effects of individual housing design and size on behavior and stress indicators of special-fed Holstein veal calves. *Journal of Animal Science* 77: 1341–1347.

4

Pain in Farm Animals: Nature, Recognition, and Management

G. John Benson

Dying is nothing, but pain is a very serious matter.
— Henry Jacob Bigelow, 1871

We all must die. But that I can save him from days of torture, that is what I feel as my great and ever new privilege. Pain is a more terrible lord of mankind than even death itself.
—Albert Schweitzer, 1931

Pain is perfect miserie, the worst
Of evils, and excessive, overturns
All patience.

—John Milton, *Paradise Lost*

CONCEPT AND DEFINITION OF PAIN

Pain has been a constant concern of humans throughout history. In the records of every race, there are testimonials to the omnipresence and scourge of pain from the Babylonian clay tablets, in papyri of the ancient Egyptians, in Persian leather documents, in inscriptions from Mycenae, on parchment rolls from Troy and down through the ages in every civilization and culture. What exactly is pain and how do we recognize it in people or animals incapable of speech? Pain is a perception or unpleasant sensation arising from the activation of a discrete set of neural receptors and pathways by noxious stimuli. A noxious stimulus is mechanical, chemical, or thermal activity that is actually or potentially damaging to tissues. Pain is defined introspectively by every person as that which hurts. Pain is a subjective experience accompanied by feelings of fear, anxiety, and panic. Pain elicits protective motor actions, results in learned avoidance, and may modify species-specific traits of behavior including social behavior (Kitchell, 1987). Because pain is a perception, it is subjective and has no definitive physical dimensions. A stimulus resulting in the perception of pain in a person in one circumstance may not be painful to that individual in another circumstance or to another person. The perception of pain is probably the most highly modified of any sensory system of the body. Furthermore, the conscious state of the individual is of paramount importance to the ability to perceive pain. Stimuli that are strong enough to be perceived as painful in a conscious individual will produce activity in nerve fibers and pathways and even elicit reflex movements in unconscious individuals totally unaware of the stimulus (Bonica, 1990). Thus, because of the very nature of pain as a subjective emotional and psychological experience, and because of variable responses to pain among individuals and species, pain has been difficult to recognize in people as well as animals. Because animals, like the human infant, cannot speak, the stoic individual or species, or the individual who lies quietly, is often assumed to not be experiencing pain. Furthermore, because pain is a highly subjective and emotional experience, some are reluctant to equate the pain of newborn humans and animals with that of adults. In addition, many regard anthropomorphic judgments and assumptions to be unscientific or inappropriate.

PAIN IN ANIMALS

The idea that animals have no souls and are merely machines, first espoused by St. Thomas Aquinas and later by Rene Descartes, led to the belief that animals have no moral rights or status and that humans could do with them as they wished (Rowan and Tannenbaum, 1986). In the early twentieth century, the theory of behaviorism and the rejection of consciousness in animals by early ethologists led to the denial of thought and feeling in animals (Rollin, 1987). While such philosophies have prevailed and suppressed the recognition of pain and suffering in animals, they are no longer universally accepted.

Animals, while not viewed as being equal to human beings, have been considered to be worthy of moral concern by some because they are capable of suffering. In 1789, Jeremy Bentham stated, "The question is not, can they reason? Nor can they talk? But, can they suffer?" If an animal were a sentient being, then it could suffer and therefore would have moral status. Sentience refers to the capacity to suffer pain or distress and/or enjoy pleasure. While mental activities cannot be directly measured, animals have at least some of the same features of consciousness as people. Animals display distinct preferences when presented with choices in such things as diet and temperature. Numerous examples suggest that animals consciously interact with their environment and, if given the opportunity, will alter it. For example, if allowed to manipulate a thermostat, pigs will control environmental temperature such that early afternoon temperatures on average are 11°C higher than in early morning (Curtis and Morris, 1982). Veal calves will control illumination to provide light 67 percent of the day, while chickens will choose illumination 80 percent of the day (Mench and van Tienhoven, 1986). Recently, lame broiler chickens demonstrated a preference for medicated feed containing carprofen over nonmedicated feed. As severity of lameness increased, so did the consumption of medicated feed (Danbury et al., 2000). This is potent evidence not only of the ability to suffer pain but of the birds' ability to self-medicate to achieve relief. Psychological stimuli such as frustration or conflict are as effective as physical stimuli in activating the pituitary-adrenal stress response in both animals and people (Levine, 1985; Wylie and Gentle, 1998; Gentle and Coor, 1995).

Comparative studies have revealed that the anatomic structures and neurophysiologic mechanisms leading to the perception of pain are remarkably similar in human beings and animals, as is the pain detection threshold (Zimmerman, 1984; Bonica, 1990). Therefore, it is reasonable to assume that if a stimulus were painful to people, were damaging or potentially damaging to tissues, and induced escape and emotional responses in an animal, it must be considered to be painful to that animal (Rowan and Tannenbaum, 1986). That animals exhibit signs of distress, learn avoidance behavior, and vocalize in response to (painful) stimuli is further evidence of their capacity to suffer pain. Further, it may be argued that any being with the capacity to suffer, to reason and display purposeful behavior, and to develop self-awareness has a life that matters to it and has a "right" to live a life free of unnecessary suffering. Thus, people have moral obligations regarding animals and their treatment (Rowan and Tannenbaum, 1986; Rollin, 1987)

Society has not achieved a consensus regarding our moral obligations to animals. There is no agreement on the value of animal life or our obligations to animals similar to the one that is shared on the value of human life and our obligations to our fellow humans. The moral code of society recognizes the essentials of individual human nature, that is, we are thinking, social beings, who feel pleasure and pain, value freedom, and so on. From this recognition comes legal and moral protection of the individual, called rights, which protect the individual as an object of moral concern. Just as human beings have needs and interests that are essential to their nature, animals have certain basic needs that are genetically encoded, environmentally modified, and expressed that are essential to the survival of their species. Fulfillment of their needs is attended by joy and comfort, and thwarting these needs induces fear, pain, and anxiety. Their needs are as essential to them as ours are to us. What we do to animals matters to them. If there were no morally relevant difference justifying our withholding of our moral concern for animals, and we protect the essential nature of human beings, then we are also obligated to do so for animals. If we are obligated to relieve human pain and suffering, then we are morally obligated to do so for animals (Rollin, 1988).

This obligation would appear to be especially true for animals with whom we establish a bond of companionship and/or stewardship, such as pets or those whose health and well-being are under our personal care. Being animals ourselves, we can understand the perception of pain in our animal charges. Thus, we sympathize with them when they are in pain. Does the existence of sympathy entail an obligation to relieve the pain? As human beings, we are capable of feeling and appreciating sympathy and framing an ideal of behavior. An ideal is a standard by which we judge how we should behave. To have ideals is essential to morality itself. Human beings are capable of possessing ideals; other animals are not. Our capability for sympathy and for articulating it as an ideal is sufficient reason for pursuing it. The obligation springs from the ideal itself. Therefore, if we understand that animals suffer from pain, and understand that our pain and theirs are the same, then it is incumbent on us to relieve their pain, especially if we have been the cause of it. Sympathy is not the only human ideal, but it is one that we neglect at the cost of some portion of our humanity (Warnock, 1982).

If one accepts that animals are sentient beings capable of feeling pain and having basic needs and interests peculiar to their species, then they do indeed have moral status that we are morally obligated to recognize. Further, if we subscribe to the ideal for human behavior of being caring and compassionate, we are obligated by that ideal to strive to provide relief from pain in animals. This is particularly true of those animals that have been en-trusted to our care or for whose pain we are responsible. While pain may not always be overtly expressed and may be evidenced only by subtle changes in behavior or posture, one should be vigilant, especially in situations that are known to cause pain in people. Thus, a degree of anthropomorphism is appropriate and desirable (Soma, 1985; Breazile, Kitchell, and Naitoh, 1963).

The administration of analgesic agents should not be reserved for only those animals displaying obvious signs of severe pain and suffering, but should be administered to any animal under circumstances in which the observer would desire an analgesic himself. Just as vaccines and antibiotics are administered prophylactically to prevent infection, it is ap-propriate to administer analgesics to prevent pain where it is likely to occur. Pain-induced alterations in metabolism, endocrine, and cardiopulmonary function are well recognized and of serious consequence to the animal (Russell and Burch, 1959).

Pain, like other subjective judgments, is known by experience and described by illus-tration (Lewis, 1942). Much of our knowledge of human pain perception is by description. Someone else's toothache is understood by verbal description. However, in humans, as well as in animals, communication can be by other than verbal methods—by behavior and physiological reactions to certain stimuli. That animals respond to stimuli known to be both painful to people and damaging or potentially damaging to tissue by escape behavior, emotional responses, learned avoidance, and vocalization is evidence of their capacity to suffer pain. Because the ascription of pain perception to animals is feasible only by anal-ogy, knowledge about pain in animals remains a probable inference. When considering pain in animals, analogies that indicate a similarity of perception in animals and humans must be made through comparative anatomy, physiology, and behavior (Kitchell et al., 1962; Breazile et al., 1963).

DIMENSIONS OF PAIN

The pain experience has three dimensions: sensory-discriminative, motivational-affective, and cognitive-evaluative. Each is subserved by physiologically distinct neural systems (Melzack and Casey, 1968; Melzack, 1986). The sensory-discriminative dimension pro-vides information on the onset, location, intensity, type, and duration of the pain-inducing stimulus. This allows one to recognize the intensity and rate of onset of a painful stimulus. It also allows one to accurately locate the painful area and, at least in people, characterize or describe the pain as stabbing, cutting, crushing, burning, aching, and so on. This aspect is subserved primarily by the lateral ascending nociceptive tracts of the spinal cord, thala-mus, and somatosensory cortex of the cerebrum. People having lesions of the lateral as-cending spinal tracts have a diminished ability to recognize the type of painful stimulus being applied and to accurately identify which area of the body is being stimulated while the aversive and emotional aspects of pain are not obtunded. The motivational-affective di-mension disturbs the feeling of well-being of the individual resulting in the unpleasant af-fect of pain, provides information as to the severity of injury, produces the suffering aspect of the pain experience, and triggers the organism to action to avoid further injury and to conserve resources for healing. This dimension is closely linked to the autonomic nervous system and the associated cardiovascular, respiratory, and gastrointestinal responses. It is subserved by the medial ascending spinal nociceptive tracts, reticular formation of the brain stem, and limbic system of the midbrain and cerebrum. Lesions of medial ascending nociceptive tracts result in a person who is able to perceive pain, localize it precisely, recognize the type of stimuli, but who finds it to be tolerable. They do not suffer. Animals with similar lesions demonstrate greatly reduced aversive behavior as compared to normal animals (Mitchell and Kaebler, 1966; 1967; Kaebler et al., 1975). The cognitive-evaluative dimension encompasses the effects of prior experience, social and cultural values, anxiety, attention, and conditioning. These activities are largely due to cerebrocortical activity and are dependent on reticular activity (Melzack,1986; Melzack and Casey, 1968). Cognitive-evaluative activity in animals was demonstrated by Pavlov. He conditioned dogs by repeatedly feeding them after a specific area of skin was cut, burned, or shocked. Soon the dogs responded to these stimuli as food signals and would salivate but not show signs of pain, but would howl if the stimuli were applied to other areas (Pavlov, 1928). That nonprimate mammals share in common with humans the underlying spinal and brain structures subserving these functions indicates that animals would experience pain in a manner similar to people. There is, however, a structural difference between humans and nonprimate mammals. In humans, the lateral spinal tracts and the thalamocortical areas subserving the sensory-discriminative aspects of pain are highly developed and have more nerve fibers than are present in other mammals, whereas in nonhuman mammals, the medial spinal tracts, reticular and limbic systems subserving the motivational-affective aspects are comparable if not larger than those of primates (Dennis and Melzack, 1983). Thus, it would appear that nonhuman mammals may experience a greater degree of suffering and stronger motivational drive from noxious stimuli while being less able to precisely locate and characterize the type of pain. In people whose lateral tracts were severed to alleviate intractable pain, the pain often reappeared a year later and was reported as being even more disagreeable than before. The return of pain was attributed to medial tracts taking over the functions of the lateral tracts (White and Sweet, 1969).

PHYSIOLOGY OF PAIN

Nociception is the reception, conduction, and central nervous processing of nerve signals generated by the stimulation of nociceptors. It is the physiologic process that when carried to completion results in the conscious perception of pain. Nociceptors are free nerve ending receptors preferentially sensitive to a noxious stimulus or to a stimulus that would become noxious if prolonged. The nociceptor threshold is the minimum strength of stimulus that will cause a nociceptor to generate a nerve impulse. The nociceptor threshold is essentially the same in all species including humans. The pain detection threshold is the least amount of pain that a subject can recognize. The pain detection threshold is relatively constant among individuals and species. In most cases, it is higher than the nociceptor threshold (Zimmermann, 1984). Pain tolerance is the greatest level of pain that a subject will tolerate. Pain tolerance varies considerably among individuals, both human and animal. It is influenced greatly by the individual's prior experience, environment, stress, and drugs. Thus, there is no evidence based on nociceptor threshold or pain detection threshold that animals are any less sensitive or less capable of responding to noxious stimuli than people. If something is painful to a person, it will in all likelihood be equally painful to an animal (Breazile et al., 1963)

Noxious stimuli activate nociceptors, resulting in the generation of impulses in afferent A-delta and C nerve fibers. Both A-delta and C fiber nociceptors are essential for perception of acute pain. A-delta receptors appear to be specialized for detection of dangerous mechanical and thermal stimuli and for triggering rapid nociceptive responses. C polymodal receptors respond to strong mechanical, thermal, and chemical stimuli, are sensitized by chemicals released in damaged or inflamed skin, and mediate slow pain (La Motte and Campbell, 1978; Perl, 1976). C fibers reinforce the immediate response of A-delta fibers, signal the presence of damaged or inflamed tissue, and promote their protection and rest. Nociceptors in both humans and animals encode the intensity of noxious stimuli by increasing their frequency of discharge. In people, the rate of frequency of discharge is highly correlated with the magnitude of the pain sensation (Torebjork and Hallin, 1974). Animals appear to be able to detect differences in severity of noxious stimuli as well. Animals react faster and more vigorously on a learned escape task to terminate a moderately noxious stimulus than a mildly noxious stimulus (Dubner et al., 1977; Vierck, Cooper, and Cohen, 1983). All nociceptors become sensitized following injury resulting in hyperalgesia, that is, an increased response to stimuli that are normally painful (Bonica, 1990, 159).

Innervation of the internal organs (i.e., viscera) is different from skin in that it is primarily mediated by C polymodal receptors. Visceral C-fiber axons are primarily associated with sympathetic pathways, are relatively few in number compared to cutaneous afferents, and have large overlapping receptor fields. Mesenteric stretching, inflammation, ischemia, and dilation or spasm of hollow organs result in severe pain, whereas burning, clamping, or cutting do not stimulate visceral pain (Cervero, 1983; Janig and Morrison, 1986).

Nociceptors do not demonstrate fatigue with repeated stimulation, but rather display enhanced sensitivity and prolonged and enhanced response to stimulation (after discharge). Enhanced sensitivity is induced by endogenous algogenic substances released into the extracellular fluid by damaged, diseased, or inflamed tissues. These substances include H^+, K^+, serotonin, histamine, prostaglandins, bradykinin, substance P, and many others. Although the mechanisms are not well understood, injured primary afferents develop a sensitivity to norepinephrine that can be released from sympathetic postganglionic neurons (sympathetic-dependent hyperalgesia) (Bonica, 1990, 159; Perl, 1976; Brodal, 1981; Langford and Coggeshal, 1981; Hokfelt et al., 1983; Keele and Armstrong, 1964; Morrison and Henson, 1978).

Nociceptive impulses generated by the nociceptors are carried to the central nervous system by afferent A-delta and C fibers whose cell body is in the dorsal root ganglion. Afferents enter the spinal cord via the dorsal nerve root and terminate on cells in the dorsal horn of the grey matter (Willis, 1985; Coggeshall et al., 1975). Nociceptive specific cells (NS) receive excitatory input only from nociceptive afferents. Wide dynamic range (WDR) neurons receive convergent input from primary afferents innervating skin, subcutaneous tissue, muscle, and viscera. This convergence is the neural basis for referred pain (Pomeranz, Wall, and Weber, 1968; Price and Dubner, 1977). Wide dynamic range neurons can respond to hair movement and weak mechanical stimuli (touch) but respond maximally to intense potentially or actually damaging stimuli.

The ascending spinal tracts are bundles of nerve fibers whose cell bodies are located in the grey matter of the spinal cord or brain stem and terminate in the brain. The neurons in the dorsal horn whose axons form the fibers of the ascending tracts (NS and WDR neurons) are called relay or transmitter (T) cells because when excited by afferent nociceptive impulses, they relay or transmit the activity to other parts of the nervous system. Nociceptive information is conveyed from the spinal cord to the brain by multiple tracts, which can be divided into lateral and medial groups.

There are differences in these systems among species; however, the similarities outweigh the differences. The lateral ascending pathways (spinothalamic tracts) transmit nociceptive information leading to the sensory-discriminative aspects of pain. They terminate in the ventrobasal thalamus, which in turn relays the activity to the somatosensory cortex. The medial pathways (spinoreticular) subserve the motivational-affective aspect of pain. They terminate in the reticular formation, the periaqueductal gray matter, hypothalamus and thalamus (Dennis and Melzack, 1977).

The lateral tracts are not as effective as the medial tracts in mediating reflexes or in altering generalized brain function, that is, general arousal or alertness. The terminations of the medial pathways in the reticular formation and thalamus establish connections with the hypothalamus and limbic system. The limbic system includes the amygdala, hippocampus, septal nuclei, the preoptic region, hypothalamus, parts of the thalamus, and the epithalamus. The limbic system is concerned with mood and incentives to action (i.e., motivational interactions and emotions). The limbic system endows information derived from internal and external events with its particular significance to the individual and thus determines purposeful behavior. The hypothalamus and limbic structures have an important role in motivated, emotional, and affective behaviors, which are integral parts of the pain experience. Observation of these behaviors allows us to recognize the presence of pain in animals and nonverbal people. The hypothalamic-limbic system mediates emotional states and reactions. Limbic structures provide the neural basis for the aversive drive and affect that comprise the motivational dimensions of pain. Lesions of the limbic system in both humans and animals markedly obtund the aversive quality of noxious stimuli without interfering with the discriminative aspects of bodily sensation. The ability of opioids to reduce pain-induced suffering while preserving discriminative function is attributed to their effects on reticular and limbic neurons (Dennis and Melzack, 1983; Cassem, 1983).

The thalamus serves as the relay for ascending sensory information entering the cerebral cortex. The somatosensory cerebral cortex plays a major role in providing the sensory-discriminative dimension of pain. Neocortical processes subserve cognitive-evaluative aspects of pain including prior experience, conditioning, anxiety, attention, background, and evaluation of the pain-producing situation. The frontal cortex appears to play a significant role in mediating between cognitive activities and motivational-affective features of pain (Bowser, 1976; Casey, 1980a,b; Kitchell and Guinan, 1990).

The reticular formation consists of a core of neurons organized to distribute information rapidly, extending from the spinal cord to the cerebral cortex. Reticular function appears to be critical to integration of the pain experience and behavior. Ascending reticular neurons mediate the affective/ motivational aspects of pain via their input into the medial thalamus, hypothalamus, and limbic system (Casey, 1980b; Melzack and Casey, 1968)

A significant portion of central nervous system activity is concerned with selection, modulation, and control of ascending sensory information by descending fibers. The descending inhibitory system has been described as being activated centrally by enkephalins and opioids and sending serotonergic and noradrenergic fibers to terminate in the spinal and medullary dorsal horn. In addition, noradrenergic neurons arising from the locus ceruleus and other brain stem nuclei contribute to the endogenous system (Kerr, 1975; Gebhart, 1986; Hammond, 1986; Westlund and Coulter, 1980).

RESPONSES TO INJURY AND PAIN

Injury to tissues results in local biochemical changes and autonomic reflex responses intended to be protective. Release of intracellular substances from damaged tissue into the extracellular fluid induces local pain, tenderness, and hyperalgesia. Transmitted impulses evoke somatomotor and sympathetic segmental autonomic nocifensive reflex responses. Impulses reaching the brain stem initiate suprasegmental reflex responses and activate the descending modulating system, while those reaching the cortex stimulate cortical responses (Bonica 1990,159; Morrison and Henson, 1978; Kitchell and Johnson, 1985).

Segmental reflexes can enhance nociception and produce alterations of ventilation, circulation, and gastrointestinal and urinary functions. Stimulation of somatosensory pathways induce increased skeletal muscle tone or spasm, decreasing thoracic and abdominal wall compliance (splinting). In addition, positive feedback loops that initiate nociceptive impulses from the muscles result in reflex spasm and pain (Bonica, 1990, 159; Zimmermann, 1979).

Stimulation of sympathetic preganglionic neurons causes increased heart rate and stroke volume and increases myocardial work and oxygen consumption. If pain is severe enough, it can cause severe cardiac dysrythmias. Sympathetic hyperactivity causes decreased gastrointestinal and urinary function, which can lead to ileus and reduced urinary output (Bonica, 1990, 159).

Massive nociceptive input has profound effects on dorsal horn neurons, interneurons, and anterior motor neurons. C fibers from muscles, joints, and periosteum can produce long-latency long-duration facilitation and very prolonged increased excitability of dorsal horn cells ("wind-up"). Receptive fields are expanded and nociceptive cells become sensitive to nonnoxious stimuli such as light touch. Cells with receptive fields distant from that of the stimulated nerve are also affected. This facilitation, while triggered by peripheral C fibers, is maintained by intrinsic spinal cord processes. This facilitated activity appears to be the basis for widespread prolonged tenderness, hyperalgesia, and bouts of intense skeletal muscle spasm associated with excruciating pain that may persist for days or weeks following injury (Bonica, 1990, 159; Zimmermann, 1979; Thompson, King, and Woolf, 1990; Cook et al., 1987; Woolf and Wall, 1986).

Nociceptive stimulation of medullary centers of circulation and ventilation, hypothalamic centers of neuroendocrine function (primarily sympathetic), and limbic structures results in suprasegmental reflex responses. These consist of hyperventilation, increased hypothalamic neural sympathetic tone, and increased secretion of catecholamines and other endocrine hormones. Increased neural sympathetic tone and catecholamine secretion add to that induced segmentally to further increase cardiac output, peripheral resistance, blood pressure, cardiac work, and myocardial oxygen consumption. In addition, there is increased secretion of cortisol, ACTH, glucagon, cAMP, ADH, growth hormone, renin, and other catabolically active hormones and a concomitant decrease in insulin and testosterone. These responses, characteristic of the stress response, cause increased blood glucose, free fatty acids, blood lactate, and ketones, as well as increased rate of metabolism and oxygen consumption. These responses cause substrate mobilization to central organs and injured tissues and lead to a catabolic state and negative nitrogen balance. The magnitude and duration of these changes parallel that of the degree of tissue damage and may last for days (Bonica, 1990, 159; Melzack and Wall, 1982; Kehlet, 1986; Wilmore et al., 1976; Bessman and Renner, 1982). These responses can be obtunded or largely prevented by the preoperative administration of analgesic agents (preemptive analgesia) (Woolf and Chong, 1993). Intense anxiety and fear are an integral part of the pain response/experience. They greatly enhance the hypothalamic responses through cortical stimulation. In addition, anxiety causes cortically mediated increases in blood viscosity, clotting time, fibrinolysis, and platelet aggregation (Hume and Egdahl, 1959; Hume, 1969). Clinical signs of pain are summarized in table 4.1.

These responses induced by tissue damage and pain while immediately protective for short-term survival can be deleterious if prolonged. Indeed, in the hospital setting and specifically in a surgical environment, they may be more deleterious than helpful. More specifically, the stress response results in increased cardiac output, cardiac work, and oxygen consumption at a time when cardiac reserve is diminished. Intense vasoconstriction, especially of the splanchnic beds, leads to ischemia, tissue hypoxia, and release of substances toxic to the myocardium. Renal failure may ensue as a result of intense vasoconstriction and the release of ADH and aldosterone. Stress-induced metabolic changes lead to a catabolic state with negative nitrogen balance. In many patients with severe posttraumatic or postsurgical pain, these neuroendocrine responses are of sufficient magnitude to initiate and maintain shock (Hume and Egdahl, 1959; Hume, 1969; Schneider, 1950; Dreyfuss, 1956; Ogston, McDonald, and Fullerton, 1962; Zahavi and Dreyfus, 1971; Roizen, 1988).

Attenuation of the stress response through adequate pain relief and supportive therapy should result in improved patient outcome. Preemptive analgesia has been shown to be highly effective in preventing wind-up and in reducing the amount of postoperative pain and requirement for analgesics. In addition, the nonsteroidal anti-inflammatory agents may be useful in relieving pain resulting from the continued release of algogenic substances from injured and inflamed tissues. Pain can be controlled initially through systemic administration of analgesics, primarily opioids and alpha-2 adrenergic agonists. Long-term control of pain may include epidural or spinal administration of these agents. Local and regional nerve blocks can play an important role in the perioperative period and as a part of a balanced anesthetic protocol. Nonpharmacologic treatments such as supportive bandages and splinting should not be overlooked.

Table 4.1.   Signs of Pain

Acute pain
Guarding of affected area
Crying or vocalizing on movement or palpation
Mutilation—excessive licking, biting, scratching
Restlessness—pacing, lying down, getting up
Sweating
Recumbency
Heavy breathing
Defense reactions including freezing
Aggressive reactions
Avoidance learning

Chronic pain
Limping or carrying limb
Licking area of body
Reluctance to move; changes in exploratory activity
Loss of appetite
Change in personality
Dysuria (painful urination)
Bowel lassitude
Animals not up 24 hours postsurgery
Avoidance of pain-aggravating influences
Seeking of pain-relieving factors and environments
Self-mutilation
Changes in sleeping behavior
Changes in feeding behavior, e.g., decrease of food intake

ACUTE PAIN

Acute pain is the result of a traumatic, surgical, or infectious event that is abrupt in onset and relatively short in duration. Acute pain has a biologic function (i.e., is physiologic), in that it serves as a warning that something is wrong and leads to behavioral changes and limits of activity that are protective. Acute pain is a symptom of disease, whereas chronic pain itself is a disease. Acute pain is generally alleviated by analgesic drugs. The most common cause of acute pain in agricultural animals is the result of management practices thought to benefit the producer, herd or flock, and/or the individual animal. Examples include castration, dehorning, branding, tail docking of sheep and pigs (and more recently dairy cattle), and debeaking of chickens. These are elective procedures in that they are not necessary for the health and well-being of the individual animal. Such surgical procedures will be painful. The severity of the pain and its duration will depend on the procedure, the efficiency and skill of the operator, and the age of the animal. As producers and caregivers, we are obligated both ethically and morally to carry out these procedures when they are the least traumatic to the individual and with due attention to minimizing pain. For example, castrating should be done early rather than waiting until the animal approaches sexual maturity. Disbudding a baby calf entails much less tissue damage and pain than does dehorning when the horn is fully developed. In any case, humane treatment dictates that analgesia be provided for the procedure itself and, if justified, for a period postoperatively. When dehorning, local blockade of the cornual nerves is easy, cheap, and effective in rendering the horn analgesic (insensible) so that removal is painless. An injection of an analgesic drug such as ketoprofen will reduce the postoperative pain and discomfort that arises when the nerve block wears off.

PAIN IN NEWBORNS

In an effort to minimize pain and distress, common elective management practices, such as castration, disbudding (dehorning), ear notching, and tail docking, are performed within the first days or weeks following birth. The underlying assumption is that due to the animal's small size and immaturity, these procedures will result in less tissue trauma and pain than if delayed until later in life. Further, it has been believed that neonates do not perceive or react to painful stimuli as do adults, thus precluding or minimizing the use of anesthetics or analgesics. Such an attitude has until fairly recently been the case in human medicine as well. Beginning in the late 1800s with the emergence of developmental embryology and neuroscience, it was thought that unmyelinated nerves were not functional at birth and, as a result, newborns were not sufficiently developed to perceive pain. In 1872, Charles Darwin stated in *The Expression of Emotions in Animals and Man* that children's facial expressions, cries, convulsive movements, and vascular and breathing changes were only reflex actions and did not reflect the sensory and emotional aspects of pain. He further contended that the expressions of pain in animals, children, savages, and the insane did not imply awareness of pain (Cope, 1998). Because infants were believed incapable of experiencing pain due to their immature nervous systems, the use of minimal or no anesthesia/analgesia was often the standard of care through the mid-1980s (Mather and Mackie, 1995). Surgical procedures ranging from circumcision and hernia repair to thoracotomy for correction of congenital vascular anomalies were performed with little or no anesthesia and analgesia. A series of studies in England changed the concept of pain perception and management in infants. These studies showed that infants receiving minimal anesthesia and analgesia mounted a markedly increased hormonal stress response. Subsequent studies showed that the massive hormonal and metabolic stress responses were blunted by potent anesthetics (Anand, Brown, Causon, et al., 1985; Anand, 1986; Anand, Brown, Bloom, et al., 1985; Anand and Aynsley-Green, 1985; Anand et al., 1988; Anand, Sippell, and Aynsley-Green, 1987).

Neonatal pain research has involved the rat pup model. Rat pups, like human infants, have complete peripheral and spinal cord sensory connections at birth. However, maturation of C-fiber synapses in the spinal cord, development of inhibitory neurons in the substantia gelatinosa of the spinal cord, and functional maturation of the descending inhibitory systems from supraspinal centers all take place postnatally. Thus, the newborn nervous system is capable of mounting a response to painful stimuli but the response is un-predictable and not well organized. More important, because descending inhibition is lacking, the response is exaggerated. Both human and animal studies have shown that the neonate's spinal sensory cells are more excitable than those of adults, with a greater and more prolonged response as well as a larger receptive field. Infants and neonatal rat pups demonstrate hyperresponsivity to noxious stimuli that may result in hyperalgesia. After birth, peripheral cutaneous innervation, neuroendocrine function, and mechanisms of inflammation still undergo developmental changes (Franck, Greenberg, and Stevens, 2000; Fitzgerald, 1995; Fitzgerald and Jennings, 1999; Fitzgerald, 1991; Fitzgerald, Millard, and McIntosh, 1988, 1989; Fitzgerald and Lynn, 1977; Fitzgerald and Beggs, 2001). The neurotransmitters of descending inhibition develop late or postnatally (Kostarczyk, 1999). The response to tissue injury includes sensitization of peripheral nociceptors and central neuronal pathways. In addition, tissue damage leads to sprouting of sensory nerve terminals in the area of injury. This response is particularly intense in neonates as compared to adults. The resulting hyperinnervation and hypersensitivity cannot be prevented by regional analgesia (De Lima et al., 1999). Thus, it would appear that the potential for central sensitization (i.e., wind-up) would be greater than following full development. In neonates, pain transmission is primarily by C fibers, and reflex responses are less precisely located and involve a greater body area. Neonates can perceive pain at birth and have a functionally mature hypothalamic-pituitary axis capable of mounting a stress response.

Recent studies in children have shown that perinatal and neonatal pain can result in altered pain sensitivity, stress disorders, increased anxiety, and other behavioral disorders. Boys circumcised without analgesia had differences in sleeping and feeding behavior and displayed anxiety after the surgery. In another study, circumcised boys displayed more pain behavior during vaccinations at four and six months than did uncircumcised boys (Taddio et al., 1995). In a prospective study in 1997, Taddio et al. reported that during vaccinations at four and six months, uncircumcised boys had the lowest pain scores while boys circumcised with analgesia had a lower pain score than did those in a placebo group. This suggested that infants retain a memory of painful experiences and response to subsequent pain is altered.

PAIN RESULTING FROM PRODUCTION PRACTICES

Calves and Cattle

Just as studies of pain in nonverbal infants and children have been based on behavior and stress responses, so have those in agricultural animals. In calves 4 to 11 weeks of age, surgical castration induced more agitation during the operation than the application of a rubber ring. However, both groups resumed normal behavior soon after the operation was completed. Salivary cortisol concentrations were significantly higher in surgically castrated calves than those castrated by rubber ring and both were greater than in control calves. Cortisol concentrations had returned to control levels by four hours (Fell, Wells, and Shutt, 1986). The data would support the contention that in these small calves, rubber ring castration is less distressing than surgical castration. Subsequently, in 1994, Robertson, Kent, and Molony compared the behavioral and cortisol responses in bull calves of 6, 21, and 42 days of age induced by either surgical, Burdizzo, or rubber ring castration. When compared to handled but unoperated controls, and calves castrated by surgical or Burdizzo methods, the rubber ring caused significant increases in active behavior and abnormal postures for two hours following application. Surgical techniques resulted in abnormal standing for 30 minutes. Abnormal behaviors and postures were least frequent in the 6-day-old calves. Cortisol was increased significantly in all castrated calves compared to the control (handled) group. Greatest cortisol response occurred in 42-day-old calves following surgical castration. The cortisol response induced by Burdizzo castration was of shorter duration than that induced by rubber ring or surgical castration. It was concluded that all methods were acutely painful irrespective of age but that the Burdizzo method appeared to be least painful, particularly in young calves. In 1998, Obritzhauser, Deutz, and Kofer compared the stress responses and behavioral changes following either surgical castration or castration by the Burdizzo method. Plasma cortisol was increased for three hours following castration with either method, and behaviors indicative of pain were similar between groups. They concluded that both methods were equally painful. Fisher et al. (2001) compared the effects of surgical castration to those of latex-banding methods of castration in 9- and 14-month-old bulls following local analgesia. In the hours following castration, surgically castrated 14-month-old bulls exhibited more leg stamping and tail swishing than did unoperated controls or those banded. Surgical castrates had elevated haptoglobin concentrations that returned to control levels in four days. Plasma cortisol was generally unaffected by castration in this study. Surgical castrates grew more slowly than did intact control bulls, but faster than banded castrates. In addition, the banded castrates developed persistent wounds above the band, which did not close for several weeks after scrotal dehiscence. This did not occur in those banded at nine months. It was concluded that while banding may induce fewer acute effects, banding suppressed growth and caused prolonged wound formation in the older animals, suggesting that this method would be better used on animals less than a year old. Early and Crowe (2002) evaluated the use of ketoprofen, a nonsteroidal anti-inflammatory-analgesic drug, alone or in combination with local analgesia for surgical castration of bull calves. In Holstein bull calves weighing 215 kg, plasma cortisol concentrations were increased for 12 hours following castration, castration with local anesthesia, and castration with local anesthesia plus ketoprofen compared to unoperated controls. Calves receiving ketoprofen prior to castration had total cortisol responses not different from controls. In calves castrated with local anesthesia, the peak cortisol response was delayed but the total response was not suppressed. In addition, ketoprofen had a beneficial effect on acute-phase proteins not observed in the other groups. It was concluded that ketoprofen was more effective than local anesthesia at suppressing the pain-induced stress response to castration. In light of the foregoing studies, it would appear that all methods of castration are painful to calves of any age. Furthermore, castration should be done early. Burdizzo and surgical methods appear to be least distressful. Latex bands should not be used on bulls greater than a year old. Regardless of the method chosen, local anesthesia will decrease the pain of castration and administration of ketoprofen will diminish postoperative pain and stress responses.

Dehorning is a common practice. In 1997, Taschke and Folsch determined histologically that the horn buds and surrounding area are well innervated in calves ranging from newborn to four months of age. Thermal disbudding without anesthesia resulted in distinct pain and defense behaviors. Salivary cortisol concentration was significantly increased following disbudding. They concluded that calves should only be dehorned using anesthesia. In adult cows dehorned using a wire saw, anesthesia did not prevent the increase in salivary cortisol probably due to the stress induced by restraint. While anesthesia prevented pain responses during dehorning, the cows were painful upon recovery from neural blockade. Milk production was diminished transiently. McMeekan et al. (1998) demonstrated that scoop dehorning without anesthesia induced a significant increase in plasma cortisol that lasted seven hours. In calves undergoing neural blockade with bupivacaine, a local anesthetic that induces analgesia lasting three to four hours, cortisol concentrations were similar to those of undehorned controls. As neural blockade waned at four hours, cortisol concentrations increased dramatically returning to control levels at nine hours. Similarly, calves receiving a bupivacaine block prior to dehorning and again at four hours had normal cortisol concentrations until eight hours. This study demonstrated the efficacy of cornual nerve blockade in anesthetizing the horn and preventing the pain-induced stress response. It further demonstrated that postoperative pain is still present and significant following recovery from neural blockade and needs to be addressed. In 1999, Grondahl-Nielsen et al. investigated the behavioral, endocrine, and cardiac responses of young calves to thermal dehorning. They found that cornual blockade prevented the immediate behavioral response to dehorning and prevented short-term increases in plasma cortisol concentration and long-term increases in heart rate. Dehorning without cornual block or sedation-analgesia (dehorned control) resulted in significant behavioral and cortisol responses. Heart rate was increased for 213 minutes and rumination was significantly decreased. Conscious sedation-analgesia induced by xylazine-butorphanol without cornual block did not prevent behavioral responses to dehorning but did prevent increases in cortisol similar to cornual blockade. The combination of cornual blockade and xylazine-butorphanol sedation-analgesia resulted in lowest cortisol concentration at four hours. Grondahl-Nielsen concluded that dehorning was painful and that cornual blockade was indicated and improved the welfare of calves being dehorned. In a similar study, Faulkner and Weary (2000) reported the behavioral effects of dehorning in Holstein calves. All calves were sedated with xylazine and the cornual nerves anesthetized. Half of the calves received ketoprofen prior to dehorning and again at 2 and 7 hours postoperatively. Calves treated with ketoprofen demonstrated little head shaking or ear flicking behavior, while those that did not receive ketoprofen had higher frequencies of these pain-related behaviors, which peaked at 6 hours. Differences between the two groups were significant for 12 hours for head shaking and 24 hours for ear flicking. Weight gain was greater in ketoprofen-treated calves in the 24 hours following dehorning. These results indicate that ketoprofen effectively mitigates pain induced by hot-iron dehorning. In summary, these studies document the need for and efficacy of cornual blockade in preventing the pain of dehorning. Furthermore, they demonstrate that local anesthesia does not diminish pain upon recovery from the block. Thus, the concurrent use of systemic analgesics such as ketoprofen are indicated to ensure adequate analgesia and promote welfare in the immediate postoperative period.

Branding is a means of permanently identifying cattle. Traditionally this has involved the use of a hot iron. Recently this practice has been called into question on the grounds that it would be quite painful. As a result of these concerns, freeze branding has been suggested as a more humane alternative. In 1992, Lay et al. compared the behavioral and physiologic effects of hot and freeze branding in crossbred calves. In a carefully controlled study, they were unable to demonstrate any differences between the freeze- and hot-branding methods with respect to behavior. The only significant difference was greater plasma epinephrine concentrations in the hot-branded calves at 0.5 minutes postbranding. In a similar study in adult dairy cows, they were unable to demonstrate any difference in the stress response induced by the two branding methods. However, in these cows, hot branding caused greater escape-avoidance reactions and heart rates. Therefore, Lay et al. concluded that freeze branding was preferable where feasible. There can be little doubt that either method is painful. It would seem that, at the very least, where branding is deemed necessary, some type of systemic analgesic should be administered to diminish discomfort as for castration or dehorning.

Lambs

Local anesthesia has been shown to eliminate the behavioral and cortisol responses induced by castration and tail docking in lambs. Administration of naloxone, a mu-opioid antagonist, intensified the behavioral responses indicating that endogenous opioid release mitigates pain in young lambs (Wood et al., 1991). Molony, Kent, and Robertson (1993, 95) compared the response to castration and tail docking by rubber ring, Burdizzo and rubber ring, and surgical castration at 5, 21, and 42 days. All methods caused behaviors associated with considerable [sic] pain. Rubber rings were associated with the most severe signs at all ages. Least responses were observed in the Burdizzo-rubber ring group. They concluded that the use of the Burdizzo with the rubber ring may provide the least painful method when local anesthesia is not used and that age of the lambs in this study had little effect on responses. Behavioral and cortisol responses were used to compare pain induced by tail docking with a heated docking iron, Burdizzo and rubber rings, or rubber ring alone. Docking with the heated iron resulted in responses not different from those of handled controls. The rubber ring caused the greatest increase in cortisol and behavioral responses. Subcutaneous bupivacaine, a local anesthetic, administered immediately prior to application of the ring was more effective at reducing these responses than epidural injection of bupivacaine, topical cold analgesic spray, or diclofenac, a nonsteroidal anti-inflammatory analgesic drug (Graham, Kent, and Molony, 1997). For castration, injection of local anesthetic is more effective if injected into the neck of the scrotum at the site of the ring than injection into the testes prior to ring application. Alternatively, while slightly less effective than local anesthetic, a bloodless castrator applied just proximal to the ring also reduced behavioral and cortisol responses induced by castration or tail docking (Kent, Molony, and Graham, 1998; Sutherland et al., 1999). Last, Kent et al. (2000) compared be-havioral changes in 2-day-old lambs castrated and tail docked with rubber rings with and without local anesthetic and Burdizzo-rubber ring. Castration and tail docking did not af-fect body weight with or without pain reduction methods. However, when evaluated at 10, 20, 31, and 41 days following treatment, lambs that were castrated and tail docked with rubber rings without local anesthetic or Burdizzo displayed significantly more pain-related abnormal behavior. The unexpected duration of these behaviors appeared to be evidence of long-lasting increases in pain sensitivity (wind-up) induced by an episode of acute in-tense pain in a young animal. It would appear based on these studies that castration and tail docking should be done with local anesthetic injected at the site of ring application. Alternatively, the combined use of a Burdizzo applied proximal to the ring to destroy the nerves may be used.

Pigs

McGlone et al. (1993) examined the development of castration-induced behavior changes, the effect of castration age on weight gain, and the efficacy of analgesics for use in cas-trated pigs. Castration caused changes in behavior (reduced suckling time and increased lying times, decreased standing) in castrated versus intact pigs at all ages (i.e., 1, 5, 10, 15, or 20 days of age). In a second experiment, pigs castrated on day 1 were compared with those castrated on day 14. Birth weight, weaning weight, and mortality were recorded. Pigs castrated on day 1 had lower weaning weight and gained less weight during lactation than did those castrated on day 14. Mortality was the same between groups. Last, the ef-fect of aspirin or butorphanol were evaluated on castration-induced behavioral changes in 8-week-old pigs. While castration reduced feeding time and weight gain, neither aspirin nor butorphanol influenced castration-induced behaviors. The authors concluded that pigs had similar behavioral changes and, by inference, pain perception when castrated at all ages studied. However, performance data favored castration at day 14 rather than day 1. This may be due to greater wind-up occurring in the 1-day-old pigs similar to the results reported in 2-day-old lambs (Kent et al., 2000).

Chickens

Debeaking is a common management practice in the poultry industry. Trimming the beak by 3 mm results in a prolonged increase in heart rate as compared to handled nontrimmed control birds. This prolonged tachycardia is thought to be pain induced. Trimming by 3 mm does not affect body weight or rate of lay but does decrease food consumption and mean egg weight for nine to ten days (Glatz, 1987). Debeaking results in behavioral changes. There are short-term decreases in time spent feeding, drinking, and preening. Longer term, preening time and cage pecking behaviors decreased and time spent stand-ing inactive increased without returning to pretreatment levels after five weeks. For two weeks following debeaking, time spent eating and drinking decreased and time spent doz-ing increased, returning to pretreatment levels after five weeks. It is probable that these changes are pain induced. The authors concluded that the pain induced by debeaking de-creased welfare of the individual bird. The decrease in individual welfare conflicts with the increase in welfare to the flock brought about by debeaking. The balance between the two should be considered before any decision to beak trim is taken (Duncan et al., 1989).

CHRONIC PAIN IN FOOD ANIMALS

Chronic pain is that which persists beyond the usual course of an acute disease or beyond a reasonable time for an injury to heal or that is associated with a chronic pathologic process that causes continuous pain or pain that recurs for months or years. Chronic pain is seldom alleviated by analgesics, but frequently responds to tranquilizers or psychotropic drugs combined with environmental manipulation and behavioral conditioning. Chronic pain never serves a biologic function, is considered to be pathologic in and of itself, and imposes severe detrimental stresses on the patient. Chronic pain is most commonly asso-ciated with arthritis or other chronic degenerative conditions or with lesions resulting in dysfunction of the nociceptive system at any point from the periphery to the cerebral cor-tex. In food animals, the best recognized and studied chronic pain is that induced by in-fections (footrot, abscesses) and/or trauma to the feet of sheep, cattle, and pigs. Numerous studies have demonstrated the long-term effects of these conditions on chronic lameness and decreased mechanical threshold that persist beyond resolution of the inciting condi-tion. In 1996, Ley, Waterman, and Livingston demonstrated that the threshold response to a noxious mechanical stimulus was lower in lame cattle than in nonlame cattle. However, there was no difference in plasma catecholamine or cortisol concentrations. Whay et al. (1998) reported that lame cattle had lower nociceptive thresholds than did nonlame cattle. In cattle with acute digital infection, the mechanical threshold was no different from that in sound cattle 28 days following successful treatment. However, cattle with chronic sole ulcers and white line disease still had decreased nociceptor thresholds at 28 days.

In sheep, footrot has been shown to decrease the threshold to noxious mechanical (pres-sure) stimuli but not to noxious thermal (heat) stimuli. Treatment of sheep with low-sever-ity footrot resulted in a return to normal threshold values, while those of sheep with highly severe lesions required up to three months to return to normal values (Ley, Waterman, Liv-ingston, 1989, 95). Subsequently, Brandt and Livingston (1990) demonstrated that the hy-persensitivity induced by chronic footrot in sheep was associated with an increase in the number of alpha-2 adrenergic receptors and mu-opioid receptors in areas of the sheep spinal cord associated with nociception. The analgesic potency of xylazine was signifi-cantly reduced in chronically painful sheep and this effect persisted beyond resolution of the clinical lameness (Ley, Waterman, Livingston, 1991). Chronic pain causes plasma cor-tisol to be increased but the increase does not correlate with the severity of lameness. Fur-thermore, plasma cortisol remains elevated up to three months following resolution of clinical signs (Ley et al., 1994). Plasma epinephrine and norepinephrine are similarly af-fected (Ley, Livingston, Waterman, 1992).

A common chronic condition occurring in broiler chickens is lameness caused by arthritis. This lameness has been shown to be relieved by carprofen, a nonsteroidal anti-inflammatory drug, indicating that the condition is in fact painful to the chicken (McGeowen et al., 1999). Subsequent studies demonstrated that lame chickens preferred feed containing carprofen over nonmedicated feed, and that as severity of lameness increased, the birds consumption of medicated feed increased (Danbury et al., 2000).

In pets, chronic pain can be treated in much the same manner as in people (e.g., nonsteroidal anti-inflammatory drugs). In livestock production, long-term administration of drugs is uneconomical and not approved under the present regulations in most countries. Agricultural animals suffering from intolerable chronic pain resulting in decreased productivity, weight loss, or inability to thrive as a result of degenerative conditions should be salvaged as soon as possible or euthanatized.

DRUG USE IN FOOD ANIMALS

The use of anesthetics and analgesics in food animals is somewhat problematic at this time. In North America and Europe, there are few anesthetic or analgesic drugs approved for use in food animals. Extra-label use of drugs in the United States in food producing animals is allowed under the Animal Medicinal Drug Use Clarification Act (AMDUCA) if they are intended for the medical treatment of the animal and don't create a risk to public safety, if adequate records are kept, and if the veterinarian has established an adequate withdrawal period. Because very few drugs used for anesthesia or analgesia are labeled for use in food producing animals, there is little information available to guide the establishment of appropriate withdrawal periods. The Food Animal Residue Avoidance Databank (FARAD) has been used to estimate the appropriate meat and milk withdrawal times to give veterinarians a starting point to be in compliance with AMDUCA (Craigmill et al., 1997). An alternative approach when considering withdrawal times for anesthetics and analgesics would be to delay slaughter or marketing of milk until the surgical site has healed. Anesthetics or analgesics administered to young animals for routine procedures such as castration, tail docking, or disbudding would pose little threat of residues since the time to marketing would be months. In addition, the use of nonsteroidal anti-inflammatory analgesics such as carprofen and ketoprofen would appear to present little danger to the consumer since these drugs are available over the counter for unrestricted use in people. However, injectable general anesthetics, especially drugs such as ketamine, Telazol, and xylazine have caused adverse reactions in people consuming meat from animals immobilized or anesthetized for slaughter. In any case, the producer should consult with a veterinarian for the proper drug(s), dosage, and withdrawal times of anesthetics and analgesics. The AMDUCA regulation can be found at http://www.fda.gov/cvm/index/amduca/amducafr.htm.

REFERENCES

Anand KG. The stress response to surgical trauma: from physiologic basis to therapeutic implications. Prog Food Nutr Sci 10: 67, 1986.

Anand KG, Aynsley-Green A. Metabolic and endocrine effects of surgical ligation of patent ductus arteriosus in the human preterm neonate: are there implications for further improvement of postoperative outcome? Mod Prob Pediatr 23: 143, 1985.

Anand KG, Brown MJ, Bloom SR, et al. Studies on the hormonal regulation of fuel metabolism in the human newborn infant undergoing anesthesia and surgery. Horm Res 22: 115, 1985.

Anand KG, Brown MJ, Causon RC, et al. Can the human neonate mount an endocrine and metabolic response to surgery? J Pediatr Surg 20: 41, 1985.

Anand KG, Sippell WG, Aynsley-Green A. Randomized trial of fentanyl anesthesia in preterm babies undergoing surgery: effects on the stress response. Lancet 1: 62, 1987.

Anand KG, Sippell WG, Schofield NM, et al. Does halothane anesthesia decrease the metabolic and endocrine stress responses of newborn infants undergoing operation? Br Med J (Clin Res Educ) 296: 668, 1988.

Bessman FP, Renner VJ. The biphasic hormonal nature of stress. In: RA Crowley and BF Trump, eds. Pathophysiology of shock, anoxia and ischemia. Baltimore: Williams and Wilkens, 1982: 60–65.

Bonica, JJ. General considerations of acute pain. In: JJ Bonica, JD Loeser, CR Chapman, and WE Fordyce, eds. The management of pain, 2nd ed. Philadelphia: Lea and Febiger, 1990: 159–179.

Bowser D. Role of the reticular formation in response to noxious stimuli. Pain 2:361, 1976.

Brandt SA, Livingston A. Receptor changes in the spinal cord of sheep associated with exposure to chronic pain. Pain 42: 323, 1990.

Breazile JE, Kitchell RL, Naitoh Y. Neural basis of pain in animals. In: Proc 15th Res Conf American Meat Institute Foundation, Chicago, 1963, 53.

Brodal A. Neurological anatomy in relation to clinical medicine, 3rd ed. New York: Oxford University Press, 1981.

Casey KL. The reticular formation and pain: towards a unifying concept. In: JJ Bonica ed. Pain research publications: association for research in nervous and mental disease. New York: Raven Press, 1980a: 63.

——. Supraspinal mechanisms and pain. The reticular formation. In: HW Kosterlitz and LY Terenius, eds. Pain and society. Verlag Weinheim Chemie, 1980b: 183–200.

Cassem NH. Current topics in medicine, II. Pain. In: E Rubinstein and DD Fedderman, eds. Scientific American Medicine, November 1983. New York: Scientific American, 1987: 1.

Cervero F. Mechanisms of visceral pain. In: Persistent pain, vol.4. New York: Grune and Stratton, 1983: 1–19.

Coggeshall RE et al. Unmyelinated axons in human ventral roots. A possible explanation for the failure of dorsal rhizotomy to relieve pain. Brain 98: 157, 1975.

Cook AJ et al. Dynapic receptive field plasticity in rat spinal cord dorsal horn following C-primary afferent input. Nature 325: 151, 1987.

Cope D. Neonatal pain: the evolution of an idea. Am Soc Anesthesiol Newslett 1998: Sept, 6.

Craigmill AL, Rangel-Lugo M, Damian P, Riviere JE. Extralabel use of tranquilizers and general anesthetics. JAVMA 211: 302, 1997.

Curtis SE, Morris GL. Operant supplemental heat in swine nurseries. In: Proc 2nd Int Livestock Symp, Ames: Iowa State University Press, 1982: 295.

Danbury TC, Weeks CA, Chambers JP, Waterman-Pearson AE, Kestin SC. Self-selection of the analgesic drug carprofen by lame broiler chickens. Vet Rec 146: 307, 2000.

De Lima J, Alvares D, Hatch DJ, Fitzgerald M. Sensory hyperinnervation after neonatal skin wounding: effect of bupivacaine sciatic nerve block. Br J Anaesth 83: 662, 1999.

Dennis SG, Melzack R. Pain signaling systems in the dorsal and ventral spinal cord. Pain 4: 97, 1977.

——. Perspectives on phylogenetic evolution of pain expression. In: RL Kitchell, HH Erickson, E Carstens, and LE Davis, eds. Animal pain: perception and alleviation. Bethesda MD: American Physiological Society, 1983, 151.

Dreyfuss F. Coagulation time of the blood, level of blood eosinophils and thrombocytes under emotional stress. J Psychosom Res 1: 252, 1956.

Dubner R, Price DD, Beital RE, Hu, JW. Peripheral neural correlates of behavior in monkey and human related to sensory-discriminative aspects of pain. In: DJ Anderson, B Mathews, eds. Pain in the Trigeminal Region. Amsterdam, Elsevier, 1977: 57.

Duncan IJ, Slee GS, Seawright E, Breward J. Behavioral consequences of partial beak amputation (beak trimming) in poultry. Br Poult Sci 30: 479, 1989.

Early B, Crowe MA. Effects of ketoprofen alone or in combination with local anesthesia during castration of bull calves on plasma cortisol, immunological and inflammatory responses. J Anim Sci 80: 1044, 2002.

Faulkner PM, Weary DM. Reducing pain after dehorning in dairy calves. J Dairy Sci 83: 2037, 2000.

Fell LR, Wells R, Shutt DA. Stress in calves castrated surgically or by the application of rubber rings. Aust Vet J 63: 16, 1986.

Fisher AD, Knight TW, Cosgrove GP, Death AF, Anderson CB, Duganzich DM, Matthews LR. Effects of surgical or banding castration on stress responses and behavior of bulls. Aust Vet J 79: 279, 2001.

Fitzgerald M. Development of pain mechanisms. Br Med Bull 47: 667, 1991.

——. Developmental biology of inflammatory pain. Br Anaesth 75: 177, 1995.

Fitzgerald M, Beggs S. The neurobiology of pain: developmental aspects. Neuroscientist 7: 246–2001.

Fitzgerald M, Jennings E. The postnatal development of spinal sensory processing. Proc Natl Acad Sci USA 96: 7719, 1999.

Fitzgerald M, Lynn B. The sensitization of high threshold mechanoreceptors with myelinated axons by repeated heating. J Physiol 265: 549, 1977.

Fitzgerald M, Millard C, McIntosh N. Hyperalgesia in premature infants. Lancet 1: 292, 1988.

——. Cutaneous hypersensitivity following peripheral tissue damage in newborn infants and its reversal with topical anaesthesia. Pain 39: 31, 1989.

Franck LS, Greenberg CS, Stevens B. Pain assessment in infants and children. Pediatr Clin North Am 47: 487, 2000.ebhart GF. Modulatory effects of descending systems on spinal dorsal horn neurons. In: TL Yaksh, ed. Spinal afferent processing. New York: Plenum Press, 1986: 391–416.

Gentle MJ, Corr SA. Endogenous analgesia in the chicken. Neursci Lett 201: 211, 1995.

Gentle MJ, Hunter LN, Waddington D. The onset of pain related behaviors following partial beak amputation in the chicken. Neurosci Lett 128: 113, 1991.

Glatz PC. Effects of beak trimming and restraint on heart rate, food intake, body weight and egg production in hens. Br Poult Sci 28: 601, 1987.

Graham MJ, Kent JE, Molony V. Effects of four analgesic treatments on the behavioral and cortisol responses of 3-week-old lambs to tail docking. Vet J 153: 87, 1997.

Grondahl-Nielsen C, Simonsen HB, Lund JD, Hesselholt M. Behavioral, endocrine and cardiac responses in young calves undergoing dehorning without and with use of sedation and analgesia. Vet J 158: 14, 1999.

Hammond DL. Control systems of nociceptive afferent processing: the descending inhibitory pathways. In: TL Yaksh, ed. Spinal afferent processing. New York: Plenum Press, 1986: 363–390.

Hokfelt T et al. Neuropeptides and pain pathways. In: JJ Bonica, U Lindblom and A Iggo, eds. Advances in pain research and therapy, vol. 5. New York: Raven Press, 1983: 227–246.

Hume DM. The endocrine and metabolic response to injury. In: SE Schwartz, ed. Principles of surgery. New York: McGraw-Hill, 1969.

Hume DM, Egdahl RH. The importance of the brain in the endocrine response to injury. Ann Surg 150: 697, 1959.

Janig W, Morrison JFB. Functional properties of spinal visceral afferents supplying abdominal and pelvic organs with special emphasis on visceral nociception. In: F Cervero and JFB Morrison, eds. Visceral sensation. Amsterdam: Elsevier, 1986: 87–114.

Kaebler WW, Mitchell CL, Yarmat AJ, Affifi AK, Lorens SA. Centrum medianum-parafasciculus lesions and reactivity to noxious and non-noxious stimulus. Exp Neurol 46: 282, 1975.

Keele CA, Armstrong D. Substances producing pain and itch. In: H Barcroft, H Davson and WDM Paton, eds. Monographs of the physiological society, vol. 12. London: Edward Arnold, 1964: 1–374.

Kehlet H. Pain relief and modification of the stress response. In: MJ cousins and GD Philips, eds. Acute pain management. New York: Churchill Livingstone, 1986: 49–65.

Kent JE, Jackson RE, Molony V, Hosie BD. Effects of acute pain reduction methods on the chronic inflammatory lesions and behavior of lambs castrated and tail docked with rubber rings at less than two days of age. Vet J 160: 33,2000.

Kent JE, Molony V, Graham MJ. Comparison of methods for the reduction of acute pain produced by rubber ring castration or tail docking of week-old lambs. Vet J 155: 39, 1998.

Kerr FWL. Neuroanatomical substrates of nociception in the spinal cord. Pain 1: 325, 1975.

Kitchell R. Problems in defining pain and peripheral mechanisms of pain. J Am Vet Med Assoc 191: 1195, 1987.

Kitchell RL, Guinan MJ. The nature of pain in animals. In: BE Rollin and MS Kesel, eds. The experimental animal in biomedical research. Boston: CRC Press, 1990: 85.

Kitchell RL, Johnson RD: Assessment of pain in animals. In: Animal stress. Bethesda MD: American Physiological Society, 1985: 113.

Kitchell RL, Naitoh Y, Breazile JE, Lagerwerff JM. Methodological considerations for assessment of pain perception in animals. In: CA Keele, R Smith, eds. The assessment of pain in man and animals. Edinburg: Churchill Livingstone, 1962: 244.

Kostarczyk E. Recent advances in neonatal pain research. Folia Morphol (Warsz) 58: 47, 1999.

La Motte RH and Campbell JN. Comparison of responses of warm and nociceptive C-fiber afferents in monkey with human judgements of thermal pain. J Neurophysiol 41: 509, 1978.

Langford LA, Coggeshal RE. Branching of the sensory axons in the peripheral nerve of the rat. J Comp Neurol 203: 745, 1981.

Lay DC, Friend TH, Bowers CL, Grissom KK, Jenkins OC. A comparative physiological and behavioral study of freeze and hot-iron branding using dairy cows. J Anim Sci 70: 1121, 1992.

Lay DC, Friend TH, Randel RD, Bowers CL, Grissom KK, Jenkins OC. Behavioral and physiological effects of freeze or hot-iron branding on crossbred cattle. J Anim Sci 70: 330, 1992.

Lee HL. Managing pain in human neonates—applications for animals. JAVMA 221: 233, 2002.

Levine S. A definition of stress? In: GP Moberg, ed. Animal stress. Bethesda, Md, American Physiological Society, 1985: 51.

Lewis T. Pain. New York: Macmillan, 1942.

Ley SJ, Livingston A, Waterman AE. Effects of clinically occurring chronic lameness in sheep on the concentrations of plasma noradrenaline and adrenaline. Res Vet Sci 53: 122, 1992.

Ley SJ, Waterman AE, Livingston A. The effect of chronic clinical pain on thermal and mechanical thresholds in sheep. Pain 39: 353, 1989.

Ley S, Waterman A, Livingston A. The influence of chronic pain on the analgesic effects of the alpha-2 adrenoceptor agonist xylazine in sheep. J Vet Pharmcol Ther 14: 141, 1991.

——. A field study of the effect of lameness on mechanical nociceptive thresholds in sheep. Vet Rec 137: 85, 1995.

——. Measurement of mechanical thresholds, plasma cortisol and catecholamines in control and lame cattle: a preliminary study. Res Vet Sci 61: 172, 1996.

Ley SJ, Waterman AE, Livingston A, Parkinson TJ. Effect of chronic pain associated with lameness on plasma cortisol concentrations in sheep: a field study. Res Vet Sci 57: 332, 1994.

Mather L, Mackie J. The incidence of postoperative pain in children. Pain 15: 271, 1983; in boys. Lancet 345: 291, 1995.

McGeown D, Danbury TC, Waterman-Pearson, AE, Kestin SC. Effect of carprofen on lameness in broiler chickens. Vet Rec 144: 668, 1999.

McGlone JJ, Nicholson RI, Hellman JM, Herzog DN. The development of pain in young pigs associated with castration and attempts to prevent castration-induced behavioral changes. J Anim Sci 71: 1441, 1993.

McMeekan CM, Mellor DJ, Stafford KJ, Bruce RA, Ward RN, Gregory NG. Effects of local anesthesia of 4 to 8 hours duration on the acute cortisol response to scoop dehorning in calves. Aust Vet J 76: 281, 1998.

Melzack R. Neurophysiological foundations of pain. In: RA Sternbach, ed. The psychology of pain. New York: Raven Press, 1986: 1.

Melzack R, Casey KL. Sensory, motivational and central control determinants of pain. In: D Kenshalo, ed. The skin senses. Springfield, IL: Charles C. Thomas, 1968: 423.

Melzack R, Wall PD. The challenge of pain. New York: Basic Books, 1982.

Mench JA, van Tienhoven A. Farm animal welfare. Am Sci 74: 598, 1986.

Mitchell CL, Kaebler WW. Effect of medial thalamic lesions on responses elicited by tooth pulp stimulation. Am J Physiol 210: 263, 1966.

——. Unilateral vs bilateral lesions and reactivity to noxious stimuli. Arch Neurol 17: 653, 1967.

Molony V, Kent JE, Robertson, IS. Behavioral responses of lambs of three ages in the first three hours after three methods of castration and tail docking. Res Vet Sci 55: 236, 1993.

Morrison DC, Henson PM. Release of mediators from mast cells and basophils induced by different stimuli. In: MK Bach, ed. Immediate hypersensitivity: modern concepts and developments. New York: Marcel Decker, 1978: 431–511.

Obritzhauser W, Deutz A, Kofer J. Comparison of two castration methods in cattle: plasma cortisol levels, leukocyte count and behavioral changes. Tierarztl Prax AUSG Grosstiere Nutztiere 26: 119, 1998.

Ogston D, McDonald GA, Fullerton HW. The influence of anxiety in tests of blood coagulability and fibrinolytic activity. Lancet 2: 521, 1962.

Pavlov IP. Lectures on conditioned reflexes. New York: International Publishers, 1928.

Perl ER. Sensitization of nociceptors and its relation to sensation. In: JJ Bonica and D Albe-Fessard, eds. Advances in pain research and therapy, vol 1. New York: Raven Press, 1976: 17–28.

Pomeranz B, Wall PD, Weber WV. Cord cells responding to fine myelinated afferents from viscera, muscle and skin. J Physiol 199: 511, 1968.

Price DD, Dubner R. Neurons that subserve the sensory-discriminative aspects of pain. Pain 3: 307, 1977.

Robertson IS, Kent JE, Molony V. Effect of different methods of castration on behavior and plasma cortisol in calves of three ages. Res Vet Sci 56: 8. 1994.

Roizen MF. Should we all have a sympathectomy at birth? Or at least postoperatively? [Editorial] Anesthesiology 68: 482, 1988.

Rollin B. Animal pain, scientific ideology and the reappropriation of common sense. J Am Vet Med Assoc 191: 1222, 1987.

Rollin BE. Veterinary and animal ethics. In: JF Wilson, ed. Law and ethics of the veterinary profession. Yardley, PA: Priority Press, 1988: 24.

Rowan A, Tannenbaum J. Animal rights, in National Forum 66: Phi Kappa Phi, 30, 1986.

Russell WMS, Burch RL. The principles of humane experimental techniques. London: Metheune, 1959: chap.3.

Schneider RA. The relation of stress to clotting time, relative viscosity and certain biophysical alterations of the blood in normotensive and hypertensive subjects. In: HG Wolff, SG Wolff, CC Hare, eds. Life stresses and bodily disease. Baltimore: Williams and Wilkens, 1950: 818–831.

Soma LR. Behavioral changes and the assessment of pain in animals. In: J Grandy, S Hildebrand, W McDonnell, eds. Proc 2nd Int Cong of Veterinary Anesthesia. Sacramento: American College of Veterinary Anesthesiologists, 1985: 38.

Sutherland MA, Mellor DJ, Stafford KJ, Gregory NG, Bruce RA, Ward RN, Todd SE. Acute cortisol responses of lambs to ring castration and docking after the injection of lignocaine into the scrotal neck or testes at the time of ring application. Aust Vet J 77: 738, 1999.

Taddio A, Goldbach M, Ipp M, et al. Effect of neonatal circumcision on pain responses during vaccination in boys. Lancet 345: 291, 1995.

Taddio A, Katz J, Ilersich AL, et al. Effect of neonatal circumcision on pain response during subsequent routine vaccination. Lancet 349: 599, 1997.

Taschke AC, Folsch DW,. Ethological, physiological and histological aspects of pain and stress in cattle when being dehorned. Tierarztl Prax 25: 19, 1997.

Thompson SWN, King AE, Woolf CJ. Activity-dependent changes in rat ventral horn neurons in vitro; Summation of prolonged afferent evoked postsynaptic depolarizations produce a D-2-amino-5-phosphonovaleric acid sensitive windup. Eur J Neurosci 2: 638, 1990.

Torebjork HE, Hallin RG. Identification of afferent C units in intact human skin nerves. Brain Res 67: 387, 1974.

Vierck CJ, Cooper BY, Cohen RH. Human and nonhuman primate reactions to painful electrocutaneous stimuli and to morphine. In: RL Kitchell, HH Erickson, E Carstens, LE Davis, eds. Animal pain: perception and alleviation. Bethesda, MD, American Physiological Society, 1983: 117.

Warnock M. The philosophical approach to pain and pain relief. In: PM Taylor, ed. Proc First Int Cong of Veterinary Anaesthesia, Cambridge, Association of Veterinary Anaesthetists of Great Britain and Ireland, 1982: 6.

Westlund KN, Coulter JD. Descending projections of the locus coeruleus and subcoeruleus/medial parabrachial nuclei in the monkey: Axonal transport studies and dopamine-beta-hydroxylase immunocytochemistry. Brain Res Rev 2: 235, 1980.

Whay HR, Waterman AE, Webster AJ, O'Brien JK. The influence of lesion type on the duration of hyperalgesia associated with hindlimb lameness in dairy cattle. Vet J 156: 23, 1998.

White JC, Sweet WH. Pain and the neurosurgeon: a forty year experience. Springfield, IL: Charles C Thomas, 1969: 850.

Willis WD. The pain system: the neural basis of nociceptive transmission in the mammalian nervous system. Basel: S Karger, 1985.

Wilmore DW, Long JM, Mason AD, Pruitt BA. Stress in surgical patients as a neurophysiologic reflex response. Surg Gynecol Obstet 142: 257, 1976.

Wood GN, Molony V, Fleetwood-Walker SM, Hodgson JC, Mellor DJ. Effects of local anesthesia and intravenous naloxone on the changes in behavior and plasma concentrations of cortisol produced by castration and tail docking with tight rubber rings in young lambs. Res Vet Sci 51: 193, 1991.

Woolf CJ, Chong MS. Preemptive analgesia-treating postoperative pain by preventing the establishment of central sensitization. Anesth Analg 77: 362, 1993.

Woolf CJ, Wall PD. The relative effectiveness of C-primary afferents of different origins in evoking a prolonged facilitation on the flexor reflex in the rat. J Neurosci 6: 1433, 1986.

Wylie LM, Gentle MJ. Feeding-induced tonic pain suppression in the chicken: reversal by naloxone. Phsiol Behav 64: 27, 1998.

Zahavi J, Dreyfuss F. Adenosine diphosphate-induced platelet aggregation in myocardial infarction and ischemic heart disease. Presented at Second Congress of Thrombosis and Hemostasis, Oslo, July 13, 1971.

Zimmerman M. Peripheral and central mechanisms of nociception, pain and pain therapy; Facts and hypotheses. In: JJ Bonica, JC Liebeskind, and DC Albe-Fessard, eds. Advances in pain research and therapy, vol 3. New York: Raven Press, 1979: 3–32.

——. Neurobiological concepts of pain, its assessment and therapy. In: B Bromm, ed. Neurophysiological correlates of pain. Amsterdam: Elsevier, 1984: 15.

5

A Concept of Welfare Based on Feelings

Ian J. H. Duncan

INTRODUCTION

When scientists first started to investigate animal welfare in the late 1960s and 1970s, it was generally accepted that an animal's welfare would be a reflection of how physiologically stressed it was; an animal that was not stressed would have good welfare and an animal that was highly stressed would have poor welfare (Bareham, 1972; Bryant, 1972; Wood-Gush, Duncan, and Fraser, 1975; Freeman, 1978). In the 1970s, it seemed that assessing welfare was simply a matter of finding a reliable measurement of stress. The argument was convincing. "Welfare," whatever that might be, was a consequence of certain physiological processes, and the most likely physiological processes to be involved were those connected with stress.

It is interesting that when Ruth Harrison set the ball rolling a little earlier with her pivotal book *Animal Machines*, she, as a layperson, laid much more emphasis on animal suffering than on the physiological stress response of animals in intensive agriculture, in biomedical research, and in product testing (Harrison, 1964). The Brambell Committee, which was set up by the British government in response to the public outcry following the publication of *Animal Machines*, also acknowledged that feelings were an important feature of welfare (Command Paper 2836, 1965). In my view, the Brambell Committee was very farsighted in claiming that, "welfare is a wide term that embraces both the physical and mental well-being of the animal. Any attempt to evaluate welfare, therefore, must take into account the scientific evidence available concerning the feelings of animals that can be derived from their structure and functions and also from their behaviour." Nevertheless, in spite of these allusions to the feelings of animals in general and the suffering of animals in particular, the widespread view within the scientific community at that time was that welfare was intimately connected with stress.

As the number of investigations into animal welfare increased through the 1970s, different scientists came up with many different definitions of welfare. Duncan and Dawkins (1983) reviewed this whole field in order to see if there were any common threads in these definitions. They decided that it was impossible to give welfare a precise scientific definition. A broad working description would be one that encompassed the notions of the animal in complete mental and physical health, the animal in harmony with its environment, the animal able to adapt to an artificial environment provided by human beings without suffering, with the animal's feelings, somehow, taken into account. It should be noted that this broad working description includes both the physical aspects of welfare as well as the psychological aspects of subjective feelings. Duncan and Dawkins (1983) also proposed that a broad working description of suffering would be "a wide range of unpleasant emotional states."

A DIVISION OF OPINION

For a period, this broad description of "animal welfare" worked quite well. Scientists investigating a variety of problems saw some advantage to using a range of physiological and behavioral indicators of welfare (e.g., Warnier and Zayan, 1985; Mormède, 1990; Barnett et al., 1991; Lay et al., 1992). However, as the number of investigations into welfare expanded, examples were found in which there was disagreement among the list of descriptors of welfare. For example, animals were identified that gave all the outward signs of being in good welfare but had subclinical disease. Did these animals actually have good welfare, or did the disease compromise their welfare? Sows confined in dry sow stalls commonly performed stereotyped movements and looked distressed although they appeared to be healthy and physiologically normal (Terlouw et al., 1991). Is their welfare reduced or not? And what of an animal such as a male rat (Szechtman et al., 1974) or a stallion (Colborn et al., 1991) that actively seeks to participate in mating, an apparently rewarding activity, and then shows symptoms of stress as a consequence of this participation? Is the animal's welfare good or poor? These discrepancies in the evidence led to a prolonged debate within the scientific animal welfare community. When the strands of evidence regarding physical and psychological well-being diverge, which should take precedence? Is animal welfare really to do with physical health and good biological functioning, or is more to do with psychological health and how the animal feels? From this debate, emerged two distinct schools of thought: the "biological functioning" school and the "feelings" school.

THE BIOLOGICAL FUNCTIONING SCHOOL

The biological functioning school believes that animal welfare is all to do with good biological functioning, with the absence of a stress response, or at least with the absence of a large stress response (Broom, 1986; Wiepkema, 1987; Barnett and Hemsworth, 1990; Broom and Johnson, 1993), with the animal being able to "cope" (Fraser and Broom, 1990; Broom and Johnson, 1993), and with the satisfaction of the animal's biological needs (Curtis, 1987; Hurnik and Lehman, 1988). As was stated at the start of this chapter, linking welfare to stress makes intuitive sense. However, when the arguments are examined in more detail, the link is not so clear-cut. For example, Broom and Johnson (1993, p. 72) state, "Therefore, we reach the conclusion that stress is an environmental effect on an individual which overtaxes its control systems and reduces its fitness or appears likely to do so." However, these authors also suggest that if control systems are overtaxed the organism will not survive. So, linking welfare to stress (defined in this way) means the situation is so serious that, if nothing is done, the animal will die. Also, in none of these studies is fitness actually measured; it is just assumed that fitness will be reduced. So the clause linking fitness to the definition of welfare would seem to be unwarranted. Moreover, this approach cannot deal adequately with cases in which participation in a rewarding activity results in a stress response (Szechtman et al., 1974; Colborn et al., 1991). The concept of coping is also unclear. Broom and Johnson (1993, p. 49) state,

> An important concept . . . is [that of] coping. In the scientific literature the ability to tolerate different degrees of stimulation, particularly noxious stimulation, is embodied in the concept of coping. Coping is defined as having control of mental and bodily stability (Fraser and Broom, 1990). In an account of human adaptation to various stimuli, Lazarus and Folkman (1984) suggest that it is the extent of the ability to cope that ultimately determines whether the individual survives in unfavorable conditions.

This definition of "coping" runs into the same problem encountered by the concept of "stress": the animal either copes and survives, or does not cope and dies. There is, however, a chink in the biological functioning school's armor. Broom and Johnson (1993, p. 73) say,

> There are many occasions when individuals find coping difficult, but succeed without long-term adverse consequences by, for example, using a brief adrenal response or a behavioural change of some kind. A minor injury or a period of illness might have no effect on the fitness of an individual. In each of these situations and on all occasions in which there is any kind of suffering, there is an effect on welfare even if there is no likely effect on individual fitness. Hence stress invariably implies poor welfare, but welfare can be poor without stress.

Therefore, having spent 70 pages building the case that welfare is to do with the absence of a stress response (or absence of a large stress response) and with the animal being able to "cope," Broom and Johnson (1993, p. 73) concede that reduced welfare is *actually* about suffering! They move from the position that stress is necessary and sufficient for reduced welfare to one that it is sufficient only. In light of the evidence showing that some animals show a stress response to an enjoyable activity, I would argue that stress is neither necessary nor sufficient for reduced welfare.

The importance of an animal's biological needs in determining its welfare has been described by Hurnik and Lehman (1988). They proposed that an animal's welfare is governed by a hierarchy of needs that are, in order of importance, life-sustaining needs, health-sustaining needs, and comfort-sustaining needs. For example, animals need food and water, and if deprived of food and water, their welfare will be reduced; if the deprivation is prolonged, the animals will die. Of secondary importance are the animal's "health needs" and of tertiary importance, its "comfort needs." If these are not met, welfare will also be reduced, but not so severely as when life-sustaining or health-sustaining needs are not met. Intuitively, this scheme seems to make sense. However, closer examination reveals that not all "life-sustaining needs" result in suffering if they are not satisfied. For example, in most terrestrial species, lack of oxygen is *not* accompanied by suffering. Human beings subjected to low oxygen tension simply become unconscious (sometimes reporting pleasant feelings). Most animals also subside into unconsciousness without any symptoms of suffering. Is welfare reduced in these cases? Hurnik and Lehman (1988) would argue that it is, since the animal is deprived of a life-sustaining requirement. I would contend that welfare is not reduced since an animal deprived of oxygen does not suffer (Raj, 1998). Curtis (1987) has proposed a very similar scheme to that of Hurnik and Lehman (1988), with physiologic needs as the most important followed by safety needs and behavioral needs.

THE FEELINGS SCHOOL

In contrast to the biological functioning school, the feelings school believes that welfare is all to do with what the animal feels, with the absence of negative subjective emotional states that are usually called "suffering" and probably with the presence of positive subjective emotional states that are usually called "pleasure." After Harrison (1964) and the Brambell Committee (Command Paper 2836, 1965) had alluded to the importance of subjective feelings as a component of welfare, the idea was given more scientific credibility by Marian Dawkins in her influential book *Animal Suffering* (Dawkins, 1980). The idea of feelings being important for welfare was gradually developed (Duncan, 1981; Duncan and Dawkins, 1983), and then the suggestion was made that, in fact, feelings were the only thing that mattered (Duncan and Petherick, 1991; Duncan, 1993).

The argument was developed in the following way. All living organisms have certain needs that have to be satisfied in order for the organism to survive, grow, and reproduce. This is as true for pine trees as it is for protozoa as it is for pigs. If these needs are not met, the organism will show symptoms of atrophy, ill-health, and stress (in a general sense), and it may even die. In the animal kingdom, the lower invertebrates satisfy their needs by means of simple, hard-wired, stimulus-response behavior. If a fly lands on my arm and I try to swat it, the fly avoids my hand moving toward it. This behavior is of the stimulus-response type; the fly will avoid any large shape rushing toward it, will not habituate to mock swats, will not avoid a stationary flyswatter, and will not learn to anticipate from my behavior that I am going to swat it. In contrast to this, the higher organisms (the vertebrates and the higher invertebrates) have evolved "feelings," subjective affective states, to motivate behavior in a much more flexible way. If a cat moves toward a bird, the bird will avoid the cat, but its avoidance is governed by fear. The bird will avoid stationary cats and, in fact, anything with catlike properties. It may also learn the habits of local cats and so be able to anticipate where and when they are likely to appear and so avoid them without actually seeing them. This difference between the mechanisms by which the "lower" and "higher" animals operate is crucial in the animal welfare debate. The lower invertebrates are responding to their environment by simple stimulus-response mechanisms, with no (or very little) conscious awareness of what is going on. These mechanisms can be linked to give quite complex chains of behavior, but there is a limit to their flexibility. Robots can be programmed to perform quite complex tasks and to change their behavior as their environment changes—but only within limits. The higher invertebrates and the vertebrates have solved the problem of dealing with a constantly changing environment, not by adding to stimulus-response chains, but by evolving the higher mental processes of cognition and consciousness.

The importance of feelings in motivating behavior has been recognized for hundreds of years. Even René Descartes, the person commonly blamed for promoting the idea of animals as machines, seems to have accepted that animals have feelings. He wrote, "Similarly of all the things which dogs, horses and monkeys are made to do are merely expressions of their fear, their hope, or their joy; consequently they can do these things without any thought" (Kenny, 1970, p. 207). This certainly suggests that Descartes accepted that animals have feelings or sensations while denying that they have language or thought. In the eighteenth century, the Scottish philosopher David Hume had this to say on feelings in animals: "Is it not experience which renders a dog apprehensive of pain, when you menace him, or lift up the whip to beat him?" (Hume, 1739, pp. 397–398). And in the nineteenth century, Jeremy Bentham, the English social reformer, discussed why animals at that time were not receiving much protection from the law, and said "the question is not, Can they *reason*? nor Can they *talk*? but, Can they *suffer*?" (Bentham, 1823). By the middle of the nineteenth century, feelings were being viewed as adaptations that allowed animals to substitute flexible adaptive responses for reflexive ones (Spencer, 1855). So, by the time of Darwin's *The Origin of Species by Means of Natural Selection*, it was widely accepted that animals had feelings, and within a short time they came to be viewed as adaptations to pressures of natural selection. For example, George John Romanes (1884) wrote,

> Pleasures and pains must have been evolved as the subjective accompaniment of processes which are respectively beneficial or injurious to the organism, and so evolved for the purpose or to the end that the organism should seek the one and shun the other. . . . Thus, then, we see that the affixing of painful or disagreeable states of consciousness to deleterious changes of the organism, and the reverse states to reverse changes, has been a necessary function of the survival of the fittest.

The actual evolutionary "path" (Ruse, 1984) that may have been followed by feelings is discussed by Humphrey (1986, 1992). He uses the metaphor of consciousness being an "inner eye" that allows the organism awareness of certain inner states such as hunger and fear.

OPPOSITION TO FEELINGS

It seems strange that a concept that was well accepted by the late nineteenth century should generate such debate as that which occurred between the biological functioning school and the feelings school in the late twentieth century. Romanes's (1884) view is exactly my view (Duncan, 1996) more than one hundred years later. The reason for the reluctance to accept feelings or consciousness as a legitimate subject for scientific investigation was the rise of Behaviorism, a very important school of psychology, especially in North America. Behaviorists were vehement in their campaign against paying any attention to feelings or consciousness through the twentieth century into the 1970s. For example, one of the founders of Behaviorism, William James (1904), wrote, "Consciousness . . . is the name of a non-entity, and has no right to a place among first principles. Those who still cling to it are clinging to a mere echo, the faint rumor left behind by the disappearing 'soul' upon the air of philosophy. . . . It seems to me that the hour is ripe for it to be openly and universally discarded." One of the most influential proponents of Behaviorism was J. B. Watson. He stated, "The behaviorist sweeps aside all medieval conceptions. He drops from his scientific vocabulary all subjective terms such as sensation, perception, image, desire and even thinking and emotion" (Watson, 1928). A later adherent, B. F. Skinner, the inventor of the "Skinner box" or operant conditioning chamber, wrote, "We seem to have an inside information about our behavior—we have feelings about it. And what a diversion they have proved to be! . . . Feelings have proved to be one of the most fascinating attractions along the path of dalliance" (Skinner, 1975).

These strongly expressed views against the scientific study of consciousness had a profound effect on the whole of psychology. Only a few brave souls, such as McDougall (1926) and Young (1959), dared to discuss consciousness and subjective affective states in their writings. Even the European-founded discipline of ethology shunned a consideration of feelings, until Donald Griffin broached the subject in his book *The Question of Animal Awareness* (Griffin, 1976), since then there has been a burgeoning of literature on this topic (e.g., Radner and Radner, 1989; Ristau, 1991; Damasio, 1999).

Against this antagonistic background, fostered by the Behaviorists, the reluctance to consider feelings in any way by the rest of the scientific community is perhaps understandable. However, even if studies of feelings were to be universally acknowledged as creditable, this still leaves unanswered the question of whether feelings are what welfare is all about, and that will be tackled now.

FEELINGS AND WELFARE

If we start with introspection and consider our own welfare, it certainly seems that it is how we feel that affects our welfare. Sudden danger elicits feelings of fear, a visit to the dentist raises feelings of apprehension, loss of a loved one makes us feel very sad, good social interaction produces feelings of happiness, and so on. We also carefully separate out health and welfare in our everyday conversation. Being able to say of someone with terminal cancer "But they don't seem to be suffering" or "But they seem to be happy within themselves" gives us tremendous solace. We can be upset that their health is terrible, but we get great comfort from knowing that they are not suffering or even that they seem to be enjoying what life they have. The opposite relationship between welfare and health can also hold true. Thus, we may be in excellent health, but if we *think* that we have contracted some serious disease (possibly by receiving a false positive result from a diagnostic test) then our welfare may be devastated as we worry about our future.

We can argue, by analogy, that surely it must be the same for animals. Veterinarians and owners often have very difficult decisions to make about when to euthanize terminally ill companion animals. They normally use quality-of-life indicators to help them with these decisions and these are generally indicators of how the animal is feeling. Thus, the decision would normally be delayed in the case of a terminally ill dog that is, on balance, getting more pleasure from life than it is suffering. Of course, this is a very difficult decision for human beings to make, especially since the veterinarian might be better qualified to judge the suffering and the owner better qualified to judge the dog's positive emotions. Nevertheless, how the dog feels would be the critical question.

There is also general agreement that the concept of welfare can only be applied to sentient animals, that is, animals that are capable of feeling. Thus, among rational people, there is no concern for the welfare of plants, protozoa, or the lower invertebrates. I would argue that if sentience is necessary for a consideration of welfare, surely it is sentience that welfare is all about. The animal protection laws of most developed countries reflect this view and cover the vertebrates and sometimes the higher invertebrates such as the cephalopods. It is interesting that many of these countries are now struggling with the thorny problem of when in development should embryonic life get protection. The simple answer "when sentience begins" is not really tenable, since different aspects of sentience probably appear gradually and at different times.

WHAT ARE FEELINGS?

According to Bunge (1980) and Bunge and Ardilla (1987), a sensory system of an animal is a subsystem of its nervous system, composed of neurosensors and neural pathways leading to the corresponding primary sensory cortical area in the brain. "Sensing" or "detecting" is a specific activity in a sensory system. This should be distinguished from a "feeling," which is a specific activity in a sensory system of which an animal is aware. An animal is aware of only a small proportion of the sensory input that is entering its central nervous system at any particular time. Awareness has a lot to do with paying attention. Thus, a person approaching a lime tree could be asked to look at the beautiful blossom, or smell the scent of the blossom drifting on the wind, or listen to the buzz of thousands of bees working the blossoms. All three of the person's sensory systems would be working at the same time, but the person would only be aware of the stimulus he or she was paying attention to at any one time.

I have used the term *feelings* in this chapter, but other names are also used. *Emotions* is often used interchangeably with feelings, but Crooks and Stein (1988, p. 310) have pointed out that subjective feelings are only one component of the emotions. In addition, the emotions are composed of physiological arousal, cognitive processes, and behavioral reactions. The more technical, perhaps more neutral and certainly more long-winded term *affective subjective states* is sometimes used instead of feelings or emotions. As previously stated, the term *sentient* means capable of feeling.

In summary, in the course of evolution, the vertebrates and higher invertebrates have evolved feelings or affective subjective states to motivate behavior in a more flexible way than is possible with simple stimulus-response mechanisms. The positive states are usually called states of pleasure and the negative states, states of suffering. The argument being made by the feelings school is that welfare is all to do with these subjective states, that is, with the absence of states of suffering and (probably) with the presence of states of pleasure. I say "probably" because, although certain states of suffering can be recognized throughout the vertebrates and higher invertebrates, recognizing states of pleasure is much more of a challenge when one moves away from the common companion animals with which human beings have been coevolving for thousands of years. This may be simply a case of these states being difficult to recognize, but there is also the possibility that many species may have a fairly meager repertoire of states of pleasure. Fraser and Duncan (1998) proposed that negative and positive subjective feelings may be two very different states that have evolved to solve two different types of motivational problem. They suggested that negative feelings have evolved to motivate behavior in "need situations" where an immediate solution is required because there is a threat to the animal's survival or reproductive success. In contrast, positive feelings have evolved to motivate behavior in "opportunity situations" in which there will be a long-term benefit from performing the behavior but no immediate need. So behavior motivated by pleasure is likely to occur when all other need-motivated behavior is satisfied and the fitness cost of performing the pleasure-motivated behavior has declined. It may be that behavior driven by negative states is more primitive in evolutionary terms than that driven by positive states. If this were the case, it might explain why negative states seem to be more widespread within the vertebrates and higher invertebrates than positive states.

Table 5.1 shows a list of some primary needs or deficiencies of animals together with the secondary subjective feelings that might have evolved to protect these primary needs.

Table 5.1. Primary Needs or Deficiencies and Associated Secondary Feelings in Animals

Primary need or deficiency	Secondary feeling
Having a nutrient deficiency	Feeling hungry
Having a fluid deficiency	Feeling thirsty
Avoiding a predator	Feeling frightened
Being ill	Feeling ill
Being stressed	Feeling stressed
Being injured	Feeling pain
Maintaining social contact	Feeling lonely
Learning social graces in a young animal	Play-fighting leads to feelings of pleasure
Maintaining social bonds	Grooming (or being groomed by) a herd- or flock-mate leads to feelings of pleasure
Keeping plumage or pelage in good order	Bathing leads to feelings of pleasure

Source: Fraser and Duncan (1998).

Note: The first seven needs in the table require an immediate solution and therefore the secondary feelings that have become linked to them are negative feelings. The last three examples are of behavior that will have a long-term benefit but can be performed at any time when all other urgent needs are satisfied. The feelings associated with these motivational systems are positive.

The first seven are examples of needs or deficiencies that are linked to negative subjective states, and the last three are suggestions of the types of behavior that might be linked to feelings of pleasure. I say "suggestions" because states of pleasure in animals have been investigated very little. However, dog and cat owners will not be in any doubt that social grooming (from the owner!) leads to feelings of pleasure in the dog or cat and many dogs and cats will actively solicit grooming.

The biological functioning school believes that welfare is principally to do with the satisfaction of the primary needs and much less to do with the satisfaction of the secondary subjective feelings. The feelings school, on the other hand, believes that welfare is *all* to do with the secondary subjective feelings, with the absence of negative feelings, particularly the strong negative feelings we call suffering and with the presence of positive feelings that we call pleasure. So, I am drawing a fine distinction between the primary need of having a nutrient deficiency and the secondary subjective feeling of hunger. I am even distinguishing being ill and feeling ill. Being ill reduces one's health and biological fitness; feeling ill (even if one is *not* ill!) reduces one's welfare. The connection between primary need and secondary subjective feeling is discussed in detail elsewhere (Duncan, 1996). Of course, usually there will be a close correspondence between the primary need and the secondary feeling, because feelings have evolved through the pressure of natural selection to protect needs. So usually an animal that is ill will also feel ill. Usually an animal with a nutrient deficiency will feel hungry. However, this is not always the case with domesticated animals. Thousands of years of artificial selection has resulted in some strains of animal in which the biological need and the corresponding feeling have become divorced. For example, many strains of meat-type chickens and fast growing pigs have huge appetites that do not correspond to their nutritional needs. They have been intensively selected for fast growth and huge appetites. This is not a big problem for the meat chickens or the fattening pigs themselves; they simply reach market-weight very quickly. It is, however, a huge problem for the parent stock, for the broiler breeders and breeding sows and boars that produce the meat animals. Since they have a very similar genetic makeup to their offspring, they too have huge appetites, and if allowed to satisfy these appetites, they would become obese, unable to breed, and suffer from diseases of obesity. On the other hand, if their food intake is very severely restricted, they function fairly well, their nutritional needs are met, and they are biologically fitter than if not deprived. However, it is quite obvious in the case of both broiler breeders (Mench and Falcone, 2000) and breeding sows (Appleby and Lawrence, 1987) that their welfare is severely compromised by the food restriction. Using the criteria of the biological functioning school to judge welfare, one would conclude that the severely restricted parent stock have good welfare because they are functioning reasonably well and they have good biological fitness. The feelings school, on the other hand, would argue that the continuous severe hunger felt by the restricted animals greatly reduces their welfare. Nor is the answer to allow these animals to eat to appetite, since very quickly this would result in obesity and feelings of malaise. It should be pointed out that there is no solution to this welfare problem with these particular breeding animals. Although it may be possible to alleviate the situation by, say, allowing the animals to fill their guts with a low-density ration that contains lots of cellulose, this does not eliminate hunger.

MEASURING FEELINGS AND THUS WELFARE

One of the big advantages of assuming that biological functioning and primary needs are the important features of welfare is that the associated physiological states are (1) substantial and (2) possible to measure directly and accurately. For example, heart rate could be measured as an indicator of the alarm reaction or level of plasma glucocorticoids could be measured as an indicator of the general adaptation syndrome. Feelings, on the other hand, are (1) ill defined, (2) impossible to measure directly, and (3) difficult to measure indirectly. Nevertheless, I would argue strongly that if feelings are what welfare is all about then it is feelings that we should be attempting to measure. There is now evidence that an increasing number of welfare scientists are agreeing with this thesis, and even sometime hard-line biological functioning adherents are softening their approach (e.g., Broom, 1998).

The argument has been made that animal welfare is all to do with what animals feel. At this point we appear to hit a huge obstacle. Subjective feelings are just that—*subjective*. Subjective feelings are not directly available for scientific investigation. Only I know how I feel. Therefore, no matter how convinced we are that welfare is all to do with feelings, this is of little help if an organism's feelings are locked inside its consciousness. However, in the case of human beings, this has not proved to be insuperable. We have language and can listen to others describing their feelings in certain situations. Usually, we find there is close correspondence between the descriptions we hear and how we feel ourselves. The fear of speaking in public, the frustration of missing a bus, the pain of stubbing a toe, the pleasure of good social interaction are examples of feelings commonly experienced and similarly described by a large proportion of the human population. But this is not always true. It is more difficult to empathize with individuals who enjoy giving or receiving painful stimuli or who have an extreme fear of unusual stimuli like tiny insects. The fact remains that language lets us share our feelings. Of course, we can also argue by analogy and homology that since we are built in approximately the same way, our feelings are likely to be experienced similarly. When you have a toothache, it is likely that the pain you feel will be fairly similar to the pain I feel when I have a toothache.

But what of animals? We do not have a common language with them so they cannot tell us directly what they feel. However, we are beginning to understand their systems of communication, or "languages," and it *may* be possible to gain information about their feelings from studying those. For example, Seyfarth, Cheney, and Marler (1980) have been able to tease apart vervet monkey alarm calls, which contain information about the source of the alarm, the intended audience, and the state of the monkey giving the call. On a more practical level, Weary, Braithwaite, and Fraser (1998) and Taylor and Weary (2000) have been able to assess the severity of pain experienced by piglets during castration by carefully analyzing their vocalizations. (See also figure 3.3 of this volume for vocalizations after weaning.) Therefore, a study of animal communication may open up some windows on feelings.

It is also fortunate in the animal welfare debate that we do not need to know exactly what an animal is feeling. The important thing to know is whether the animal is experiencing positive feelings or negative feelings. Thus, in the case of a piglet being castrated, it is not necessary to know if what the piglet experiences is similar to what a human being experiences with a deep cut or a severe burn or renal colic or whatever. What we need to know, in order to assess welfare, is whether or not the piglet experiences something that is negative. If the piglet does experience negative feelings, it would also be helpful to know how negative they are. It is possible to gather information of this type indirectly. The animal is allowed to choose between certain aspects of its environment and the assumption is made that it will choose in the best interests of its welfare. This technique called "preference testing," was pioneered by Barry Hughes and Marian Dawkins, both working with poultry. For example, Hughes has determined the hens' preferences for cage floor type (Hughes and Black, 1973), cage size (Hughes, 1975), and social conditions (Hughes, 1977) using this method. Dawkins has examined the hens' preferences for floor type (Dawkins, 1978), inside or outside environment (Dawkins, 1976, 1977), and cage size (Dawkins, 1978). There are certain pitfalls to be avoided when using preference tests, and these have been well elucidated (Duncan, 1978, 1992; Dawkins, 1983; Fraser and Matthews, 1997).

Carrying out a preference test is only the first step in investigating how an animal feels about its environment. It is also essential to know how important a particular choice is for the animal. A choice in one direction, even if it is consistent, may be trivial and not at all important for the animal. I tend to choose consistently one particular malt whisky over others, but my welfare is not going to be adversely affected if I am forced to take a less-preferred brand! Likewise, I prefer injections in my upper arm to my backside and, in this case, my welfare is going to be decreased (a little) by both. So a choice may represent the lesser of two evils with the subject suffering with both options.

For these reasons, therefore, it is necessary to measure the strength of preference as a follow-up to preference testing. There are various ways of doing this and often an economic analogy is used in the description of these methods. We can "increase the price" of the commodity that the animal is choosing, that is, we can see how hard the animal will "work" in order to obtain the preferred choice. Operant responding is a common method for measuring motivation (e.g., Dawkins and Beardsley, 1986), as are obstruction tests (e.g., Nicol and Guildford, 1991; Mason, Cooper, and Clarebrough, 2001) in which the animal has to push past an obstruction to reach its preferred choice. In general, motivation testing in which the animal is attempting to reach a goal is more straightforward than measuring strength of avoidance, but this methodology is also being developed (e.g., Rutter and Duncan, 1991, 1992). Fraser and Matthews (1997) discuss motivation testing in some depth and point out the pitfalls. It is also possible to investigate motivation by reducing an animal's "income" rather than increasing the "price" of the commodity, although this is rather stretching the economic analogy. The time that an animal has available to perform its various activities can be regarded as "income." The available time can be decreased until there is insufficient time for the animal to perform its full repertoire of behavior. It is assumed that "luxury" activities will then drop out and "essential" activities will remain. For example, Duncan, Widowski, and Keeling (1991) kept broiler chickens on intermittent lighting (1 hour light: 3 hours dark repeated) so that they only had 6 hours light available in 24 hours compared with 23 hours light for control birds. The chickens on intermittent light performed all of the activities that were seen in the control birds, including preening and dust bathing, but at a much faster rate. No activities dropped out, suggesting that they were all very important to the birds. There was evidence that time was limited, because feeding occurred in the dark for a few minutes each time before the lights came on and after they went off.

Pain is a state of suffering responsible for reducing welfare on a huge scale. In animal agriculture there are lots of surgical interventions practiced without analgesic or anesthetic cover. For example, piglets are commonly castrated and have their teeth trimmed and tails docked; calves are castrated and dehorned; lambs are castrated and tail docked; chicks are debeaked; turkey poults are de-beaked, de-snooded, and de-toed, all without painkillers. Apart from the possibility of immediate pain associated with the surgery, there is the post-surgical healing period, and, in some cases involving amputation of body parts, the possibility of chronic pain. In addition, many farm animals suffer abrasions through living in ill-designed environments. For example, sows housed in dry sow stalls often have pressure sores on their hips, and the incidence of lameness in dairy cows housed in intensive units seems to be increasing. In addition to all these problems, the poultry and swine sectors are running into fast-growth problems that often involve weaknesses of the skeleton, which could be painful.

How do we ask animals if they are in pain? This is more of a challenge than investigating other aversions in which use can be made of avoidance behavior. Sometimes, as in the previously described research of Dan Weary, it might be possible to make use of an animal's vocalizations to assess the acute pain of a procedure (Weary et al., 1998; Taylor and Weary, 2000). Otherwise, looking carefully at the effects of analgesics can give clues to how much pain an animal is in (e.g., Duncan et al., 1990; Molony and Kent, 1997). In a very exciting development, broiler chickens have been shown capable of self-administering a painkilling drug. When given a choice between two feeds, one of which contained an analgesic, broilers with gait abnormalities ate more of the drugged feed than did broilers with no lameness. Also, the walking ability of the lame birds was improved by this self-administered treatment (Danbury et al., 2000). This is a very clever way of asking broilers how much pain they are in—and the answer is very clear.

We are now beginning to understand the major states of suffering in farm animals. The causes of the subjective feelings of fear, frustration, pain, and discomfort are being elucidated and methods are being developed to "ask" the animals how aversive they find these states. The knowledge gained is gradually being put to use to alleviate this suffering. It is doubtful if similar progress could have been made without acknowledging the central role of feelings in animal welfare.

The emphasis to date in welfare research has been in investigating and alleviating states of suffering. However, there is a growing opinion that welfare should be more than just the absence of suffering (e.g., Mench, 1998). In human affairs, the presence of pleasure adds much to the quality of life. Why should animals be different? Surely, being able to state (and being able to back up the statement with some evidence) that a product came from contented cows or happy hens or peaceful pigs would be an extremely powerful selling point. I would argue that an understanding of pleasure is also important because we are unlikely ever to eliminate suffering completely. There will always be necessary interventions for the animals' own good that reduce welfare. It might be possible to counterbalance these unavoidable negative feelings by understanding and promoting positive feelings.

Although pleasure has been mentioned in passing by several welfare scientists, no one has investigated it in any systematic way. I suspect that it will require a new approach with different research methods from those used to measure suffering. In a recent experiment, Tina Widowski and I were investigating how hard hens would "work" (by pushing through a weighted door) to reach a dust bath when they had been deprived of the opportunity to dust bathe (Widowski and Duncan, 2000). Since hens cannot dust bathe in battery cages, we were attempting to measure what this welfare cost would be. We had assumed that deprivation would lead to a "need to dust bathe" and so to a state of suffering. Our results did not confirm this at all. They were not consistent with a "needs" model of motivation in which deprivation leads to suffering. They were more consistent with an "opportunity" model of motivation (see Fraser and Duncan, 1998) in which performance of the behavior, when the opportunity presents itself, leads to a state of pleasure.

CONCLUSIONS

An argument has been put forward that animal welfare is all to do with the subjective feelings that animals experience, with the negative feelings commonly called suffering, and with the positive feelings known as pleasure. The vertebrates and higher invertebrates have evolved feelings to protect their biological needs in a more flexible way than is possible with simple stimulus-response behavior. It is the fact that these animals are sentient that means they can experience a quality of life or, in other words, that they are capable of having welfare. So, in spite of the fact that feelings have evolved secondarily to animals' primary needs, and in spite of the fact that feelings cannot be investigated directly and are difficult to measure indirectly, nevertheless it is feelings that govern welfare, and in any research on welfare it is feelings that should be investigated. It is possible to gain information on feelings by studying animals' communication systems. Methods have also been developed to "ask" animals what they feel about aspects of the environments in which they are kept and procedures to which they are subjected. Good progress is being made in investigating the major states of suffering in our farm animals—the states of fear, frustration, pain, and discomfort—and methodologies are being improved and refined all the time. A watch needs to be kept for the possibility of other states of suffering, perhaps states not experienced by human beings and therefore difficult to recognize in animals. Also, the time is now ripe for a systematic investigation of pleasure in animals. I look forward to the day when it can be said not only that our farm animals do not suffer (or seldom suffer), but also that they are contented or happy.

REFERENCES

Appleby, M. C. and Lawrence, A. B., 1987. Food restriction as a cause of stereotypic behaviour in tethered gilts. *Animal Production*, 45: 103–110.

Bareham, J. R., 1972. Effects of cages and semi-intensive deep litter pens on the behaviour, adrenal response and production in two strains of laying hens. *British Veterinary Journal*, 128: 153–163.

Barnett, J. L. and Hemsworth, P. H., 1990. The validity of physiological and behavioural measures of animal welfare. *Applied Animal Behaviour Science*, 25: 177–187.

Barnett, J. L., Hemsworth, P. H., Cronin, G. M., Newman, E. A. and McCallum, T. H., 1991. Effects of design of individual cage-stalls on the behavioural and physiological responses related to the welfare of pregnant pigs. *Applied Animal Behaviour Science*, 32: 23–33.

Bentham, J., 1823. *An Introduction to the Principles of Morals and Legislation*. Oxford, Clarendon Press.

Broom, D. and Johnson, K., 1993. *Stress and Animal Welfare*. London, Chapman and Hall.

Broom, D. M., 1986. Indicators of poor welfare. *British Veterinary Journal*, 142: 524–526.

——. 1998. Welfare, stress and the evolution of feelings. *Advances in the Study of Behaviour*, 27: 371–403.

Bryant, M. J., 1972. The social environment: Behaviour and stress in housed livestock. *Veterinary Record*, 90: 351–359.

Bunge, M., 1980. *The Mind-Body Problem*. Oxford, Pergamon Press.

Bunge, M. and Ardilla, R., 1987. *Philosophy of Psychology*. New York, Springer-Verlag.

Colborn, D. R., Thompson, D. L., Roth, T. L., Capehart, J. S. and White, K. L., 1991. Responses of cortisol and prolactin to sexual excitement and stress in stallions and geldings. *Journal of Animal Science*, 69: 2556–2562.

Command Paper 2836, 1965. *Report of the Technical Committee to Enquire into the Welfare of Animals Kept under Intensive Livestock Husbandry Systems*. London, Her Majesty's Stationery Office.

Crooks, R. L. and Stein, J., 1988. *Psychology: Science Behavior and Life*. New York, Holt, Rinehart and Winston.

Curtis, S. E., 1987. Animal well-being and animal care. *Veterinary Clinics of North America: Food Animal Practice*, 3: 369–382.

Damasio, A., 1999. *The Feeling of What Happens: Body, Emotion and the Making of Consciousness*. London, Vintage Random House.

Danbury, T. C., Weeks, C. A., Chambers, J.P. Waterman-Pearson, A. E. and Kestin, S. C., 2000. Self-selection of the analgesic drug Carprofen by lame broiler chickens. *Veterinary Record*, 146: 307–311.

Dawkins, M. S., 1976. Towards an objective method of assessing welfare in domestic fowl. *Applied Animal Ethology*, 2: 245–254.

——. 1977. Do hens suffer in battery cages? Environmental preferences and welfare. *Animal Behaviour*, 25: 1034–1046.

——. 1978. Welfare and the structure of battery cages: size and cage floor preferences in domestic hens. *British Veterinary Journal*, 134: 469–475.

——. 1980. *Animal Suffering*. London, Chapman and Hall.

——. 1983. The current status of preference tests in the assessment of animal welfare. In: *Farm Animal Housing and Welfare* (Eds. Baxter, S. H., Baxter, M. R. and MacCormack, J. A. C.), pp. 20–26. The Hague, Martinus Nijhoff.

Dawkins, M. S. and Beardsley, T. M., 1986. Reinforcing properties of access to litter in hens. *Applied Animal Behaviour Science*, 15: 351–364.

Duncan, I. J. H., 1978. The interpretation of preference tests in animal behaviour. *Applied Animal Ethology*, 4: 197–200.

——. 1981. Animal rights—animal welfare: a scientist's assessment. *Poultry Science*, 60: 489–499.

——. 1992. Measuring preferences and the strength of preference. *Poultry Science*, 71: 658–663.

——. 1993. Welfare is to do with what animals feel. *Journal of Agricultural and Environmental Ethics*, 6: Suppl. 2, 8–14.

——. 1996. Animal welfare defined in terms of feelings. *Acta Agricolæ Scandinavica, Section A, Animal Science,* Supplementum 27: 29–35.

Duncan, I. J. H. and Dawkins, M. S., 1983. The problem of assessing "well-being" and "suffering" in farm animals. In: *Indicators Relevant to Farm Animal Welfare* (Ed. Smidt, D.), pp. 13–24. The Hague, Martinus Nijhoff.

Duncan, I. J. H. and Petherick, J. C., 1991. The implications of cognitive processes for animal welfare. *Journal of Animal Science*, 69: 5017–5022.

Duncan, I. J. H., Beatty, E. R., Hocking, P. M. and Duff, S. R. I., 1990. An assessment of pain associated with degenerative hip disorders in adult male turkeys. *Research in Veterinary Science*, 50: 200–203.

Duncan, I. J. H., Widowski, T. M. and Keeling, L. J., 1991. The effect of non-traditional lighting on the behaviour of domestic fowl. In: *Applied Animal Behaviour: Past, Present and Future* (Eds. Appleby, M. C., Horrell, R. I., Petherick, J. C. and Rutter, S. M.), pp. 69–70. Potters Bar, England, Universities Federation for Animal Welfare.

Fraser, A. F. and Broom, D. M., 1990. *Farm Animal Behaviour and Welfare* (3rd ed.). London, Baillière Tindall.

Fraser, D. and Duncan, I. J. H., 1998. "Pleasures", "pains" and animal welfare: toward a natural history of affect. *Animal Welfare*, 7: 383–396.

Fraser, D. and Matthews, L. R., 1997. Preference and motivational testing. In: *Animal Welfare* (Eds. Appleby, M. C. and Hughes, B. O.), pp. 159–173. Wallingford, Oxon, CAB International.

Freeman, B. F., 1978. Stress in caged layers. In: *First Danish Seminar on Poultry Welfare in Egglaying Cages* (Ed. Sørensen, L. Y.), pp. 55–65. Copenhagen, Danish National Committee for Poultry and Eggs.

Griffin, D. R., 1976. *The Question of Animal Awareness*. New York, The Rockefeller University Press.

Harrison, R., 1964. *Animal Machines*. London, Vincent Stuart.

Hughes, B. O., 1975. Spatial preference in the domestic hen. *British Veterinary Journal*, 131: 560–564.

——. 1977. Selection of group size by individual laying hens. *British Poultry Science*, 18: 9–18.

Hughes, B. O. and Black, A. J., 1973. The preference of domestic hens for different types of battery cage floor. *British Poultry Science*, 14: 615–619.

Hume, D., 1739 (new edition edited by L. A. Selby Bigge, 1888). *A Treatise of Human Nature*. Oxford, Clarendon Press.

Humphrey, N., 1986. *The Inner Eye*, London, Faber & Faber.

——. 1992. *A History of the Mind: Evolution and the Birth of Consciousness*. New York, Springer-Verlag.

Hurnik, J. F. and Lehman, H., 1988. Ethics and farm animal welfare. *Journal of Agricultural Ethics*, 1: 305–318.

James, W., 1904. Does "consciousness" exist? *Journal of Philosophy, Psychology and Scientific Method*, 1: 477–491.

Kenny, A., 1970. *Descartes' Philosophical Letters*. Oxford, Clarendon Press.

Lay, D. C., Friend, T. H., Bowers, C. L., Grissom, K. K. and Jenkins, O. C., 1992. A comparative physiological and behavioral study of freeze and hot-iron branding using dairy cows. *Journal of Animal Science*, 70: 1121–1125.

Lazarus, R. S. and Folkman, S., 1984. *Stress, Appraisal and Coping*. New York, Springer.

Mason, G. J., Cooper, J. and Clarebrough, C., 2001. Frustrations of fur-farmed mink. *Nature*, 410: 35–36.

McDougall, W., 1926. *An Introduction to Social Psychology* (rev. ed.). Boston, John W. Luce and Co.

Mench, J. A., 1998. Thirty years after Brambell: Whither animal welfare science? *Journal of Applied Animal Welfare Science*, 1: 91–102.

Mench, J. A. and Falcone, C., 2000. Welfare concerns in feed-restricted meat-type poultry parent stocks. *Proceedings of the 21st World's Poultry Congress*. Montreal. Paper S3.3.03.

Molony, V. and Kent, J. E., 1997. Assessment of acute pain in farm animals using behavioural and physiological measurements. *Journal of Animal Science*, 75: 266–272.

Mormède, P. 1990. Neuroendocrine responses to social stress. In: *Social Stress in Domestic Animals* (Eds. Zayen, R. and Dantzer, R.), pp. 203–211. Dordrecht, Kluwer.

Nicol, C. J. and Guildford, T., 1991. Exploratory activity as a measure of motivation in deprived hens. *Animal Behaviour*, 41: 333–341.

Radner, D. and Radner, M., 1989. *Animal Consciousness*. Buffalo, Prometheus Books.

Raj, M., 1998. Welfare during stunning and slaughter of poultry. *Poultry Science*, 77: 1815–1819.

Ristau, C. A. (Ed.), 1991. *Cognitive Ethology: The Minds of Other Animals*. Hillsdale, NJ, Lawrence Erlbaum Associates.

Romanes, G. J., 1884 (reprinted 1969). *Mental Evolution in Animals*. New York, AMS Press.

Ruse, M., 1984. Is there a limit to our knowledge of evolution? *BioScience*, 34: 100–104.

Rutter, S. M. and Duncan, I. J. H., 1991. Shuttle and one-way avoidance as measures of aversion in the domestic fowl. *Applied Animal Behaviour Science*, 30: 117–124.

——. 1992. Measuring aversion in domestic fowl using passive avoidance. *Applied Animal Behaviour Science*, 33: 53–61.

Seyfarth, R. M., Cheney, D. L. and Marler, P., 1980. Vervet monkey alarm calls: Evidence for predator classification and semantic communication. *Animal Behaviour*, 28: 1070–1094.

Skinner, B. F., 1975. The steep and thorny path to a science of behaviour. In: *Problems of Scientific Revolution* (Ed. Harre, R.). Oxford, Oxford University Press.

Spencer, H., 1855. *The Principles of Psychology*, London, Longmen, Brown, Green and Longmans.

Szechtman, H., Lambrou, P. J., Caggiula, A. R. and Redgate, E. S., 1974. Plasma corticosterone levels during sexual behaviour in male rats. *Hormones and Behaviour*, 5: 191–200.

Taylor, A. A. and Weary, D. M., 2000. Vocal responses of piglets to castration: identifying procedural sources of pain. *Applied Animal Behavioural Science*, 70: 17–26.

Terlouw, E. M. C., Lawrence, A. B., Ladewig, J., de Passillé, A. M. B., Rushen, J. and Schouten, W., 1991. A relationship between stereotypies and cortisol in sows. *Behavioural Processes*, 25: 133–153.

Warnier, A. and Zayan, R., 1985. Effects of confinement upon behavioural, hormonal responses and production indices in fattening pigs. In: *Social Space for Domestic Animals* (Ed. Zayan, R.), pp. 128–150. Dordrecht, Martinus Nijhoff.

Watson, J. B., 1928. *Behaviorism*. London, Routledge and Kegan Paul.

Weary, D. M., Braithwaite, L. A. and Fraser, D. , 1998. Vocal responses to pain in piglets. *Applied Animal Behaviour Science*, 56: 161–172.

Widowski, T. M. and Duncan, I. J. H., 2000. Working for a dustbath: are hens increasing pleasure rather than reducing suffering? *Applied Animal Behaviour Science*, 68: 39–53.

Wiepkema, P. R., 1987. Behavioural aspects of stress. In: *Biology of Stress in Farm Animals: An Integrative Approach* (Eds. Wiepkema, P. R. and Van Adrichem, P. W. M.), pp. 113–133. Dordrecht, Martinus Nijhoff.

Wood-Gush, D. G. M., Duncan, I. J. H. and Fraser, D., 1975. Social stress and welfare problems in agricultural animals. In: *The Behaviour of Domestic Animals* (3rd ed.) (Ed. Hafez, E. S. E.), pp. 182–200. Baltimore, Williams and Wilkins.

Young, P. T., 1959. The role of affective processes in learning and motivation. *Psychological Review*, 66: 104–125.

6

Meeting Physical Needs: Environmental Management for Well-Being

Ted H. Friend

The first step is to measure whatever can be easily measured.
This is okay as far as it goes.
The second step is to disregard that which can't be measured or give it an
arbitrary quantitative value.
This is artificial and misleading.
The third step is to presume that what can't be measured easily isn't very
important.
This is blindness.
The fourth step is to say what can't be measured really doesn't exist.
This is suicide.

—Daniel Yankelovich

Over the last century, agricultural engineers and animal scientists carefully researched physical characteristics of animal environments. As technology developed, more aspects of the physical environments were measured more precisely. Those measurements were then correlated to production or production-related factors of various species. The term *production* traditionally refers to economically important variables that are relatively simple to measure, such as weight gain, milk production, conception rates, and incidence of disease. It is also important to realize that farmers are not usually seeking to maximize production from each animal, but rather, to reach some optimum level that will yield the greatest return for the whole enterprise. A realistic compromise is made regarding the physical needs of animals if a farm is to survive in a free-market economy.

It has been relatively easy to measure tangible aspects of an animal's environment and relate changes in those variables back to changes in economically important traits. The typical scenario assumes that farm animals respond very mechanistically to physical attributes of their environments because the intangibles of how animals perceive various aspects of their physical environments are much more difficult to measure. Also, as more and more farm animals are maintained in closer confinement, the psychological aspects of their environments become more important.

There are also several problem behaviors that are often attributed to "discomfort" that can occur in farm animals. Tail biting in swine, bulling in feedlot cattle, and stereotypic and aggressive behavior have often been linked to general discomfort relating to aspects of the physical environment (floor space, temperature, ammonia concentrations, feed bunk space). Certain health-related issues are also directly related to problems with the physical environment (e.g., hoof abscesses due to rough or wet flooring, lameness due to long-term housing on concrete, respiratory disease due to poor air quality).

The purpose of this chapter is to briefly review what we know about the physical requirements of farm animals and to stress that simple physical measurements only begin to scratch the surface in regard to determining the actual well-being of animals under the control of people.

SPACE

Recommendations for floor space for farm animals are readily available (e.g., Midwest Plan Service's Equipment Handbooks for various species of livestock [https://www.mwpshq.org/catalog.html] or state extension specialists). Most recommendations are based on the number of animals per unit floor space; however, the type of flooring, the size of the group of animals, the shape of the enclosure, the activity level of the animals, and the type of feeding system can greatly influence the amount of floor space animals require. Although most research has been oriented toward floor space requirements, there are several distinct types of space. Recommendations regarding space requirements should be broken down into categories such as social, resting, feeding, and vertical space. Lack of adequate vertical space in multideck trailers that are used to transport horses, for example, is resulting in a phaseout of these trailers for the transport of horses in the United States. Researchers have generally tackled the challenge of assessing space requirements either by placing animals in treatments consisting of different stocking densities and then examining the effects, or by measuring the size or dimensions of animals and making inferences from those measurements. M. R. Baxter (1992) published a good review of both methodologies.

Although decreased space results in increased aggression, leg problems, mastitis, bloat, and parturition-related problems (FASS, 1999), most livestock need housing during extreme weather conditions, necessitating close confinement. Keeping cows out of the mud increases their productivity and reduces endoparasitic and foot problems (FASS, 1999). Confinement housing of farm animals is also necessary to simplify the management of the large number of animals that is now needed to achieve economies of scale. There are strong economic pressures to give confined farm animals as little space as possible. However, those pressures are offset by the economic costs of poor performance and health of the animals.

To understand the complexities of space, understanding a few basic terms and principles is useful. *Density* is a simple physical measurement usually expressed as amount of floor space per animal. *Personal space* is a portable territory that an animal wears or transports as it travels. An animal will defend its portable territory from other members of its species. It will fight to keep unwelcome visitors out of that territory. Such territories are usually much larger in front of an animal than at its side or back. An example of personal space in people is the way people line up facing the door in a full elevator. Although a stranger may be within one foot of you, this is not a problem unless the person standing directly in front of you turns around. Although that person is not any closer to you, he is now violating your personal space, so you consider pushing the emergency stop button and yell for help. Although density within the elevator did not change, one person simply turning around made the elevator ride uncomfortable and stressful. Personal space in people varies with cultural background (e.g., the French are considered to have much smaller personal spaces than Americans), social relationships (boy and girl friend in private), or mood. Similarly, personal space in livestock will vary with species, breed, reproductive status, social relationships, and other factors.

Crowding is another very important consideration when studying space requirements. Crowding can occur at different densities. It is a function of density, but also includes psychological factors such as social status, communication, activity, and reproductive status. The effects of long-term crowding have been known for many years and were conceptually summarized by Christian (1961). As crowding increased in a population, maternal care, reproductive rates, fecundity, survival of the young and elderly, and maternal care decreased, while disease rates and mortality increased. Christian's observations arose from experiments with freely growing populations of house mice. They started off with several male and female mice in the room. As the mice matured and started reproducing, the population skyrocketed with most of the young that were born surviving into adulthood. Although the mice were given unlimited food and water, they did not end up knee deep in the room. The growth of the population leveled off as the mice became crowded and very few newborn mice survived to join the breeding population. At first, people in the 1970s hypothesized that that would also be the not-too-distant fate of humans as we continue to reproduce. However, it was soon discovered that one could easily get a crowded population of mice to start increasing in numbers again without increasing the size of room (i.e., the earth) or decreasing the density of mice (i.e., removing people from earth). By merely placing a number of empty flower pots or similar objects within the room, the population growth rate increased again. Reducing communication and social stress by providing small apartments was all that was needed to reduce crowding.

A very important limitation of simple density recommendations is that they usually fail to consider the size of the group of animals. As the number of animals housed at a particular density increases, the total size of the enclosure increases, giving the animals much more maneuvering room. For example, when water-deprived horses that were being transported were offered water when they were in small groups of 4 or 6 horses, 1 or more of the horses were consistently blocked from drinking by more aggressive horses (Gibbs and Friend, 2000). When the group size was increased to 12 horses and the size of the compartment doubled in size, all of the horses readily drank, although the number of water troughs and floor area remained constant per horse. The increased maneuvering room allowed the more timid horses to avoid the aggressive horses and get to an open water trough. Increasing group size beyond certain limits, however, can have disastrous effects. If you have more than five to six gestating gilts in a group and extremely cold conditions occur, the gilts are likely to lie in one large pile to keep warm, which could result in those on the bottom being suffocated by the weight of the gilts on the top. Pigs will not pile up during hot conditions; however, if the size of a group gets too large, major problems can arise during hot weather. It is possible that some members of very large groups can be crushed by their colleagues if something causes them to all go in the same direction at the same time. On rare occasions, too many cattle may be placed in an alley at a feedlot. If all of the cattle move away from something that is frightening, one or more animals at the far end of the group may be crushed by the combined force of the group. A similar problem may occur during transport if groups are too large and the driver has to stop very suddenly, throwing all the animals in a group in one direction.

Recent studies on the transport of cattle and horses have provided very useful insights in regard to problems with transporting animals at very high densities. There is a common belief among truckers who transport large groups of cattle and horses that the animals should be loaded as densely as possible for the animals' own good. The thinking is that if animals are loaded tightly enough, they will help hold each other up. The driver in the cab of a tractor that is hauling a semi load of cattle or horses can easily hear and feel the animals shifting and impacting the sides and deck of the trailer. The hard hooves of horses and cattle make it easy to tell when they are taking heavy steps to maintain their balance. There is noticeably less noise coming from the trailer when cattle or horses are tightly loaded. However, recent studies with cattle (Eldridge and Winfield, 1988; Tarrant, Kenny, and Harrington, 1988, 1992; Tarrant and Grandin, 1993) and horses (Collins et al., 2000) have found that the old anecdote is not true and that moderate density is preferable. At moderate density, horses have more opportunity to move a hoof or change their posture to compensate for changes in speed. Moving their hooves greater distances and more frequently results in the driver's hearing more impacts. When at high density, horses (Collins et al., 2000) and cattle (Tarrant and Grandin, 1993) are inhibited from shifting within trailers, and there is a corresponding increase in struggles and falls, which the driver cannot usually hear. Horses at high density constantly repositioned their feet in small increments in an attempt to maintain their balance and frequently stepped on the hooves and pasterns of other horses. The ability of horses to stand up after a fall was also hampered, causing a greater number and severity of injuries (Collins et al., 2000). When animals at high density go down due to fatigue or other causes, they are often trapped on the floor by the remaining animals "closing over" and occupying the available standing space. Although cattle and horses will attempt to avoid stepping on a colleague that goes down, a downed animal at high density will generally be trampled to death unless people promptly come to the animal's aid. Detailed observations of cattle (Friend et al., 1981) and horses (Collins, et al., 2000) during transport found that cattle and horses avoid contacting surfaces during transport and prefer to maintain their balance independent of other horses (Friend, 2001). This is further evidence that the anecdote about loading livestock as densely as possible so they hold each other up is not true.

AIR QUALITY

Providing the correct amount of ventilation is extremely important in maintaining an optimal environment for livestock in intensive animal husbandry. In confinement buildings, ventilation is needed for moisture, odor, and heat control. There is an important relationship between ventilation rate needed to control moisture, odor, and heat, and the temperature of the environment. Normally, even during the coldest weather, some ventilation is required in livestock barns to remove moisture generated by the animals themselves and from wet surfaces. It is not uncommon for moisture condensing on noninsulated ceilings to cause "rain" within a building that is not adequately ventilated. Ventilation is also needed to remove odors and gases. During cold weather, the ventilation rate needed to keep humidity between 50 and 65 percent can be too great for the heat released from the animals to maintain the temperature within the building at acceptable levels. Supplemental heat is then needed under those conditions. As the outside temperature increases, the need for supplemental heat decreases until a point is reached where ventilation rates need to be increased to prevent heat from building up within the building.

In addition to regulation of temperature and humidity, ventilation dilutes and helps disperse air pollutants within livestock housing. Air pollutants may include small physical particles or dust, small liquid particles or droplets, gases or vapors, and positive and negative ions. Proper ventilation of livestock facilities is also an important human health issue. A survey conducted in the early 1980s found that over 60 percent of the 2,459 Iowa livestock confinement workers that responded had some type of cough, sore throat, runny nose, eye irritation, headache, tightness of chest, or muscle aches and pains (Donham and Gustafson, 1982).

Physical Particles

Most dust particles range in size from 1.0 μm to over 0.1 mm in diameter. Larger particles require greater convection currents to keep them airborne. Particles less than 10 μm in size can remain airborne for hours. Dust may carry microorganisms that may make the particles hazardous to livestock and workers.

Dust particles may originate from feed, dried manure, soil, bedding, animal dander, hair, or feathers. In egg layer houses, dust originates largely from feed, but bedding and feces can be a major source in broiler houses. On dairy farms and feedlots, the major source is dried manure and soil. During dry, windy conditions, the dust from feedlots can be seen for many miles. Dust levels are much higher during periods when animals are active.

Feedlots are increasingly under pressure to control dust from lots and associated roads, especially from people in neighboring communities. As feedlots are established in drier regions, dust will become an ever-increasing problem. Feedlots attempt to control dust by removing excess manure from their lots, spraying their lots with water, and increasing stocking density. Moisture content of the pad is one of the keys to dust control. Increasing the density of cattle in a pen will cause the contribution to moisture through urine and feces to exceed evaporation rate. Such high density, however, creates a problem with mud and reduced performance during periods of rain. The roads in feedlots can be watered, oiled, or otherwise treated with chemicals to reduce dust.

Liquid Particles

Liquid droplets, or aerosols, are a very common method of transmission of disease from one animal to another. Coughs and sneezes are a frequent source of germ-laden aerosols.

When larger droplets evaporate, they become very small droplets that can remain airborne for several hours. The smaller droplets, less than 10 μm in diameter, can be transported deeper into the respiratory tract than larger droplets. The farther they are transported into the respiratory tract, the greater the health risk. Ultraviolet light in sunlight is effective in killing bacteria and viruses that are transported by droplets or dust.

Gases

Odorous air pollutants are often associated with livestock, livestock maintained in confinement buildings, and manure disposal systems. As urban sprawl encroaches on traditional farming communities and areas, undesirable odors are becoming an increasingly important issue of concern for farmers. Also, some gases generated by farming enterprises can reduce performance of livestock, increase morbidity, and even be toxic to livestock and people in high concentrations. Gases released by decomposition of livestock feces and urine may include ammonia, hydrogen sulfide, carbon dioxide, methane, and hydrogen sulfide. In addition, carbon monoxide is a potentially dangerous gas that may be released from incomplete combustion of fuels when buildings are being heated. Different gases are associated with different housing systems (table 6.1).

Ammonia

Ammonia is the most common air pollutant found in animal housing where feces and urine accumulate and decompose. Anaerobic decomposition of waste products is the primary source. Ammonia is an eye and respiratory tract irritant, and at higher concentrations, it may have metabolic effects and cause poisoning. Humans can detect ammonia at 10 ppm. Weight gain was reduced by 12 percent at 50 ppm and by 30 percent at 100 or 150 ppm in growing pigs (Drummond et al., 1980). Ammonia is much more of a potential risk in housing systems that have deep manure pits under the animals, or in housing that has manure packs. High levels of ammonia have been related to outbreaks of tail biting in pigs.

Hydrogen Sulfide

Poisoning from hydrogen sulfide is probably responsible for more livestock deaths in confinement housing than any other gas. It is formed during anaerobic decomposition of live-

Table 6.1.   Gases Found in Confinement Housing Systems

Gas	Poultry	Swine	Veal	Sheep	Cattle
Ammonia	Yes	Yes	Yes	Yes	Yes
Carbon monoxide	Yes	Yes	Yes	Yes	Yes
Carbon dioxide	Yes	Yes	Yes	Yes	Yes
Hydrogen sulfide	Found only in buildings with liquid manure systems				
Methane	Found only in buildings with liquid manure systems				

Source: Mutel et al. (1986).

stock waste and is heavier than air. Agitating the slurry prior to pumping manure storage pits can result in the rapid release of hydrogen sulfide gas.

In lower concentrations (approximately 10 ppm), hydrogen sulfide irritates eyes and the respiratory tract. At higher concentrations, respiratory tract lesions are common. Death can occur after acute exposure to concentrations of 400 ppm or more.

Carbon Monoxide

Carbon monoxide is an odorless and tasteless gas that originates from incomplete combustion of fuels. It is not usually a problem in unheated buildings, but care must be taken in heated buildings to make sure that the heater is properly vented. Carbon monoxide is also a potential problem when animals are transported in enclosed trailers and trucks during winter months. Care should be taken to ensure that the exhaust from engines is properly vented and cannot be drawn into the trailer.

Methane

Tasteless, odorless, and colorless, methane gas is not often considered a problem affecting the welfare of livestock because other gases usually reach noxious concentrations prior to methane. Methane is lighter than air at room temperatures so it can accumulate only in relatively airtight structures. It is nontoxic when inhaled, but it can cause suffocation by reducing the amount of available oxygen in the air. Methane is flammable and can be explosive in concentrations of 5 to 15 percent in air. Such concentrations have been known to accumulate under the roofs of some buildings. Although methane is produced during the anaerobic breakdown of waste, ruminant livestock produce and release considerably more methane during normal digestion.

Methane production from livestock has received considerable attention recently because methane is a potent greenhouse gas that can contribute to global climate change (EPA, 2002). Human activity accounts for 70 percent of global methane emissions, of which it is estimated that domestic livestock account for 21 percent and decomposition of manure, 5.6 percent (EPA, 2002). Manure deposited on fields and pastures, or otherwise handled in a dry form, produces insignificant amounts of methane. Given the trend toward larger and more intensive farms, however, liquid manure systems are increasing in number. The U.S. Environmental Protection Agency encourages adoption of on-farm biogas recovery techniques (EPA, 2002). The EPA and USDA also have a joint program that can help livestock managers increase their overall efficiency and reduce their methane emissions (accessible through EPA's web page).

LIGHT

Most of the interest in light (visible electromagnetic radiation) in regard to farm animals has traditionally been on the effect that photoperiod has on reproduction (e.g., Curtis, 1983). Reproductive efficiency has traditionally been considered one of the major limiting factors in livestock production, so animal, dairy, and poultry science departments have emphasized research on reproduction. Breeding is stimulated by decreasing day length in sheep and goats, while increasing day length stimulates reproductive activity in horses and poultry. Photoperiod also influences many other functions in livestock and poultry, as reviewed by C. J. C. Phillips (1992). For example, most dairy farms are now giving their milking cows 16 to 18 hours of light during the fall, winter, and spring months to stimulate milk production. The roughly 10 percent increase in milk production is thought to be due more to stimulating increased feed intake than through stimulation of the pineal gland. In general, it appears that when farm animals are given increased periods of supplemental light, increases in milk production or growth are observed, probably related to stimulating increased feeding bouts and activity. Some other factors that are influenced by photoperiod are hair coat, milk composition, growth rates, partitioning of fat and protein, general activity, and onset of puberty. As a general rule, the farther from the equator, the greater the seasonal variation in photoperiod and, hence, the greater the effect that photoperiod has on farm animals (e.g., heavier hair coat, more distinct breeding season).

The retinas of all species of farm animals (with the exception of poultry) contain both rods and cones. Rods are sensitive to lower levels of light while cones respond during higher levels of light. Thus, at lower levels of light, rods are activated. As light intensity increases, most rods have been activated, so their usefulness in discriminating between contrasts in light greatly diminishes. The less-sensitive cones then come into play, allowing high acuity under very bright conditions. Animals possessing only rods, for example many owls, will function best under lower light levels and prefer nocturnal activity. Those with purely cone retinas, such as chickens, will function best under higher light levels and will be very diurnal in activity (Piggins, 1992). The ratio of rods to cones in farm animals appears to make them more adapted to low-intensity vision and less to visual acuity than humans (Phillips, 1992). For example, in cattle the ratio of rods to cones is 15:1, compared with 20:1 in humans, giving cattle optimum *visual acuity* (Phillips's emphasis) at a light intensity as low as 120 lux (Dannenmann, Buchenauer, and Fliegner, 1985). Light intensity of 120 lux is roughly equivalent to a relatively dark, cloudy day.

The old and persistent notion that farm animals do not possess color vision was largely promulgated by a lack of data and the desire of scientists to err on the conservative side. For example, Wright (1975) commented that it would be scientifically foolhardy to infer that even if a species has a full complement of the three types of cones used by humans for perception of color, that the species perceives as colorful a world as do humans. David Piggins (1992) also concluded that the jury was still out and that it was unlikely that sheep possessed color vision. The issue, however, has evolved rapidly over recent years. Studies using operant conditioning techniques that involved training animals to choose specific colors found that at least some cattle (Arave et al., 1993; Dabrowska et al., 1981; Gilbert and Arave, 1986; Roil et al., 1989; and Soffie, Thines, and Flater, 1980), sheep (Munkenbeck, 1982), and horses (Smith and Goldman, 1999) showed no deficits in their ability to discriminate colors. Recent physiological studies (Jacobs, Deegan, and Neitz, 1998), however, found that the cones in the retinas of cattle, sheep, goats, pigs, and deer show peak sensitivity to light in the wavelength ranges of 444–455 nm and 552–555 nm, which is similar to the blue and green sensitive cones in humans. However, all the animals tested lacked cones that respond to light in the 580 nm range, indicating that they do not have cones similar to those of humans that react to red light. Farm animals appear to have dichromatic, rather than trichromatic, color vision. If this is true, and the evidence is convincing, it does not mean that yellows, oranges, and reds are invisible to livestock, but that those colors appear as different shades of other colors. The color perception of ungulates is probably similar to a person who is red color-blind.

Ungulates and many other species of animals possess a tapetum, a reflective surface behind the retina that reflects light back through the retina. A tapetum is believed to increase the amount of light available to stimulate the photopigments in the rods and cones. This reflective surface is the basis of "eye shine," the bright reflection that can be seen from the eyes of many animals when a flashlight is shone on the animal at night, when its pupil is dilated. Eye shine is not seen in poultry or humans because they lack a tapetum. Animals with a tapetum can be considered to have superior visual acuity and sensitivity in low-light conditions. The lack of a functional tapetum in humans is the cause of "red eye," seen only in flash photographs. Under dark conditions resulting in the need to use a flash to take a photograph, the subject's pupil is fully dilated, resulting in the camera catching a glimpse of the red blood vessels and tissue of the retina.

Operant conditioning studies in which animals were given control over lighting have shown that livestock and poultry prefer to have light for a major portion of each day. When livestock were trained to turn lights on and off, pigs kept the lights on 72 percent (Baldwin and Meese, 1977), sheep 82 percent (Baldwin and Start, 1981), calves 67 percent (Baldwin and Start, 1981) and poultry 80 percent of each day (Savoy and Duncan, 1982). Livestock will work for a light reward when housed in total darkness, but they have not yet been shown to be motivated to work for darkness when under conditions of continuous light that is of moderate intensity. Illumination was also found to be a reward for horses (Houpt and Houpt, 1988) maintained in darkened stalls. Evidence suggests that a lighted environment is important to livestock for at least a major portion of each day and that they do not find continuous lighting of moderate intensity to be adverse.

SOUND

Hearing sensitivity of livestock species has been well researched. Audiograms, hearing thresholds for pure tones of different frequencies, have been determined for sheep (Wollack, 1963), horses and cattle (Heffner and Heffner, 1983), and domestic pigs and goats (Heffner and Heffner, 1990). Overall, the hearing sensitivity of livestock is similar to that of humans, with the most significant difference being the ability of these animals to hear frequencies above the human upper limit of hearing (i.e., ultrasonic sounds) (Heffner and Heffner, 1992). The upper frequency limit of hearing for humans is approximately 16,000 hertz, whereas livestock are in the range of 32,000 hertz. Hence, sound that is annoying or painful to humans is probably affecting livestock similarly. Special consideration also should be given to higher frequency sound that is out of the hearing range of humans.

People have attempted to use sound to move livestock through facilities. Although sound (especially recorded human vocalizations) could be used, it had to be used at levels that were annoying to people and influenced other livestock in the facility (ARS 1966).

Cattle moved away from both steady tones and sirenlike sounds between 110 and 120 dB. However, their strongest adverse reaction was to recordings of the human voice at 110 and 120 dB (ARS, 1966). The cattle had been worked by people, suggesting that the content of the noise, and not just the intensity or frequency, is very important. Sound was less effective in eliciting responses in sheep and swine. Although the swine were aware of the sounds, they appeared to display a freezing response and did not move away. A freezing response makes interpretation of when sound is uncomfortable to livestock difficult.

The U.S. Department of Labor's Occupational Safety and Health Administration provides guidelines for humans that can also be used to make useful inferences for livestock. Both duration of exposure and the level of the sound are important factors in assessing the adverse effects of noise. According to OSHA (2002) regulations, humans should not be exposed to an average of more than 90 dB over 8 hours, 100 dB over 2 hours, or 110 dB over 30 minutes without hearing protection. The chance of livestock being exposed to continuous noise in excess of 85 dB (table 6.2) is rare. For example, 12 different livestock ventilation units ranged from 64 to 77 dB at 1 m from each unit (Guul-Simonsen and Madsen, 2000). Short-term exposure above 85 dB can occur, for example, when pigs start vocalizing in anticipation of feeding before their regular feeding time, or when certain types of machinery are used. Most loud noise in livestock facilities is most likely to be short-term exposure.

Livestock do show an amazing ability to habituate to what many people would consider to be uncomfortable levels of noise. For example, horses may be tied out to graze next to highways where the noise made by each passing automobile or truck would make people cringe, but the horses appear oblivious to the traffic. Cattle may habituate to loud, fast-moving freight trains to the extent that when they are grazing within 40 m of the tracks, they will not even look up at passing trains.

There has been considerable interest in the effects of playing music to livestock, especially dairy cattle. Dairy cattle have been the most commonly tested animals because of the ease of measuring the effects of various types of music and noise on their milk production. Experimental results suggest that music in the environment of cows can contribute to consistency in the environment and can become part of a cluster of stimuli that conditions the milk-ejection reflex (Albright and Arave, 1997). In one study, classical music appeared to have a significant effect on increasing milk yield compared to hard rock, country and western, and noise (Evans and Albright, 1989). In a follow-up study, however, the type

Table 6.2.   Noise Levels and Possible Effects on Humans

Decibels	Example	Effects in humans
85–90	Loud shout, train, subway	No pain, but may incur hearing loss over time
90–100	Jackhammer, lawn mower	Noise may be uncomfortable
100–130	Rock concert, riveter	Discomfort threshold is 120 dB, occasional ringing in ears post exposure
140+	Rifle or shotgun, jet aircraft	Pain threshold, single exposure can cause hearing loss

of music played did not matter in milk production, but any music was better than silence in making the cows less jumpy and restless (Evans, 1990). There is a confounding problem with those studies because of the effect that the music may have on the people working with the cattle. For example, Whittlestone (1960) found that the type of music had no influence on the cows but thought that the effect the music had on the milkers was very important. Placing headphones on the milkers so that different music could be played to the cows and the people working the cows would appear to correct for the confounding, but the headphones could make the humans irritable. Although the data are problematic, "easy listening" music is thought to be beneficial, if not directly by providing a consistency to the environment, then by improving the attitudes of the people working with livestock.

TEMPERATURE

Maintaining homeothermy (consistency of temperature) is one of the basic needs of all mammals. There is a very narrow range within which the physiological systems of homeotherms can operate, and there are a number of behavioral and physiological systems that enable animals to maintain homeothermy. As soon as the ambient temperature deviates from an animal's comfort (or thermoneutral) zone, the animal's initial response is behavioral. If it is too hot, an animal seeks shade to reduce radiant heating, or seeks increased airflow on the brow of a hill to increase convective cooling. If an animal is too cool, it may move into the sun, position itself perpendicular to the sun to maximize radiant heating, or position itself within a group of cohorts to conserve body heat. The behavior of livestock can be very useful in determining how they perceive a particular temperature.

When ambient temperature continues to decline and behavior is not successful in maintaining homeothermy, an animal's lower critical temperature may be reached. At temperatures below the lower critical temperature, an animal must increase its heat production in order to maintain homeothermy. Its metabolic rate will increase while it also attempts to increase its heat production by such activities as shivering and seeking shelter. If the ambient temperature continues to go down and an animal has exhausted all behavioral and physiological efforts to maintain a consistent body temperature, core body temperature will drop. A cyclic condition may then exist in which the decreasing body temperature will cause a decrease in the amount of heat an animal can produce physiologically, rather like placing something in a refrigerator will slow metabolic processes, retarding spoilage. If the animal's heat loss is not reduced or external heat put into the system (the animal is warmed up by a space heater, for example), death from hypothermia is likely.

A similar reaction will occur in animals subjected to high ambient temperatures, where behavior is no longer effective in reducing heat load. When the animal's upper critical temperature is exceeded, physiological adjustments (reduced feed intake, reduced milk production) are made to reduce heat production. Digestion of feed and lactation, for example, generate considerable body heat that a dairy cow must dissipate. If the behavioral and physiological adjustments are not adequate and the animal can no longer maintain a steady body temperature, increasing body temperature will actually stimulate the body to accelerate physiological processes that increase heat load, resulting in increasing hyperthermia and eventually death.

Historically, recommendations regarding the comfort zones of livestock were based on observations of when egg or milk production, or growth rates, were significantly reduced by extremes in temperature. Changes in milk production and growth rates do not occur until after the lower or upper critical temperature is exceeded. Thus, comfort zones were not actually the range of temperature within which an animal was "comfortable," but rather the temperature range within which production was not impaired.

Operant conditioning has been a very useful tool in refining thermal preferences for livestock. Baldwin and Ingram (1967) were among the first to use this technique. Additional studies followed, such as the series of studies conducted by Morrison et al. (1987; Morrison, Laforest, and McMillan, 1989) on pigs and chickens, that greatly increased our knowledge base. For example, pigs on bedded concrete did not push a button to receive supplemental heat as often as pigs that were on bare concrete or on raised rubber-coated metal flooring (Morrison et al., 1987) suggesting that animals with bedding prefer to have cooler quarters. Also, pigs wanted 32 percent to 40 percent less heat at night compared to day time, and smaller groups of pigs worked for more heat than pigs in groups of eight (Morrison et al., 1989).

Most introductory textbooks on the husbandry of a particular species contain recommended temperature ranges for different age classes of livestock. There are also excellent reviews on the subject (e.g., Curtis, 1983; Phillips and Piggins, 1992). When applying general guidelines, however, it is important to realize that there are many factors that can influence an animal's thermal comfort that guidelines do not take into consideration. For example, an animal that is kept on a concrete floor will need a warmer environment to counter the body heat it will lose to the concrete during cold weather, compared to an animal housed on dirt or with bedding. Concrete, however, is useful in helping animals dissipate heat during hot weather. Similarly, animals that are in a group have an advantage over individually housed animals during cold weather. During hot weather, they will space themselves out to aid in dissipating heat. Because of the wide range of facilities and conditions in which livestock may be kept, it is important that livestock managers carefully observe their animals for signs of thermal discomfort and take corrective measures. Good stockmen can tell when their livestock are uncomfortable by studying their behavior, and they will take corrective action before production is adversely impacted.

Intangible Aspects

People with good intentions may often build what engineers would consider to be ideal environments based on what is known about air quality, space, temperature, and light, only to find that something very important is lacking. For example, when the consulting veterinarian of a large and well-funded horse-breeding farm in Texas built a state-of-the-art hospital barn that had three large stalls, padded floors, a laboratory, air-conditioning during the summers, and heating during the winters, the manager of the farm found that whenever he placed an ill or injured horse in the hospital barn, the horse's condition usually worsened.

When physiological (Mal et al., 1991a) and behavioral (Mal et al., 1991b) studies were conducted, it was concluded that the isolation of the hospital barn was stressful to the horse and caused suppression of the horse's immune system. Solitary confinement is considered a severe form of punishment in most human penal systems. Similarly, although narrow calf stalls and even elevated, slatted-floor individual pens technically meet the basic physical environmental requirements of young calves, research has shown that suppression of the calves' drive to exercise (Dellmeier, Friend, and Gbur, 1985) resulted in a suppressed immune system and increased morbidity (Friend, Dellmeier, and Gbur, 1985). Although we may design what appears to be an adequate physical environment, ignoring the difficult-to-measure psychological aspects of an animal's environment is blindness, and may be fatal for the animal.

REFERENCES

Albright, J. L. and C. W. Arave. 1997. The Behaviour of Cattle. CAB International, Wallingford, Oxon, UK.

Arave, C. W., P. H. Stewart, A. L. T. Hansen and J. L. Walters. 1993. Primary color discrimination by Holstein heifers. Proc. W. Sect. Am. Soc. Anim. Sci. 44: 113.

ARS. 1966. Feasibility Tests of Selected Stimuli and Devices to Drive Livestock. Report; USDA, ARS Washington, DC: 52–11.

Baldwin, B. A. and D. L. Ingram. 1967. Behavioral thermoregulation in pigs. Physiology and Behavior. 2: 15.

Baldwin, B. A. and G. B. Meese. 1977. Sensory reinforcement and illumination preference in sheep and calves. Proc. R. Soc. London. Ser. B 211: 513.

Baldwin, B. A. and I. G. Start. 1981. Sensory reinforcement and illumination preferences in sheep and calves. Prod. R. Soc. London. Ser. B 211: 513.

Baxter, M. R. 1992. The space requirements of housed livestock. Pages 67–81. In: Farm Animals and the Environment, C. Phillips and D. Piggins ed., CAB Int., Wallingford, Oxon, UK.

Christian, J. J. 1961. Phenomena associated with population density. Proc. Nat. Acad. Sci. 47: 428–449.

Collins, M. N., T. H. Friend, F. D. Jousan, and S. C. Chen. 2000. Effects of density on displacement, falls, injuries, and orientation during horse transportation. Appl. Anim. Behav. Sci. 67: 169–179.

Curtis, S. E. 1983. Environmental Management in Animal Agriculture. Iowa State University Press, Ames.

Dabrowska, B., W. Harmata, Z. Lenkiewicz, Z. Schiffer and R. J. Wojtusiak. 1981. Colour perception in cows. Behav. Proc. 6: 1.

Dannenmann, K., D. Buchenauer and H. Fliegner. 1985. The behaviour of calves under four levels of lighting. Appl. Anim. Behav. Sci. 13: 243–258.

Dellmeier, G. R., T. H. Friend and E. E. Gbur. 1985. Comparison of four methods of calf confinement. II. Behavior. J. Anim. Sci. 60: 1102–1109.

Donham, K. J. and K. E. Gustafson. 1982. Human occupational hazards from swine confinement. Ann. Am. Conf. Governmental Ind. Hyg. 2: 137–142.

Drummond, J. G., S. E. Curtis, J. Simon and H. W. Norton. 1980. Effects of aerial ammonia on growth and health of young pigs. J. Anim. Sci. 50: 1085–1091.

Eldridge, G. A. and C. G. Winfield. 1988. The behavior and bruising of cattle during transport at different space allowances. Aust. J. Exp. Ag. 28, 695–698.

EPA. 2002. U.S. Environmental Protection Agency home page. Available at: http://www.epa.gov/ rlep/sustain.htm. Accessed Nov. 22, 2002.

Evans, A. 1990. Moosic is for cows, too. Hoard's Dairyman 135: 721.

Evans, A. and J. L. Albright. 1989. The effects of music and noise upon behavior and milk production in dairy cows. Indiana Academy of Science, Indiana State Library, Indianapolis, Indiana. 105th Annual Meeting of the Indiana Academy of Science, Indiana University Southeast, New Albany, IN: p. 88.

FASS. 1999. Guide for the Care and Use of Agricultural Animals in Agricultural Research and Teaching. FASS, Savoy, IL.

Friend, T. H. 2001. A review of the recent research on the transportation of horses. J. Anim. Sci. 79(Electronic Supplement): E32–E40.

Friend, T. H., G. R. Dellmeier and E. E. Gbur. 1985. Comparison of four methods of calf confinement. I. Physiology. J. Anim. Sci. 60: 1095 1101.

Friend, T. H., M. R. Irwin, A. J. Sharp, B. H. Ashby, G. B. Thompson and W. A. Bailey. 1981. Behavior and weight loss of feeder calves in a railcar modified for feeding and watering in transit. Int. J. Stud. Anim. Prob. 2: 129–137.

Gibbs, A. E. and T. H. Friend. 2000. Effect of animal density and trough placement on drinking behavior and dehydration in slaughter horses. J. Equine Vet. Sci. 20: 643–650.

Gilbert, B. J., Jr. and C. W. Arave. 1986. Ability of cattle to distinguish among different wavelengths of light. J. Dairy Sci., 69: 825.

Guul-Simonsen, F. and P. Madsen. 2000. Laboratory measurements of noise from livestock ventilation units. Appl. Eng. Agric. 16: 61–65.

Heffner, R. S. and H. E. Heffner. 1983. Hearing in large mammals: Horses (*Equus caballus*) and cattle (*Bos taurus*). Behav. Neuroscience, 97: 299–309.

——. 1990. Hearing in domestic pigs (*Sus scrofa*) and goats (*Capra bircus*). Hearing Research 48: 231–240.

——. 1992. Auditory perception. Pages 159–184. In: Farm Animals and the Environment, C. Phillips and D. Piggins ed., CAB Int., Wallingford, Oxon, UK.

Houpt, K. A. and T. R. Houpt. 1988. Social and illumination preferences of mares. J. Anim. Sci. 66: 2159.

Jacobs, H. J., J. F. Deegan and J. Neitz. 1998. Photopigment basis for dichromatic color vision in cows, goats, and sheep. Visual Neuroscience 15: 581–584.

Mal, M. E., T. H. Friend, D. C. Lay, S. G. Vogelsang and O. C. Jenkins. 1991a. Physiological responses of mares to short term confinement and social isolation. Equine Vet. Sci. 11: 96–102.

——. 1991b. Behavioral responses of mares to short-term confinement and social isolation. Appl. Anim. Behav. Sci. 31: 13–24.

Morrison, W. D., K. L. Laforest, and I. McMillan. 1989. Effect of group size on operant heat demand of piglets. Canadian Journal of Animal Science 69: 23

Morrison, W. D., L. A. Bate, I. McMillan, and E. Amyot. 1987. Operant heat demand of piglets housed on four different floors. Canadian Journal of Animal Science 67: 337.

Munkenbeck , N. W. 1982. Color vision in sheep. J. Anim. Sci. 55(Suppl.1): 129.

Mutel, C. F., K. J. Donham, J. A. Merchant, C. P. Redshaw, and S. D. Starr. 1986. Livestock Confinement Dusts and Gasses. Unit 4 of the Agricultural Respiratory Hazards Education Series. Iowa State University Extension, Ames.

Occupational Safety and Health Administration. 2002. Regulations (Standards—29 CFR) Occupational noise exposure. 1926.52. U.S. Department of Labor. http://www.osha.gov/pls.

Phillips, C., and D. Piggins. 1992. Farm Animals and the Environment. C.A.B. Int., Wallingford, Oxon, UK.

Phillips, C. J. C. 1992. Photoperiod. Pages 49–65. In: Farm Animals and the Environment, C. Phillips and D. Piggins ed., C.A.B. Int., Wallingford, Oxon, UK.

Piggins, D. 1992. Visual Perception. Pages 131–158. In: Farm Animals and the Environment, C. Phillips and D. Piggins ed., C.A.B. Int., Wallingford, Oxon, UK.

Roil, J. A., J. M. Sanchez, J. G. Eguren, and V. R. Gaudioso. 1989. Colour perception in fighting cattle. Appl. Anim. Behav. Sci. 23:.199.

Savory, C. J. and I. J. H. Duncan. 1982. Voluntary regulation of lighting by domestic fowls in Skinner boxes. Appl. Anim. Ethol. 9: 73.

Smith, S. and L. Goldman. 1999. Color discrimination in horses. Appl. Anim. Behav. Sci. 62: 13–25.

Soffie, M., G. Thines and U. Flater. 1980. Colour discrimination in heifers. Mammalia 44: 97.

Tarrant, P. V., F. J. Kenny, and D. Harrington, 1988. The effect of stocking density during 4-hour transport to slaughter on behavior, blood constituents and carcass bruising in Friesian steers. Meat Science 24: 209–222.

Tarrant, P. V., F. J. Kenny, D. Harrington, and M. Murphy. 1992. Long distance transportation of steers to slaughter: effect of stocking density on physiology, behavior and carcass quality. Livestock Prod. Sci. 30: 223–238.

Tarrant, V. and T. Grandin. 1993. Cattle transport, 109–126. In: Livestock Handling and Transport. T. Grandin, ed. Cab International, Wallingford, UK.

Whittlestone, W. G. 1960. What is a good milking machine? Lecture given to the Australian Agricultural Engineering Society (New South Wales Branch). Power Farming, February. Cited in J. L. Albright and C. W. Arave, 1997, The Behaviour of Cattle. CAB International, Wallingford, Oxon, UK: p. 198.

Wollack, C. H. 1963. The auditory acuity of the sheep (Ovis aries). J. Auditory Research 3: 121–132.

Wright, W. D. 1975. The Rays Are Not Coloured. Hilger, London.

7

Principles for Handling Grazing Animals

Temple Grandin

ABSTRACT

An understanding of the behavioral principles of grazing animals will improve animal welfare and reduce injuries to both people and animals. When an animal becomes agitated during restraint, fear is the most likely motivation. The animal kicks because it is scared. Handlers need to learn basic behavioral principles such as using the animal's flight zone and point of balance to quietly move animals. Another basic principle is keeping an animal calm. Calm animals are easier to handle. This chapter also contains information on training animals to cooperate with veterinary procedures. Trained animals will be less fearful and have lower stress levels. The effects of genetic factors such as temperament are also discussed. Animals with a flighty, excitable temperament are more likely than a calm placid animal to become fearful and agitated when they are suddenly confronted with something new. New procedures and other new things must be introduced more slowly to animals with a flighty temperament such as antelopes compared to calmer animals such as cattle. This chapter discusses horses, cattle, pigs, sheep, bison, elk, and antelope. Most of the basic principles apply to all species.

INTRODUCTION

The author has over 30 years of experience handling large animals. This chapter is based on both scientific literature and extensive practical experiences with cattle, pigs, sheep, bison, antelope, elk, and horse handling at ranches, feedlots, zoos, and slaughter plants throughout the United States, Canada, and other countries. The author has either observed or participated in animal handling in over three hundred different places.

Careful, quiet handling of all types of animals will help improve both productivity and animal welfare. Research in our laboratory has shown that cattle that become agitated during handling and restraint will have lower weight gains and tougher meat (Voisinet et al., 1997a,b). Progressive livestock producers have found that learning behavioral principles of animal handling helps to reduce sickness and improve productivity. Cattle will settle down and go back onto feed more quickly after quiet handling. Research studies done over 20 years ago have clearly demonstrated the bad effect of handling stresses on animal productivity (Hixon, Kesler, and Troxel, 1981; Fulkerson and Jamieson, 1982; Doney, Smith, and Gunn, 1976; Whittlestone et al., 1970). Further studies also show that handling restraint and transport stresses are detrimental to immune, reproductive, and rumen function (Blecha, Boyles, and Riley, 1984; Doney et al., 1976; Galyean, Lee, and Hubbert, 1981;

Kelly et al., 1981; Mertshing and Kelly, 1983). When animals become agitated during handling, it is usually due to fear. Fear is a very strong stressor (Boissy, 1995; Dantzer and Mormede, 1983). Reducing the animal's fear will make handling easier for both you and the animal. Australian researcher Paul Hemsworth has done many studies that show that dairy cows and pigs that fear people are less productive (Hemsworth and Barnett, 1991; Hemsworth and Coleman, 1998). Reducing negative interactions between people and dairy cows, such as hitting, improves production (Hemsworth et al., 2002).

Why do some people continue to handle animals roughly when so much research shows the detrimental effects of stressful handling practices? During my career, I have observed that people often are more willing to buy technology such as a new chute system instead of adopting better management. Management requires continuous effort whereas buying technology is a one-time investment. This chapter will cover easy-to-understand behavioral principles, which can be easily taught. People should learn to use behavior to control an animal instead of force.

An understanding of the behavior of large grazing animals such as cattle, horses, bison, and elk will reduce stress and help prevent injuries to both people and animals. They have more fear-motivated behavior compared to predatory animals such as dogs, wolves, and lions. Grazing animals are a prey species and fear motivates them to escape from perceived danger. Even though pigs are not true grazing animals, the same principles apply to them. Fear-based behavior is likely to be the main cause of accidents during handling or restraint, such as a horse kicking or a cow becoming agitated in a chute. Dangerous behavior such as kicking, biting, or charging people may be due to either fear or true aggression. A bull that charges people on an open pasture is probably showing true aggression whereas a bull that struggles in a squeeze chute is probably fearful. A basic principle is that punishing fearful behavior is likely to make it worse. This is why it is important to understand the animal's motivation.

REDUCING FEAR IMPROVES WELFARE AND MAKES HANDLING EASIER

A calm animal is much easier to handle than a fearful, agitated animal. If an animal becomes agitated, it will be easier and safer to handle if it is allowed to calm down before handling is attempted again. When a horse becomes agitated at a veterinary clinic, it is best to leave it alone for 20 to 30 minutes. Cattle will be easier to handle in corrals if they are allowed to settle down for 20 minutes after they have been brought into the corral. It takes 20 minutes for the heart rate to return to normal (Stermer, Camp, and Stevens, 1981). Groups of fearful excited animals are more difficult to separate and sort because scared animals will stick together in a bunch.

THE BIOLOGY OF FEAR

Fear is a universal emotion in the animal kingdom (LeDoux, 1996, 1994). It motivates animals to avoid predators and survive in the wild. All mammals and birds can be conditioned to fear things that are perceived as dangerous. The amygdala, a structure in the brain, is the central fear system that is involved in both fear behavior and learning to fear certain things or people. Scientists have learned that the amygdala is the brain's fear center (Davis, 1992). Stimulating the amygdala elicits responses in the nervous system that are similar to fear in humans (Redgate and Fahringer, 1973). In humans, electrical stimulation of the amygdala elicits feelings of fear (Gloor, Oliver, and Quesney, 1981). Destroying the amygdala will block both unconditioned (unlearned) and conditioned (learned) fear responses (LeDoux, 1996; Rogan and LeDoux, 1996). An example of an unlearned fear response would be a horse spooking at a firecracker. A learned fear response would have occurred if the horse now refuses to enter the place where the firecracker went off. Lesioning of the amygdala also had a taming effect on wild rats (Kemble et al., 1984). Fear learning takes place in a subcortical pathway, and extinguishing a learned fear response is difficult because it requires the animal to suppress the fear memory via an active learning process. A single, very frightening or painful event can produce a strong learned fear response, but eliminating this fear response is much more difficult (LeDoux, 1996). The animal may develop fear memories that are difficult to eliminate.

GOOD FIRST EXPERIENCES IMPORTANT

Observations by the author on cattle ranches have shown that to prevent cattle and sheep from becoming averse to and fearful of a new squeeze chute or corral system, painful or frightening procedures that cause visible signs of agitation should be avoided the first time the animals enter the facility (Grandin, 1997b). It is important that an animal's first experience with a new corral, trailer, or restraining chute is a good first experience. Practical experience has shown that if a horse has a frightening or painful experience the first time he goes into a trailer, this may make teaching him to get in a trailer difficult. This happens because he has developed a fear memory. First experiences with new things make a big impression on animals. When an animal is first brought in to a new farm or laboratory, make its first experiences pleasant by feeding it and giving it time to settle down. Nonslip flooring is essential because slipping and falling in the new facility may create a fear memory.

Experiments with rats demonstrate that a bad first experience with a new place may cause the animal to refuse to reenter it in the future. Rats that receive a strong electrical shock the first time they enter a novel alley would refuse to enter it again (Miller, 1960). However, if the rat is subjected to a series of shocks of gradually increasing intensity, it would continue to enter the alley to get a food reward. Stress in sheep during routine handling can be reduced if the animals are conditioned gradually to handling procedures (Hutson, 2000).

Less-severe procedures such as sorting or weighing should be done first, and feed rewards will motivate animals to move through a facility (Hutson, 1985; Hargreaves and Hutson, 1990). It is unfortunate that many animals learn to fear the veterinarian. This is especially evident in zoos. One zoo veterinarian quit because it upset him to have most of the animals fear him. He was associated with dart guns and other aversive procedures. This could have been avoided by making the animal's first few experiences with the veterinarian positive.

SENSORY BASED ANIMAL FEAR MEMORIES

As a person with autism, I can really relate to how an animal may think or feel (Grandin, 1996, 1997b). I think in pictures instead of thinking in language. Many practical experiences with animals indicate that fear memories are stored as pictures or sounds. Fear memories are often very specific. I observed a horse that was afraid of black cowboy hats because he was abused by a person wearing a black cowboy hat. White cowboy hats and baseball caps had no effect on this horse. The black hat was most threatening when it was on a person's head and somewhat less threatening when it was on the ground. Animals that had been darted by the zoo veterinarian were able to recognize his voice. On the other hand, ranchers have learned that fearful cattle will often quiet down when they hear the voice of a familiar person who is associated with previous positive experiences. At a zoo, the elephant became aggressive toward a new keeper who had a beard. The elephant feared bearded men. The new keeper was accepted after he shaved off the beard. My assistant has a dog that is terrified of hot air balloons. The first time she saw one, it revved up its roaring burner as it soared over her at a low altitude. Now she becomes highly agitated when she sees hot air balloons that are even several miles away. Research on animal perception indicates that cattle are able to differentiate between "good" and "bad" people. Animals have a tendency to associate bad experiences with prominent features on people such as beards or lab coats, or they will associate a scary or painful experience with a specific place. They can recognize a person by the color of their clothing (Koba and Tanida, 1999). They can also learn that some places are safe and others are scary and bad. It is also possible for an animal to associate a painful or scary experience with a prominent feature in the environment. In one case, a young stallion fell down and was whipped the first time he had to mount a dummy for semen collection. He developed a fear of overhead garage doors because he was looking at one when he fell. Future collection was done easily when it was done outdoors away from buildings and garage doors. Unfortunately, a fear of garage doors could cause many problems if the horse was ridden. Garage doors are very common and difficult to avoid.

Sometimes problems with bucking or rearing in horses can be stopped by changing the type of bridle or saddle. A different bridle or saddle feels different. In this case, the fear memory may be a "touch" picture. For example, if a horse was abused with a snaffle bit, he may tolerate a hackamore or a standard western bit. Another horse had a sound fear memory because he had a bad experience with a canvas tarp. Horse blankets that sounded like a tarp were scary, and a wool blanket that made little sound was well tolerated.

GRAZING ANIMAL VISION

Contrary to popular belief, horses and cattle can see color (Gilbert and Arave, 1986; Arave, 1996). Horses can discriminate different colors from gray and may have problems discriminating green (Pick et al., 1994). Research indicates that cattle, sheep, and goats are dichromats with eyes that are most sensitive to yellowish-green (553–555 nm) and blue-purple light (444–455 nm) (Jacobs, Deegan, and Neitz, 1998). This means that grazing animals may have a partial color blindness similar to a human dicromat. They do not have black and white total color blindness. Dichromatic vision may provide better vision at night and make the animal more sensitive to seeing motion. Possibly, dichromatic vision partially explains why horses, cattle, and other grazing animals are easily spooked and frightened by sudden movements and high contrasts such as shadows. This explains why animals will often refuse to walk over objects that have high contrast such as a sparkling reflection in a puddle, drain gates, or a shadow or bright spot of sunlight in the floor. All grazing animals have wide-angle vision because their eyes are located on the sides of their head. Wide-angle vision enables grazing animals to see all around themselves and to see predators while they are grazing. Their visual field is over three hundred degrees (Prince, 1977). There is a small blind spot immediately behind the animal's rear (Prince, 1977). If a person suddenly walks into a horses' blind spot, he or she may be kicked. Horses defend themselves from predators by running and kicking. When a person walks behind a horse, he or she should talk to it so that it knows that the person is there and it is safe. If a horse is suddenly startled by a person walking up behind it, it may kick.

Ruminants have depth perception (Lehman and Patterson, 1964). Cattle will often stop and put their heads down when they see a shadow on the ground. They may have to stop moving and put their heads down to see depth. All animals are sensitive to rapid movement (LeDoux, 1996; Rogan and LeDoux, 1996). It makes prey species such as grazing animals run away, and it often induces a predatory animal such as a dog to chase. Even people are sensitive to rapid movement. This is why used car dealers put flags up to attract attention. During handling, rapid movements are more likely to frighten grazing animals than slower, more deliberate movements. Animals with the most excitable and nervous temperaments are most likely to become fearful of a rapid movement such as arm waving. Nervous animals are more aware of small changes in their environment.

HEARING

Horses and cattle are more sensitive to high-pitched sound than people. The auditory sensitivity of cattle is greatest at 8,000 Hz and sheep are most sensitive at 7,000 Hz. The horse has a wider range of maximum hearing sensitivity than the cow (Ames and Arehart, 1972; Heffner and Heffner, 1983). It ranges from 1,000 to 16,000 Hz. The human ear is most sensitive at 100 to 3,000 Hz.

People working around large animals should speak softly with a low tone of voice. Observations by the author indicate that cattle remain calmer and handling is easier when handlers stop yelling and whistling. High-pitched noise is more disturbing to many animals. In pigs, an 8,000 Hz sound increased a pig's heart rate more than a 500 Hz sound (Talling, Waran, and Wathes, 1996; Talling et al., 1998). High-pitched sounds in the wild are used as alarm calls. They activate the amygdala more effectively than low-pitched sounds (LeDoux, 1996). People yelling at an animal may result in the animal becoming fearful, and it may kick, charge, or attempt to escape.

Recent research indicates that yelling and whistling at cows is very aversive and increases an animal's heart rate more than the sound of a gate slamming (Waynert et al., 1999). Cattle with a nervous temperament, which become agitated in an auction ring, were more sensitive to sudden movement and the sound of a person yelling than calmer cattle (Lanier et al., 2000).

TOUCH AND STROKING

Progressive horse trainers have learned that flighty horses can be calmed by massage. This is the basis of the Linden Tellington-Jones T Touch Method (Tellington-Jones and Bruns, 1985). Extremely light, tickle touches should be avoided because they may set off a flight reaction. Animals should be stroked, not patted. When stroking an animal, imitate the strokes of a mother animal's tongue. Stroke the spots where the mother animal would lick, such as the withers. Cattle and other animals that exert dominance by butting should not be stroked on the forehead because this encourages butting (Albright, 2000). Stroke them under the chin. Horses can be stroked on the forehead. Stroking an animal all over its body can help desensitize it to touch (fig. 7.1).

FLIGHT ZONE

All people handling grazing animals need to understand the flight zone. The flight zone is the animal's safety zone, and its size varies depending on how wild or tame the animal is (Grandin, 1980, 1987; Hedigar, 1968) (fig. 7.2). A show steer or a riding horse has no flight zone, but cattle that seldom see people will have a large flight zone. It may vary from a few

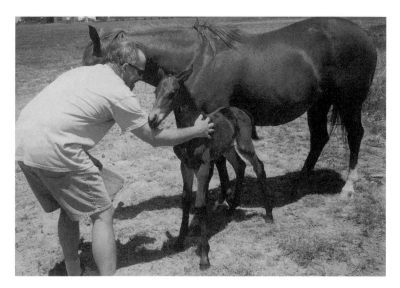

Figure 7.1.   Gently stroking a newborn filly all over its body wall desensitizes it to touch and makes it easier to train. If the mare is tame, you can usually stroke the baby after stroking the mother.

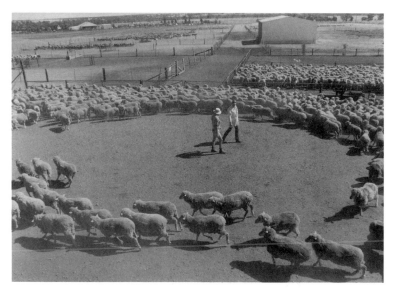

Figure 7.2.   Flight zone of a flock of extensively raised sheep in Australia.

feet to 100 yards or more. When a person enters the flight zone, the animal will turn away. If a person is outside the animal's flight zone, it will turn and look at him or her. The size of the flight zone is determined by three interacting factors: genetic traits (excitable versus calm), amount of contact with people (see them every day or only twice a year), and quality of the contact with people (aversive versus positive). Grazing animals with large flight zones may become fearful and agitated when a person deeply penetrates their flight zone when they are in a confined space and unable to move away. Cattle rearing up in squeeze chutes or single file chutes have caused many accidents. Wild cattle may do this because they are attempting to escape from a person who is deep in their flight zone. If an animal rears, people should back up and remove themselves from the animal's flight zone. When the people back away, the animal will often settle back down. Handlers should be instructed to never attempt to push a rearing animal back down. This is likely to increase its agitation and may cause injuries to either the animal or its handlers.

Grazing animals that have a large flight zone will move more quietly with less agitation if the handler works on the edge of the flight zone (fig. 7.3). The handler penetrates the edge of the flight zone to make the animal move and retreats outside the flight zone to induce the animal to stop moving. Excited, agitated animals will have a larger flight zone than calm animals. The flight zone will be bigger when a person faces an animal and smaller if he/she turns sideways. The flight zone enlarges when the handler makes herself look bigger and more intimidating. Flight zone principles may not work on completely tame animals. These animals should be led or trained to move.

Handlers also need to understand the point of balance. The point of balance is an imaginary line at the animal's shoulders. To induce the animal to move forward, the handler must be behind the point of balance. To make it move backward, he or she must be in front

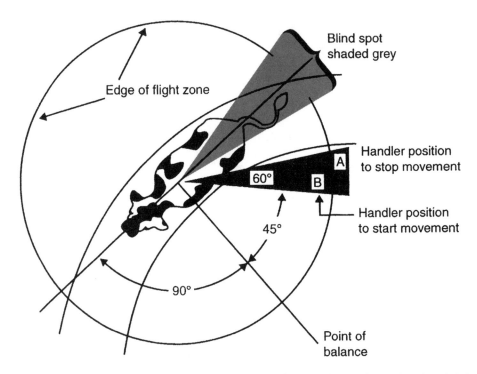

Figure 7.3. Extensively raised animals will remain calmer if the handler remains on the edge of their flight zone. The handler enters the flight zone to make the animal move and backs away to stop movement.

of the point of balance. Grazing animals will move forward when a handler walks inside the flight zone past the point of balance in the opposite direction of desired movement (fig. 7.4) (Grandin, 1998b; Kilgour and Dalton, 1984). The handler must walk quickly past the point of balance. If the handler moves too slowly, the animal will back up. Progressive people have been able to almost eliminate electric prods by using these movement patterns. On most ranches and feedlots, 99 percent of the cattle can be moved quietly and efficiently without electric prods. In large slaughter plants, 15 minutes of instruction of flight zone and movement patterns resulted in a reduction of electric prodding of beef cattle from 83 percent of the animals to 17 percent (Grandin, 1998b). To further reduce electric prod use required modifications of the facilities. The workers were able to keep up with the slaughter line with reduced prodding. The very best plants with good equipment had to use an electric prod on only 5 percent of the cattle (Grandin, 2000b). There are a few animals that refuse to move unless the electric prod is used. In this situation, the electric prod is preferable to hitting the animal or tail twisting to make it move. For both welfare and safety reasons, the use of electric prods should be avoided as much as possible. Nonelectric driving aids such as plastic paddles or a flag on the end of a stick should be used as the primary driving tools. Plastic streamers or a flag on the end of a stick can also be used to quietly turn animals. Be careful not to be too aggressive with a flag. Use it to guide an animal and

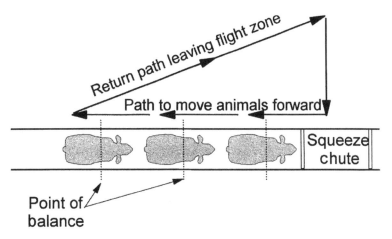

Figure 7.4.   Handler movement pattern to induce an animal to move forward. The handler moves quickly past the point of balance in the opposite direction of desired movement. An enlarged version of this pattern will work on pasture. Walking in the opposite direction of desired movement speeds groups of animals up and walking in the same direction slows them down.

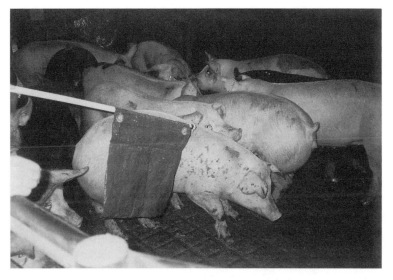

Figure 7.5.   A flag on the end of a stick works well for guiding and turning animals. Calm animals can be easily guided. Do not wildly wave the flag but use it to block vision to turn the animal.

do *not* wildly wave it (fig. 7.5). Handlers should be careful to avoid scaring the animals. It is important to get electric prods out of people's hands. Observations by the author indicate that the attitude of the people toward the cattle improved when they stopped carrying electric prods.

HANDLING IN CROWD PENS

The number-one mistake made by handlers is putting too many animals in the crowd pen that leads to the single-file chute or to a loading ramp. Animals need room to turn. When cattle or pigs are handled, the crowd pen should be filled one-half to three-quarters full. For bison and wild horses, the crowd pan should be filled half full (fig. 7.6). Do not push the crowd gate up tight against the animals. Cattle, pigs, elk, bison, deer, and wild horses should be moved in small groups. This will help keep them calm. The only exception to this rule is sheep. Sheep have such a strong following instinct that they can be moved in one continuous mob.

Animals will move through the crowd pen into a loading ramp or single-file chute more easily if the handler takes advantage of their natural following behavior. When a truck is being loaded, do not allow animals to stand in the crowd pen. They should walk through the pen and immediately go up the ramp before they have a chance to turn around. When animals are being moved into a single-file chute, the crowd pen should not be filled until there is space in the chute. The crowd pen should be renamed the "passing through pen." The animals should walk through without stopping on their way to either the loading ramp or a single-file chute. If the animals balk or turn back, distractions must be removed (see chapter 8).

All herd animals such as cattle, deer, bison, and horses will often become very agitated and stressed when a lone animal is separated from the herd (Grandin, 2000b; Boissy and LeNeindre, 1997). A single animal that is frantically attempting to rejoin its herdmates is highly stressed. The author has observed that a lone bovine left behind in a crowd pen or alley has caused several serious accidents when it jumped a fence or ran over a person. A

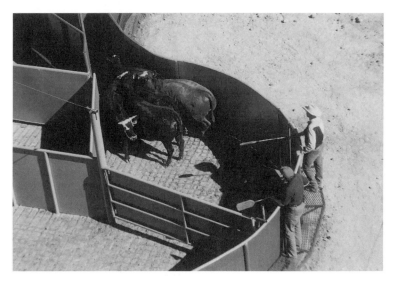

Figure 7.6.   The crowd pen that leads to the single-file chute must never be filled completely full. Half full is best because animals need room to turn.

person should never get into a confined space such as a crowd pen with a single agitated large animal. It should either be released or more animals should be put in with it. However, it is safe for experienced handlers to be in a larger pen or alley with a group of cattle. In this situation, there is sufficient room for the animals to move away. The handler is not constantly standing inside the flight zone. Calm animals can be sorted out a gate by facing and staring at the animals you want to hold in the pen and turning sideways and looking away from the animals you want to move through the gate.

HABITATION AND TEMPERAMENT

Domestic animals such as cattle will usually habituate to being quietly moved through a squeeze chute (Grandin and Deesing, 1998; Littlefield, Grandin, and Lanier, 2001). If a bovine is moved through a squeeze chute every day for several days, it will usually become calmer on each successive day because it learns that going in the squeeze chute will not hurt it (Alam and Dobson, 1986; Crookshank et al., 1979; Peischel, Schalles, and Owenby, 1980). Animals with a calm temperament will habituate to a series of forced nonpainful procedures. For example, cortisol levels in cattle decreased after they were moved through the squeeze chute a number of times over a period of days. However, extremely flighty, excitable animals such as bison and antelope may not habituate. Instead of habituating, they often react explosively to a forced handling procedure and severely injure themselves. Instead of becoming less and less fearful with each successive pass through the chute, they may become increasingly fearful. They are likely to be injured when they rear, jump out of a facility, or violently struggle. In one experiment, some pigs habituated to a series of forced swimming tasks and others responded with increasing fear (Lanier et al., 1995). A basic principle is that animals with flighty excitable genetics are less likely to habituate to a series of forced, nonpainful restraint and handling procedures. Most animals, regardless of temperament, will not habituate to a painful procedure.

EFFECTS OF PREVIOUS EXPERIENCE OF TRAINING

Previous experiences will affect how animals behave during handling. Cattle and sheep have excellent memories. They remember painful or aversive experiences, and they will be more reluctant to reenter a facility where an aversive event occurred. The author has observed that cattle that have had experiences with rough handling will have bigger flight zones and become more agitated during restraint when they are handled in the future.

Calves that have been reared in close, quiet association with people will usually be easier to handle and have a smaller flight zone when they mature. The author has also observed that cattle reared in the colder parts of the United States where they are fed every day during the winter have a smaller flight zone than cattle raised in southern states. Some southern cattle are handled only a few times each year, and they are not fed during the winter in locations where grass grows year round. There is a tendency for southern cattle to become more agitated in squeeze chutes compared to northern cattle, which are exposed to people feeding them all winter.

Australian researchers conducted some of the first training experiments in extensively used beef calves with large flight zones. These experiments were conducted to determine if training calves would make the animals easier to handle when they matured. They found that walking quietly among them and moving them quietly through the chutes produced calmer adult animals (Fordyce, Dodt, and Wythes, 1988; Fordyce, 1987; Hearnshaw, Barlow, and Want, 1979). Extensively reared Zebu calves handled ten times at one to two months of age were calmer and less likely to jump fences when handled in the future (Becker and Lobato, 1997). The calves were placed in a single-file chute and petted. Observations by the author indicated that cattle that originated from ranches where they had become accustomed to both people on foot and on horseback were calmer and easier to handle after they were shipped to a feedlot. It is important to calmly and quietly train the calves to both on-foot and on-horseback handling. Cattle that have never seen a person on foot may become fearful when they see a person walking in a pen. Frequent gentle handling and contact with people also reduces cortisol levels and stress associated with restraint in both cattle and deer (Hastings, Abbott, and George, 1992; Hopster et al., 1999). Training young cattle to the quiet presence of people walking amidst them will produce calmer adult animals. Animals need to be habituated to a variety of vehicles and people. They need to learn that some variation in their routine will not hurt them. Ried and Mills (1962) years ago found that exposing sheep to variations in routine helped to reduce stress when they were exposed to change.

Animals that have been abused can become dangerous. Pork producers have reported that boars that have been beaten by their handlers have been known to turn on them. Nervous, high-strung horses that have been subjected to overly rough training methods are more likely to suddenly spook, kick, or rear. Abuse of animals is unethical and detrimental to animal welfare. The author has observed that an animal that has been abused is more likely to panic when it sees a person that looks similar to someone who abused it in the past.

TRAINING ANIMALS TO COOPERATE WITH HANDLING

Training animals to cooperate with handling procedures will help reduce both stress and accidents to people or animals. Pigs can be trained with food rewards to stand still for various types of tests (Chilcott, Stubbs and Ashley, 2001). Sheep can be trained to voluntarily enter a restraint device (Grandin, 1989). Ferguson and Rosales-Ruiz (2001) describe behavioral methods that are positive reinforcement for training horses to load into a trailer.

We have had good success training antelope at the Denver Zoo to voluntarily cooperate with veterinary procedures such as blood sampling and injections. Training Bongo and Nyala antelope to enter a wooden crate and stand still while they were given injections improved safety for both people and animals (Phillips et al., 1998; Grandin et al., 1995) (fig. 7.7). Bongos are large, flighty animals, and if they panic, they react explosively. Training greatly reduces stress on the animal. The cortisol levels in crate-conditioned Bongos were only 2 to 9 mg/ml. This is close to resting baseline levels in cattle. Creatine phosphokinase (CPK) levels for four trained Bongos averaged 71 IU in trained animals and 288 IU in animals immobilized with dart or pole syringe. Glucose levels were 61 ml/dl in trained Bon-

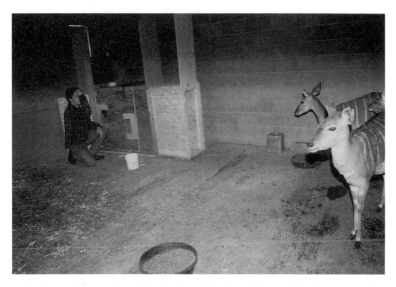

Figure 7.7.   Nyala antelope can be easily trained to allow themselves to be held in a crate for blood sampling and injections. The animal is accessed through small doors in the side of the crate.

gos and 166 ml/dl in immobilized Bongos. Since antelope are animals that survive in the wild by flight, they are very vigilant and aware of any new sight or sound. If they are suddenly confronted with a novel sight or sound, they are likely to panic. The antelopes had to be gradually habituated to each new procedure. Ten days were required to habituate the animals to the sound of the remote controlled sliding door moving on the handling crate. The first day the door was moved only two centimeters. The instant the animal turned its head toward the sound, movement was stopped. Flighty animals must never be pushed beyond this orienting response. It is very important to avoid triggering a massive flight reaction during early training. If the antelope has a scary experience associated with the handling crate, it may become impossible to train. It would be especially detrimental if it were frightened during the initial experiences with the crate. The animals were gradually habituated to all the sights and sounds associated with the crate. The next step was to entice the animals into entering the crate by placing highly palatable treats (yams or spinach), which were not part of their regular diet, at the entrance of the crate. It is important to use food that is a real treat. The food was gradually moved farther and farther into the crate. The crate was long enough that the animal had to get completely into it to get the food. The animals were then habituated to being locked in the crate for increasing lengths of time starting with one second. During the training sessions, a familiar person talked to the animal to help keep it calm.

There is a critical point during training where the purpose of the treats changes from being an enticement to enter the crate to a reward for standing still during blood sampling from the rear leg. To entice the animal into the crate, the treats were continuously available. After the animal was fully trained to enter the crate, the treats were then withheld until it kept its leg still. Each animal was then trained using operant conditioning to stand still when its leg was touched. If it stood still after its leg was touched, a treat was given immediately. Timing of giving the treat is critical. It must be given the instant the animal stands still so that it will associate the treat with standing still. It was then conditioned to tolerate increasingly hard pinches to simulate a needle. Early in the training procedure, great care was taken to avoid triggering a massive flight and panic reaction. Later on in the training program when the animals were relaxed in the crate, operant conditioning had to be used to prevent learned avoidance behavior. Some animals who were continuously fed treats learned they could avoid a needle stick by moving their leg. The treat then had to be used as a reward for not moving.

We observed that the trained antelopes still feared the veterinarian who had previously shot them with a tranquilizer or dart. He was the only person who was not able to handle the trained animals. However, a new veterinarian was able to handle the animals. For training to be successful, it must be done by people who are not associated with aversive previous experiences. Research has shown that cattle can differentiate between different people. Dairy cattle are able to cue in on either the identity of the handler or the location where an aversive event occurred as a cue to predict the type of handling they will receive. Practical experience has shown that animals can easily recognize a familiar person by their voice or recognize a type of clothing such as lab coats.

TEMPERAMENT AND TIME FOR TRAINING

A basic principle is that animals with a very flighty, excitable temperament must be trained and habituated slowly in small steps over many days (Grandin and Deesing, 1998), and animals with a placid temperament can be trained in bigger steps over a shorter period of time. It is advisable to keep training periods short. Ten to 15 minutes per day is ideal. Forcing an animal to do something over and over on the same day can cause increasing fear and agitation (Grandin et al., 1994). Even in calm animals, such as cattle, it is advisable to limit the length of a training session. Cattle can be easily trained to voluntarily enter a squeeze chute, but making the animal go through it many times in a single day may cause increasing agitation. Animals need time to calm down in between training sessions.

BISON TRAINING

Bison are not domestic cattle. They may react very violently when they are moved through a handling facility. Bison producers report that even though they try to handle their animals carefully, horns are often broken and bison gore each other during handling in corrals. Frightened bison in a confined small pen may attack both people and each other. Jennifer Lanier developed methods to train bison to handling procedures (Lanier et al., 1999). Young calves can be trained to enter the squeeze chute. Initial trials indicate that bison yearlings that had been trained to walk through and stand in the squeeze chute were less agitated when they were locked in the head gate and squeezed. An important species difference between bison and other animals such as cattle is that frightened bison will sometimes gore and injure each other when they are in a confined space. Cattle, horses, and sheep will stand quietly in a single-file queue. Bison should not be lined up in a queue to enter a squeeze chute. One or two animals at a time should be brought out of the crowd pen.

GENETIC EFFECTS ON HANDLING

Cattle with a flighty excitable temperament and flighty animals such as antelope, elk, bison, and deer are more likely to panic when they are suddenly confronted with a new experience compared to animals with a calm, placid temperament. Lawrence, Terlouw, and Illius (1991) reported that sudden stamping of a foot was one of the best tests for discriminating between calm and excitable genetic lines of pigs. Temperament in cattle is heritable (Grignard et al., 2001; Hearnshaw and Morris, 1984). Sudden exposure to a new thing is often the cause of dangerous incidents where cattle or horses have gone berserk at either a livestock show or auction. Panicked animals have injured people when they ran through crowds. They have jumped arena fences and have leaped into grandstands full of people.

Cattle and horses, which were calm and well mannered when they were in their familiar home, farm, or ranch, have been known to go berserk at shows. Ranchers, show managers, and feedlot operators have all reported that cattle and horse breeds with a more excitable temperament are more likely to become excited and difficult to handle in new surroundings. It appears that excitable animals have no tolerance for sudden new experiences. At a slaughter plant, the author observed nervous saler cross heifers that kicked at handlers with both back feet when they were touched. The novel sounds and sights at the slaughter plant caused total panic. Calmer breeds of cattle at the same plant walked quietly up the chute.

Dangerous incidents with excitable animals may be reduced by culling cattle that became highly agitated in the squeeze chute. There are some cattle that will become extremely agitated every time they are handled (Grandin et al., 1994). Genetic selection of cattle for temperament will produce calmer animals that are less likely to become agitated when handled in new surroundings.

TRAINING TO TOLERATE NOVELTY

Another approach is that animals with excitable temperaments can be trained on the home ranch or farm to tolerate the sights and sounds of a new place. A flighty horse can be gradually introduced to flags, balloons, horns, PA systems, and other stimuli that it would be exposed to at a show. A good way to habituate a horse to balloons and flags is to tie them to the fence of a large corral or pasture. The animal will be attracted to them because it can voluntarily approach them. New things are both scary and attractive. They are scary if they are suddenly shoved in the animal's face, but they are attractive if they are far away and can be cautiously approached. Bicycles are scary to animals because they move rapidly and make little noise to warn that they are coming. The new things should be introduced gradually to prevent the animal from becoming scared. If a horse is severely frightened by a flag the first time he sees one, he may develop a fear of flags for the rest of his life. The author has observed that flighty, nervous animals are more likely to develop a permanent fear of things that scared them. Accidents during loading and unloading of horse trailers can be reduced by gently training colts to load into a trailer. It is very important that the colt's first experience with a trailer be positive.

INTERACTION OF GENETICS AND TRAINING METHODS

People who use quick, forceful "breaking" methods use them because in some animals they work. They work only on the animals with calmer genetics. I was kicked by a heifer a student attempted to train to lead by tying her to a post. Tying cattle or horses to a post and letting them fight it out is not recommended. When this is done, the genetically calm animal will habituate and learn to lead, but the flighty animal may stay scared. At one junior livestock show, students trained heifers by tying them to posts. The calm Holstein heifers pulled pack, habituated, and became well-trained show cattle. However, some of the Angus heifers never habituated, and they would spin around and kick people. A few were ruined and could not be shown. This incident illustrates how genetics can interact with handling methods. Animals should be trained to lead by using the principle of pressure and release. The instant the animal steps forward it should be rewarded by releasing the lead rope. The animal learns that if it cooperates, pressure is released.

Practical experience has shown that people must be careful to avoid the formation of fear memories. This is a much greater problem in horses because horses on the average are more flighty than cattle. Horses with a more nervous temperament, such as Arabs, must be gradually introduced to new things. I have had many owners tell me stories of Arab horses that have been ruined by rough training. It is much more difficult for a horse with an excitable temperament to suppress a fear memory. A calmer quarter horse may be able to be retrained, but the fear memory may keep popping up in the Arab.

HANDLING ESCAPED ANIMALS

If horses, cattle, or other large animals escape from an auction ring, showring, or slaughter plant, they must never be chased. The author has observed several incidents where chasing escaped cattle caused them to run wildly through crowds of people and resulted in injured people and extensive property damage. If an escaped bovine or horse is located where it is not an immediate threat to people, it is usually best to leave it alone for 30 minutes to allow it to calm down. Twenty minutes is required for its heart rate to return to normal (Stermer et al., 1981). A lone animal will often return by itself to other horses and cattle. When it has calmed down, it can be quietly moved.

A panicked bovine or horse may crash through a chain-link fence because it does not see the thin mesh. The author has observed escaped cattle that knocked over a chain-link fence when people chased them. Chain-link fences will hold a calm bovine, but a frightened bovine may either knock it over or go under the bottom edge of the mesh. Fences that present a visual barrier, such as a board fence, are less likely to be broken down by charging animals. It is usually recommended to allow experienced livestock people to handle an escaped animal. The author has observed that a panicked horse, steer, or bull can sometimes be calmed when it hears its owner's familiar voice. Some of the most dangerous incidents with escaped animals have occurred when security guards or the police became involved. In one incident, a security guard almost shot a person instead of an escaped steer. Some officers make the mistake of chasing animals and making the situation worse. There was a bad incident on our own campus when campus police chased a tame, halter-broke steer and caused him to panic. He ran through a glass door into one of the dormitories and ended up in a student's room. The room was completely trashed. Fortunately, no one was hurt.

At zoos, escaped animals can often be coaxed back into their enclosures by a familiar keeper. If a dangerous animal escapes, visitors should be quietly evacuated. The John Wayne approach may make the situation worse and result in the animal escaping from the zoo property. A better approach is for an experienced person to calmly shoot the animal with a tranquilizer dart. Zoos should develop plans for dealing with escaped animals.

MOVING LARGE GROUPS ON PASTURE

Grazing animals can be easily taught to come in when called. They will often learn to associate a truck with feed. It is best to teach the animals that tooting the horn means feed instead of the sight of the truck. This will prevent the cattle from running after vehicles. When cows with young calves are being moved, it is important to control the movement of the cows so that the young calves are not left behind. This will help reduce stress on the calves. Handlers *must not* chase stragglers. Allow the motion of the herd to attract them back. When animals are moved out of a pen, the handler should stand near the gate and control their movement out of the pen. In feedlots, a lead horse should be used to prevent cattle from running down the alley.

Large groups of extensively raised cattle can be gathered by inducing their natural tendency to bunch. This method will not work on very tame cattle with little or no flight zone. Tame cattle should be led, not driven. Figure 7.8 illustrates a windshield wiper pattern in which the handler walks barely on the edges of the collective flight zone of the group (Grandin, 2000b; Smith, 1998). The handler walks quietly back and forth until the bunching instinct is triggered. The principle is to induce the bunching instinct before any attempt is made to move the cattle. Attempting to move the cattle too soon will cause them to scatter. All cattle movements should be at a walk or a slow trot. Bud Williams, a cattle-handling specialist in Texas, warns that the handler must not circle around the cattle. This will make them cut back. He prefers to use a straight zigzag line (Smith, 1998; Grandin, 2000b).

When additional pressure is applied to the flight zone to make the animals move, the handler must practice the principle of pressure and release. When the animals start moving in the desired direction, the handler should reward them by backing off and reducing pressure on the collective flight zone. Continuous pressure will cause the herd to run. When the herd slows down, pressure should be reapplied.

ACCLIMATING GROUPS OF ANIMALS TO HANDLING

Feedlot cattle, cattle on pasture, and pigs that live in indoor pens will be easier to handle and less stressed if they become accustomed to people moving through their pens or pasture. Pigs will be easier to sort and load into trucks if people walk through the pens

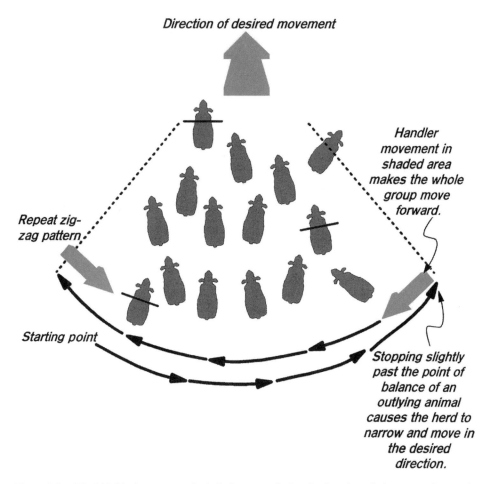

Direction of desired movement

Handler movement in shaded area makes the whole group move forward.

Repeat zig-zag pattern

Starting point

Stopping slightly past the point of balance of an outlying animal causes the herd to narrow and move in the desired direction.

Figure 7.9.   Windshield wiper pattern for inducing extensively raised cattle and sheep to gather on the range. The principle is to trigger the natural bunching instinct before any attempt is made to move the animals. This will not work on completely tame animals, so they should be either led or called in.

(Grandin, 1987, 1993). The person should move through the pens every day and train the pigs to quietly get up and flow around the the person (fig. 7.9). Walking pigs in the aisle will make them easier to handle (Geverink et al., 1998; Abbott et al., 1997; Grandin, Curtis, and Taylor, 1987). Bud Williams is using similar procedures on newly arrived feedlot calves to help reduce stress and encourage the calves to eat (Maday, 2002). He is also giving cattle walks in the alleys. When these activities are done carefully, they may help improve weight gain.

HANDLING QUALITY CONTROL

Managers need to constantly monitor handling to prevent rough practices, such as excessive electric prod use, from returning. Standards need to be upheld to prevent "bad from becoming normal." One of my biggest frustrations was teaching people how to handle cat-

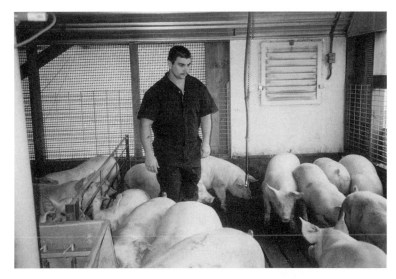

Figure 7.8. Walking through pens of pigs every day will acclimate them to people and make them easier to handle. The handler should walk through the pen in a different random pattern each day to teach the animals to calmly get up and flow around him. Similar principles can be used to get cattle accustomed to people.

tle quietly, and having them revert back, a year later, to screaming, yelling, and whips. To prevent this, different parts of handling procedures must be measured against an objectively defined standard. People manage the things they measure.

Measurement of the percentage of animals that vocalize, fall, or receive electric prods has been successfully used to greatly improve handling in slaughter plants (Grandin, 1998a, 2001). Each variable is measured on a yes/no basis for each animal. In a plant with well-designed facilities and trained people, 95 percent of the cattle can be moved without an electric prod and three or less animals per hundred (3 percent) will vocalize (moo or bellow). On feedlots and ranches, the best variables to measure are (1) percentage of animals prodded with an electric prod; (2) percentage that fall down; and (3) exit speed from the squeeze chute, such as walk, trot, or run. Australian research has shown that animals that run out of the squeeze chute have lower weight gains compared to animals that walk or trot out (Fell et al., 1999). In a feedlot that has worked hard to improve handling, it is possible to move 99 percent of the cattle without an electric prod, to have 0 percent falling down, and to have 90 percent exiting from the squeeze chute at a walk or trot. In wild horses, the number of horses that rear or kick can be easily quantified. Regular audits of handling with objective scoring will help prevent people from reverting back to old, rough methods.

AGGRESSIVE BEHAVIOR

A bull often attacks a person because he perceives the person as a conspecific (herdmate) that he attempts to dominate. This is true aggression and it is not motivated by fear. Why is the dairy bull more dangerous than most beef bulls? The difference in beef and dairy bull behavior may be explained by differences in rearing methods. Beef bull calves are reared on the mother cow and most dairy bull calves are bucket-fed by people. Research by Edward Price and his associates at the University of California found that Hereford bulls reared in groups were less likely to attack people than bulls bucket-fed in individual pens (Price and Wallach, 1990). Seventy-five percent of the individually reared bulls threatened handlers. In one thousand dam-reared bulls, only one bull attacked. Bulls that grow up with other cattle learn that they are bulls. Individually reared bulls may think they are people and when they become sexually mature they may challenge a person to exert dominance. Bull calves reared with other cattle usually direct their challenges toward other bulls instead of people. Similar problems with aggression toward humans have been reported in hand-reared deer and llamas (Reinken, 1988; Tillman, 1981).

A bull will challenge another bull or a person by making a broadside threat (Albright, 2000; Smith, 1998). He will face sideways and flex his neck to show how big he is. The bull will often not look at a person he is threatening. Bulls that make broadside threats toward people should be culled because they may charge people. The threat will be made before the bull charges. (More information on bull behavior can be found in Albright [2000] and Smith [1998].)

To reduce risk on beef cattle operations, an orphan bull calf should be either castrated or placed on a nurse cow. Castration at a young age will reduce aggression toward people. Practical experience in dairies indicates that six-week-old bull calves reared together in large groups are less likely to attack people. After a short period of individual rearing, six-week-old bull calves reared together can help reduce risks. Orphan male calves, llamas, and buck deer have also been known to attack people. The problem of attacking bulls is not due to tameness, it appears to be due to the bull mistaking a human for their own species. A basic principle is that in most grazing animals intact males will have less of a tendency to attack people if young males are reared by their own species. This is especially important very early in life. On the other hand, the strategy for working with predatory animals such as dogs, wolves, cats, and lions is different. People need to become the dominant alpha male or matriarch female. Humans become the leaders of the pack. Exerting dominance is not beating an animal into submission. It is using the animal's natural behavior pattern to become dominant. Dogs are so social that obedience training and making it very clear that people control their food works well. It is best for grazing animals to perceive people as a "higher power" instead of a fellow grazing animal. The problem with grazing animals is that their natural behaviors for exerting dominance are dangerous. Bulls establish dominance by head butting.

People working with boars have learned that attacks can often be prevented by handling the most dominant boar first. A dominant boar will sometimes attack a handler if he smells the smell of a subordinate animal that is lower in the dominance hierarchy (pecking order). In most species, individuals will fight to determine which animal will be the "boss." Attacks can also sometimes be provoked if a person uses a piece of equipment that has the subordinate animal's smell on it.

In many species, the mother animal is more likely to be dangerously aggressive when she has newborn babies. Producers have observed that sows with newborn piglets may be more aggressive toward handlers than sows with slightly older piglets. Ranchers and pork producers have observed that the tame pet cow or sow may be the most aggressive when she has newborn babies. Tame animals have less fear. Low-fear animals often have more true aggression. They are more likely to attack a person to exert dominance. High-fear animals are more likely to panic and kick or struggle during forced handling procedures.

CONCLUSIONS

Animals will be easier to handle and welfare will be improved if handlers understand their natural behavior patterns. It is also important to understand the animals' motivation. Fear is the most likely motivator of kicking or other agitated behavior during restraint or handling. Handlers should respond to fearful animals in a calm manner to calm them down. A familiar "safe" person can often calm down an agitated animal. True aggression is the most likely motivation of behaviors such as a mother protecting her young or a bull charging on a pasture. If a bull charges in a pasture, the best response would be to make yourself look big and yell at him to intimidate. The best way to handle the situation depends on the animal's motivation.

REFERENCES

Abbott, T. A., E. J. Hunter, J. H. Guise, and R. H. C. Penny. 1997. The effect of experience of handling on pig's willingness to move. Appl. Anim. Behav. Sci. 54:371–375.

Alam, M. G. S., and H. Dobson. 1986. Effects of various veterinary procedures on plasma concentrations of cortisol, luteinizing hormone and prostaglandin E2 metabolite in the cow. Vet. Rec. 118:7–10.

Albright, J. L. 2000. Dairy cattle behavior, facilities, handling and husbandry. In: T. Grandin (Ed.), Livestock handling and transport, 2nd Ed. CAB International, Wallingford, Oxon, UK; 127–174.

Ames, D. R., and Arehart, L. A. 1972. Physiological response of lambs to auditory stimuli. J. Anim. Sci. 34:994–998.

Arave, C. W. 1996. Assessing sensory capacity of animals using operant technology. J. of Anim. Sci. 74:1996–2000.

Becker, B. G., and J. F. P. Lobato. 1997. Effect of gentle handling on the reactivity of zebu cross calves to humans. Appl. Anim. Behav. Sci. 53:219–224.

Blecha, F., S. L. Boyles, and J. G. Riley. 1984. Shipping suppresses lymphocyte blastogenic responses in Angus and Brahman × Angus feeder calves. J. Anim. Sci. 59:576.

Boissy, A., and P. LeNeindre. 1997. Behavioral cardiac and cortisol responses to brief peer separation and reunion in cattle. Physiol. and Behavior 61:693–699.

Boissy, A. 1995. Fear and fearfulness in animals. Q. Rev. Biol. 70:165.

Chilcott, R. P., Stubbs, B. and Ashley, Z. 2001. Habituating pigs from in pen, non-invasive biophysical skin analysis. Lab Animal 35:230–235.

Crookshank, H. R., M. H. Elissalde, R. G. White, D. C. Clanton, and H. E. Smalley. 1979. Effect of transportation and handling of calves upon blood serum composition. J. Anim. Sci. 48:430–435.

Dantzer, R., and P. Mormede. 1983. Stress in farm animals: A need for re-evaluation. J. Anim. Sci. 57:6–18.

Davis, M. 1992. The role of the Amygdala in fear and anxiety. Ann. Rev. Neurosci. 15:353.

Doney, J. M., R. G. Smith, and F. G. Gunn. 1976. Effects of postmating environmental stress on administration of ACTH on early embryonic loss in sheep. J. Agric. Sci. 87:133.

Fell, L. R., I. G. Colditz, K. H. Walker, and D. L. Watson. 1999. Associations between temperament, performance and immune function in cattle entering a commercial feedlot. Aust. J. Exp. Agric. 39:795–802.

Ferguson, D. L., and Rosales-Ruiz J. 2001. Loading the problem loader: The effects of target training and shaping on trailer loading behavior in horses. J. Applied Behavior Analysis 34:409–423.

Fordyce, G. 1987. Weaner training. Queensland Agric. J. 6:323–324.

Fordyce, G., R. M. Dodt, and J. R. Wythes. 1988. Cattle temperaments in extensive herds in northern Queensland. Australian. J. Exp. 28:683–688.

Fulkerson, W. J., and P. A. Jamieson. 1982. Pattern of cortisol release in sheep following administration of synthetic ACTH or imposition of various stress agents. Australia J. Biol. Sci. 35:215.

Galyean, M. L., R. W. Lee, and M. W. Hubbert. 1981. Influence of fasting and transit on rumen blood metabolites in beef steers. J. Anim. Sci. 53:7.

Geverink, N. A., A. Kappers, E. Van de Burgwal, E. Lambooij, J. H. Blokhuis, and V. M. Wiegant. 1998. Effects of regular moving and handling on the behavioral and physiological responses of pigs to preslaughter treatment and consequences for meat quality. J. of Anim. Sci. 76:2080–2085.

Gilbert, B. J., and C. W. Arave. 1986. Ability of cattle to distinguish among different wavelengths of light. J. of Dairy Sci. 69:825–832.

Gloor, P., A. Oliver, and L. F. Quesney. 1981. The role of the amygdala in the expression of psychic phenomenon in temporal lobe seizures. In The Amygdaloid complex, Y. Ben Avi. (Ed.), 62. Elsevier, New York, NY.

Grandin, T. 1980. Observations of cattle behavior applied to the design of handling facilities. Appl. Anim. Ethol. 6:9.

——. 1987. Animal handling. In: Veterinary clinics of North America, Vol. 3, E. O. Price (Ed.), 323. W.B. Saunders, Philadelphia, PA.

——. 1989. Voluntary acceptance of restraint in sheep. Appl. Anim. Behav. Sci. 23:257.

——. 1993. Environmental and genetic factors which contribute to handling problems at pork slaughter plants. In: Livestock environment IV, E. Collins and C. Boone (Eds.). Am. Soc. Ag Enc., St. Joseph, MI.

——. 1996. Thinking in pictures. Doubleday, New York; Vintage Press, New York.

——. 1997a. Assessment of stress during handling and transport. J. Anim. Sci. 74:249.

——. 1997b. Thinking the way animals do. Western Horseman, November, 140–145.

——. 1998a. The feasibility of using vocalization scoring as an indicator of poor welfare during slaughter. Appl. Anim. Behav. Sci. 56:121–128.

——. 1998b. Handling methods and facilities to reduce stress on cattle. Vet. Clinics of North America: Food Animal Practice 14:325–341.

——. 1998c. Objective scoring of animal handling and stunning practices in slaughter plants. J. of the Am. Vet. Med. Assoc. 212:36–93.

——. 2000a. Behavioural principles of cattle handling under extensive conditions. In: Livestock handling and transport, T. Grandin (Ed.), 11. CAB International, Wallingford, UK.

——. 2000b. Livestock handling and transport. CAB International, Wallingford, Oxon, UK.

——. 2001. Welfare of cattle during slaughter and the prevention of nonambulatory (downer) cattle. J. Am. Vet. Med. Assoc. 219:1377–1382.

Grandin, T., and M. J. Deesing. 1998. Genetics and behavior during handling, restraint and herding. In: Genetics and the behavior of domestic animals, T. Grandin (Ed.). Academic Press, San Diego, CA.

Grandin, T., K. G. Odde, D. N. Schutz, and L. M. Behrns. 1994. The reluctance to change a learned choice may confound choice tests. Appl. Anim. Behavior. Sci. 39:21–28.

Grandin, T., M. B. Rooney, M. Phillips, R. C. Cambre, N. A. Irlbeck, and W. Graffam. 1995. Conditioning of Nyala (*Tragelaphus angasi*) to blood sampling in a crate with positive reinforcement. Zool. Biol. 14:261–273.

Grandin, T., S. E. Curtis, and I. A. Taylor. 1987. Toys, mingling and driving reduce excitability in pigs. J. Anim. Sci. 65 (Suppl. 1):230 (Abs.).

Grignard, L., Boivin, X., Boissy, A., and LeNeindre. 2001. Do beef cattle react consistently to different handling situations. Appl. Anim. Behav. Sci., 71:263–276.

Hargreaves, A. L., and G. D. Hutson. 1990. The stress response in sheep during routine handling procedures. Appl. Anim. Behav. Sci. 26:83.

Hastings, B. E., D. E. Abbott, and L. M. George. 1992. Stress factors influencing plasma cortisol levels and adrenal weights in Chinese water deer (*Hydropotes inermis*). Res. Vet. Sci. 53:375.

Hearnshaw, H., and C. A. Morris. 1984. Genetic and environment effects on a temperament score in beef cattle. Australian J. Agric. Res. 35:723.

Hearnshaw, H., R. Barlow, and G. Want. 1979. Development of a temperament or handling difficulty score for cattle. Proc. Australian Assoc., Anim. Breeding Genet. 1:164.

Hedigar, H. 1968. The psychology and behavior of animals in zoos and circuses. Dover Publications, New York.

Heffner, R. S., and H. E. Heffner. 1983. Hearing in large mammals: Horses (*Equus caballus*) and cattle (*Bos taurus*). Behav. Neurosci. 97(2):299–309.

——. 1992. Hearing in large mammals: sound-localization acuity in cattle. (*Bos taurus*) and goats (*Capra hircus*). J. of Comparative Psychology 106:107–113.

Hemsworth, P. H., and G. J. Coleman. 1998. Human-livestock interactions: The stockperson and the productivity of intensively farmed animals. CAB International, Wallingford, Oxon, UK.

Hemsworth, P. H., and J. L. Barnett. 1991. The effects of aversively handled pigs either individually or in groups on their behavior, growth and corticosteroids. Appl. Anim. Behav. Sci. 30:61.

Hemsworth, P. H., G. J. Coleman, J. C. Barnett, S. Borg, and S. Dowling. 2002. The effect of cognitive behavioral interventions on the attitude and behavior of stockpersons and the behavior and productivity of commercial dairy cows. J. Anim. Sci. 80:68–78.

Hixon, D. L., D. K. Kesler, and T. R. Troxel. 1981. Reproductive hormone secretions and first service conception rate subsequent to ovulation control with Synchromate B. Theriogenology 16:219.

Hopster, H., J. T. vanderWert, J. H. Erkens, and H. J. Blokhuis. 1999. Effects of repeated jugular puncture on plasma cortisol concentrations in loose housed dairy cows. J. Anim. Sci. 77:708–714.

Hutson, G. D. 1985. The influence of barley food rewards on sheep movements through a handling system. Appl. Anim. Behav. Sci. 14:263.

——. 2000. Behavioral principles of sheep handling. In: Livestock handling and transport, T. Grandin (Ed.), 127. CAB International, Wallingford, UK.

Jacobs, G. H., J. F. Deegan, and J. Neitz. 1998. Photopigment basis for dichromatic colour vision in cows, goats and sheep. Visual Neuroscience 15:581–584.

Kelly, K. W., C. Osborn, J. Evermann, S. Parish, and D. Hinrichs. 1981. Whole blood leukocytes vs. separated mononuclear cell blastogenis in calves, time dependent changes after shipping. Can. J. Comp. Med. 45:249.

Kemble, E. D., D. C. Blanchard, R. J. Blanchard, and R. Takushi. 1984. Taming in wild rats following medial amygdaloid lesions. Physiol. Behav. 32:131.

Kilgour, R. and D. C. Dalton. 1984. Livestock behaviour. University of New South Wales Press, Sydney, NSW, Australia.

Koba, Y. and H. Tanida. 1999. How do miniature pigs discriminate between people. The effect of exchanging cues between a non-handler and their familiar handler on discrimination. Appl. Anim. Behav. Sci., 61:239–252.

Lanier, E. K., T. H. Friend, D. M. Bushong, D. A. Knabe, T. H. Champney, and D. G. Lay. 1995. Swine habituation as a model for eustress and distress in the pig. J. Anim. Sci. 73(Suppl. 1):126 (Abs.).

Lanier, J. L., T. Grandin, A. Chaffin, and T. Chaffin. 1999. Training American bison calves. Bison World, October-November, 94–99.

Lanier, J. L., T. Grandin, R. D. Green, and K. McGee. 2000. The relationship between reaction to sudden intermittent movements and sounds to temperament. J. Anim. Sci. 78:1467–1474.

Lawrence, A. B., E. M. C. Terlouw, and A. W. Illius. 1991. Individual differences in behavioral responses to pigs exposed to non-social and social challenge. Appl. Anim. Behav. Sci. 30:73–78.

LeDoux, J. E. 1994. Emotion, memory and the brain. Sci. Am. 271:50.

——. 1996. The emotional brain. Simon and Schuster, New York.

Lehman, W. B., and G. H. Patterson. 1964. Depth perception in sheep effects of interrupting the mother–neonate bond. Science 145:835–836.

Littlefield, V., Grandin, T., and Lanier, T. L. 2001. Quiet handling reduces aversion to restraint. J. Anim. Sci. 79:277 (Suppl.) (Abstract).

Maday, J. 2002. Pressure not stress. Drover's Journal, February, Feeder Management, 1–5.

Mertshing, H. J., and A. W. Kelly. 1983. Restraint reduces the size of thymus gland and PHA swelling in pigs. J. Anim. Sci. 57 (Suppl. 1):175.

Miller, N. E. 1960. Learning resistance to pain and fear effects of over-learning, exposure and reward exposure in context. J. Exp. Psycholo. 60:137.

Peischel, P. A., R. R. Schalles, and C. E. Owenby. 1980. Effect of stress on calves grazing Kansas hills range. J. Anim. Sci. Suppl. 24:25 (Abstract).

Phillips, M., T. Grandin, W. Graffam, N. A. Irlbeck, and R. C. Cambre. 1998. Crate conditioning of bongo (*Tragelaphus eurycerus*) for veterinary and husbandry procedures at Denver Zoological Garden, Zoo Biology 17:25–32.

Pick, D. F., G. Lovell, S. Brown, and D. Dail. 1994. Equine color vision revisited. Appl. Anim. Behav. Sci. 42:61–65.

Price, E. O., and S. J. R. Wallach. 1990. Physical isolation of hand reared Hereford bulls increases their aggressiveness towards humans. Appl. Anim. Behav. Sci. 27:263–267.

Prince, J. H. 1977. The eye and vision. In: M. J. Swenson (eds.), Dukes physiology of domestic animals. Cornell University Press, Ithaca, NY; 696–712.

Redgate, E. S., and E. E. Fahringer. 1973. A comparison of pituitary adrenal activity elicited by electrical stimulation of preoptic amygdaloid and hypothalamic sites in the rat brain. Neuroendocrinology, 12:334.

Reinken, G. 1988. General and economic aspects of deer farming. In: H. W. Reid (ed.), The management and health of farmed deer. London; 53–59.

Ried, R. L., and S. C. Mills. 1962. Studies of carbohydrate metabolism of sheep. XVI. The adrenal response to physiological stress. Australian Journal of Agricultural Research, 13:282–294.

Rogan, M. T., and J. E. LeDoux. 1996. Emotion: Systems, cells and synaptic plasticity. Cell 85:369.

Smith, B. 1998. Moving 'em: A guide to low stress animal handling. Graziers Hui. Kamuela, Hawaii.

Stermer, R., T. H. Camp, and D. G. Stevens. 1981. Feeder cattle stress during transportation, Paper No. 81–6001. Am. Soc. of Ag. Engineers, St. Joseph, MI.

Talling, J. C., N. K. Waran, and C. M. Wathes. 1996. Behavioral and physiological responses of pigs to sound. Appl. Anim. Behav. Sci., 48:187–202.

Talling, J. C., N. K. Waran, C. M. Watheres, and J. A. Lines. 1998. Sound avoidance by domestic pigs depends upon characteristics of the signal. Applied Animal Behavior Sci. 58(3–4):255–266.

Tellington-Jones, L., and Bruns, L. 1985. An introduction to the Tellington-Jones Equine Awareness Method. Breakthrough Publications, Millwood, NY.

Tillman, A. 1981. Speechless brothers: The history and care of llamas. Early Winters Press, Seattle, WA.

Voisinet, B. D., T. Grandin, J. D. Tatum, S. F. O'Connor, and J. J. Struthers. 1997a. Feedlot cattle with calm temperaments have higher average daily weight gains than cattle with excitable temperaments. J. Anim. Sci. 75:892–896.

Voisinet, B. D., T. Grandin, S. F. O'Connor, J. D. Tatum, and M. J. Deesing. 1997. *Bos indicus* cross feedlot cattle with excitable temperaments have tougher meat and a higher incidence of borderline dark cutters. Meat Sci. 46:367.

Waynert, D. E., J. M. Stookey, J. M. Schwartzkopf-Gerwein, C. S. Watts, and C. S. Waltz. 1999. Response of beef cattle to noise during handling. Appl. Anim. Behav. Sci. 62:27–42.

Whittlestone, W. G., R. Kilgore, H. deLangren, and G. Duirs. 1970. Behavioural stress and the cell count of bovine milk. J. Milk Food Technol. 33:217.

8

Principles for the Design of Handling Facilities and Transport Systems

Temple Grandin

INTRODUCTION

Simple changes in an animal handling facility will often greatly facilitate the movement of animals through the facility. This chapter will cover ways to make improvements in existing facilities and the design of new facilities for handling cattle, horses, deer, and other grazing animals. Pigs will also be covered. An understanding of the behavioral principles of facility design will make it easy to design efficient facilities for handling animals during vaccinations, veterinary work, sorting, weighing, and other procedures. Facilities based on behavioral principles will improve animal welfare and help prevent injuries to both animals and people.

REMOVE DISTRACTIONS THAT IMPEDE ANIMAL MOVEMENT

Animals notice little details and distractions that people do not notice, such as moving objects or shadows with harsh contrasts of light and dark. A small, swinging piece of chain hanging down in the entrance of a chute may cause animals to balk and refuse to enter (Grandin, 1980b, 1996; fig. 8.1). Animals should move through a facility easily. Quiet handling is impossible if animals constantly balk, back up, or turn back. The distractions that cause balking and backing up should be located and removed instead of resorting to more force to move the animals. Handlers need to carefully observe to see what is causing an animal to balk (Grandin, 1998b,c). A calm animal will look right at the thing it is afraid of. It will show you the distraction that needs to be removed. If removal is not possible, the animal should be allowed to slowly investigate the distraction. Most animals will be willing to move forward after they have looked at or sniffed a distraction such as a shadow or drain grate on the floor.

To find distractions that impede animal movement, you need to walk through the chutes and pens to see what the animals are seeing. It is important to bend down and get your eyes at the same level as the animal's eyes. Reflections on wet floors often cause animals to refuse to move. A reflection that is visible at the animal's eye height may not be visible when you are standing up.

Anything that makes rapid movement is likely to make animals stop. Look for swinging chains, people moving outside the chute, vehicles, shiny metal that jiggles, a flapping

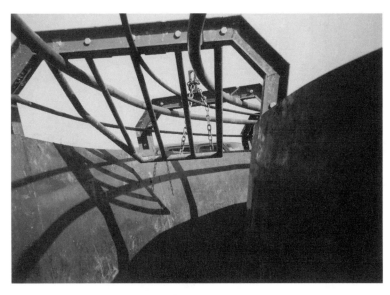

Figure 8.1.   The loose chain end dangling in their chute must be removed because it will make animals balk. The shadows may also cause balking and refusing to move.

piece of plastic, or fan blades turning in the wind. Air blowing into the faces of approaching animals will also cause them to back up. Ventilation systems must be designed so that air does not blow into the faces of approaching animals.

Sensitive to Contrasts of Light and Dark

All grazing animals are sensitive to harsh contrasts of light and dark. Facilities should be painted a single, solid color to prevent balking at contrasts of light and dark. Shadows will often cause animals to stop (Hutson, 1980b; Kilgour, 1971). Balking due to shadows is often worse on a bright, sunny day. Changing shadows can cause a facility to work well at one time of day and poorly at another time. Figure 8.1 shows shadows in a chute.

Drain grates in the middle of the floor will often make animals balk (Grandin, 1982; Lynch and Alexander, 1973). A good drainage design is to slope the concrete floor in the working area toward an open drainage ditch located outside the fences. The open drainage ditch outside the fences needs no cover, and it is easier to clean. Animals are sensitive to changes in flooring type or texture. They may refuse to move from a dirt floor onto concrete. Balking can often be reduced by putting some dirt on the concrete floor. Animals will also balk if they see a high-contrast object. A coat flung over a chute fence or the shiny reflection off a car bumper will cause balking. A bright yellow raincoat is very likely to cause animals to refuse to move. Dairy cows that move through a facility every day will learn to walk over shadows and drains because they are no longer novel. However, a dairy cow will balk if she sees a strange piece of paper on the floor or a coat hung over a fence. The new

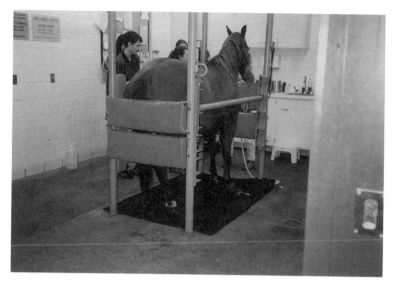

Figure 8.2.   Well-designed padded horse stock with nonslip floor. If the horse refuses to step onto the mat, it should be allowed to sniff and investigated it. Animals will often balk when flooring color, type, or texture changes.

heifers will balk at drains that the experienced cows will ignore. Figure 8.2 shows a horse stock with a black mat on a concrete floor. If the horse balks and refuses to step onto the new floor surface, it should be given an opportunity to investigate and sniff the mat.

Effects of Light

Many species of animals have a tendency to move toward the light but they will not approach blinding light (Van Putten and Elshof, 1978; Grandin, 1980b). If you ever have to handle livestock at night, it is strongly recommended that indirect lighting that does not glare in the animal's face be positioned inside of the truck or building. However, loading ramps and squeeze chutes should face either north or south; this is because animals may balk if they have to look directly into the sun. Sometimes it is difficult to persuade animals to enter a darker roofed working area. Persuading animals to enter a dark building from an outdoor pen in bright sunlight is often difficult. In some cases, animals will enter if doors are opened up so that incoming animals can see daylight through the other side of the building. Movement into a building can often be improved by installing white translucent panels in the walls or roof so that the animals will be attracted toward the light (Grandin, 1998a)(fig. 8.3). Translucent panels let in lots of shadow-free light. Problems with getting animals to move into a darker building are most likely to occur on a bright, sunny day. A facility that works poorly on a bright, sunny day may work well at night or on a cloudy day. The ideal illumination inside a building for moving animals should resemble a bright, cloudy day (fig. 8.3).

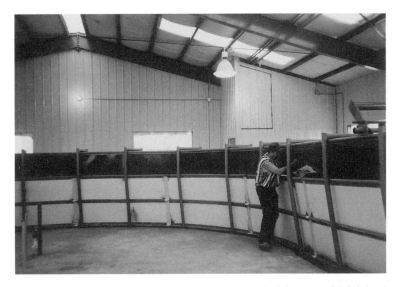

Figure 8.3.   Cattle handling facility with white translucent plastic skylights to provide bright, shadow-free light. Solid sides on the single-file chute keep cattle calmer. To move the animals, the handler lifts up the rubber curtain along the top of the chute.

Many people make the mistake of placing the single-file chute and squeeze chute entirely inside a building and the crowding pen outside. Balking will be reduced if the single-file chute is extended 10 ft. to 15 ft. (3 m to 4.5 m) outside the building. The animals will enter more easily if they are lined up single file before they enter the dark building. The wall of the building should *never* be placed at the junction between the single-file chute and the crowding pen.

In indoor facilities, lamps are effective for attracting animals into chutes. Animals will often refuse to enter a dark place. Handling was greatly improved in several slaughter plants when lights were installed on the entrance of chutes and restrainers (Grandin, 1996, 2000b). In one place, the pigs stopped balking and backing up when a ceiling lamp was moved two feet. Moving the lamp eliminated a reflection on the wet floor. Lighting works best when it is indirect. It must not shine directly into the eyes of approaching animals.

Visual Cliff Effect

Animals will often refuse to walk over a floor grating if they see the visual cliff effect. This is why a cattle guard works. The animals see the steep drop off under the bars. Ruminants can perceive depth (Lehman and Patterson, 1964). Sheep will balk and may refuse to move over a slatted floor if they can see light coming up between the slats. This is a common problem in Australian shearing sheds. When conveyor restrainers are used for handling animals in slaughter plants or on farms, a false floor should be installed to prevent entering animals from seeing the visual cliff effect under the conveyor (Grandin, 1991, 2000a,b, 2003). The false floor is installed so that it provides the optical illusion of a solid floor to walk on, but it is about 8 in. (20 cm) below the feet of an animal that is riding on the conveyor.

Solid Sides and Blocking Vision

Solid sides are recommended on chutes, restrainers, crowd pens, and loading ramps for cattle, deer, wild horses, bison, and other grazing animals (Grandin 1980a,b, 1997; Rider, Butchbaker, and Harp, 1974). Solid sides prevent animals from seeing distractions outside the chute such as moving people or vehicles. Grazing animal behavior is controlled by the animal's vision. Adding solid sides to a chute will often help keep animals quieter. Solid sides are especially important when animals with a large flight zone are handled, such as bison and wild mustang horses. They should be placed on the single-file chute that leads to the squeeze chute, crowd pen, crowd gate, and the loading ramp. A solid crowd gate prevents the animals from turning back to the pens where they came from (fig. 8.4). Solid sides make little difference if animals are completely tame and have no flight zone. A tame, halter-broke cow or horse does not need solid sides. A basic principle is that the bigger the flight zone and the wilder the animal, the more you need a visually solid barrier.

A solid side placed in between a person and cattle, sheep, wild horses, or bison will reduce the size of the flight zone (Hutson, 1980b; Grandin, 2000b). Even a partial solid side has some effect. It appears that animals feel safer when they have something solid between themselves and a person. Nyala and Bongo antelopes at the Denver Zoo were trained to enter a box for blood testing and veterinary treatments. A box with solid sides was used to handle the antelopes (Grandin et al., 1995; Phillips et al., 1998). The technician reached through openings in the box to take blood samples. Even though the antelope could see the

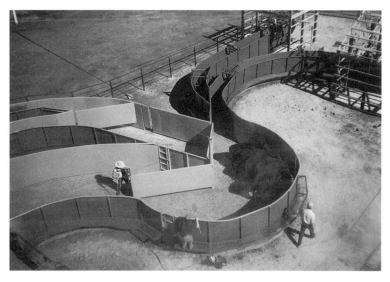

Figure 8.4.   Curved handling facility with solid sides. Handler works on catwalks alongside the cattle. Catwalks should not be placed overhead.

person through the openings, the size of the flight zone was decreased to zero. Large Bongo antelopes with a 30-ft. (10 m) flight zone could be touched and manipulated in the box. They would even eat from the handler's hand when a treat was held at the opening.

Solid shields can be strategically placed to prevent approaching animals from seeing people ahead (Kilgour, 1971). In several facilities where I have worked, building shields for people to stand behind greatly improved animal movement through the chutes. The principle of blocking vision explains why a solid panel works well for moving pigs. Animals respect a solid barrier even if it is a flimsy piece of plastic. If they cannot see through it, then they usually do not attempt to go through it. A belly rail that presents a visual barrier at animal eye height will prevent excited grazing animals from running through a cable fence (Ward, 1958). Wild ungulates and horses can be controlled in pens constructed from canvass or plastic sheets (Fowler, 1995; Wyman, 1946; Amaral, 1977). On pig farms and in packing plants, heavy stiff pig boards can often be replaced with a plastic flag. Pigs will usually not attempt to run through the flag because they cannot see through it. In some pork plants, a curtain made from conveyor belting has been used to replace steel sliding gates. This design prevents injuries caused by steel gates.

CHUTE DESIGN

For cattle, sheep, and wild horses, a single-file curved chute leading up to a squeeze chute, truck, or stunning box works better than a straight chute for three reasons. First, it prevents the animal from seeing the truck, the squeeze chute, or people until it is almost in the truck or squeeze chute. A curved chute also takes advantage of the animal's natural tendency to circle around the handler (Grandin, 1987; Barber and Freeman, 2000). When you enter a pen of cattle or sheep, you have probably noticed that the animals will turn and face you but maintain a safe distance. As you move through the pen, the animals will keep looking at you and circle around you as you move. A curved chute also takes advantage of the natural behavior of cattle to go back to where they came from.

A well-designed, curved, single-file chute has a catwalk for the handler to use beside the inner radius. Working along the inner radius puts the handler in the best position to move the animals (fig. 8.4). Another design that is getting popular is to make the outer radius of the single-file chute completely solid to block vision and the inner radius has a 4-ft. (1.2 m) high solid side, which allows the cattle to see out. The catwalk is eliminated and the handler works on the ground by penetrating and then retreating from the flight zone. Walking back by the point of balance works well in this type of facility. Another alternative is to block the opening along the top of the chute with a flexible rubber curtain made from conveyor belting. If an animal stops moving, a handler on the ground can lift up the curtain (fig. 8.3).

For all species, the crowd pen or "tub" should have a solid fence that prevents the animals from seeing out. Circular crowd pens should be laid out to take advantage of the animal's natural tendency to go back to where it came from (figs. 8.4 and 8.5). This will require at least a half circle. The ideal radius (gate length) for round crowd pens is 12 ft. (3.5 m) for cattle, wild horses, and bison; 8 ft. (2.5 m) for pigs; and 10 ft. (3 m) for sheep.

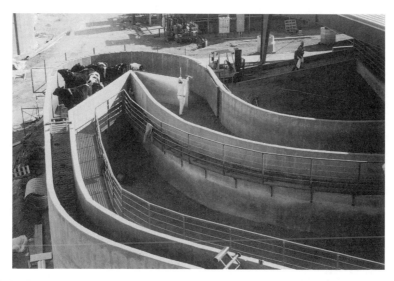

Figure 8.5.   Curved chutes and round crowd pens work efficiently because they take advantage of the natural tendency of animals to go back to where they came from. This facility has a straight section of single-file chute so that the cattle see a place to go before going around the herd.

Animals will be more difficult to handle if the pen is too small or too big. Catwalks should never be placed overhead. People walking over the animals frightens them. The best catwalk design is to locate the catwalk at 42 in. (76 cm) from the top of the fence to the catwalk. The chute or crowd-pen fence should be at waist height on the average person.

Using single-file chutes and making animals stand in a queue works well for cattle, wild horses, and sheep. Lining up in single file is natural for these species. These animals will stand quietly in a queue as long as they can see the next animal in front of them less than 3 ft. (1 m) away. American bison and elk (wapiti) often become severely agitated and injure themselves while waiting in a single-file line. For these species, the single file can be greatly shortened or even eliminated. Canadian elk producers have designed handling facilities where small groups of animals are moved through a series of small pens. The pens have solid sides and the handler works from the ground (Matthews, 2000). Similar designs have been used successfully with bison. Pigs also become agitated standing in a single-file queue. Some of the best systems are designed so that the pigs can move through without having to wait in line.

Tie Open Backstop Gates to Reduce Balking

Many cattle, pig, and sheep facilities have too many backstop gates in the single-file chute to prevent animals from backing up. Too many backstop gates can increase balking because the animals may refuse to walk through the devices. If cattle or other animals constantly back up, this is a symptom of a problem that needs to be corrected. The distractions discussed previously should be removed. If cattle balk at a backstop gate at the single-file chute entrance, it should be either tied open or equipped with a remote control rope so that it can be held open for the cattle. In a well-designed beef cattle facility with a curved, single-file chute, the only backstop gate that is really needed should be located two body lengths behind the squeeze chute. This will prevent the leaders from backing out.

Problems with balking tend to come in bunches; when one animal balks, the tendency to balk seems to spread to the next animals in line (Grandin, 1980b). When an animal is being moved through a single-file chute, the animal must never be urged forward unless it has a place to go. Once it has balked, others will start balking.

Do Not Dead-End Your Curved Chute

All species of grazing animals will balk if the entrance to a single-file chute appears to be a dead end (Barber and Freeman, 2000; Grandin, 1987, 1998b). Sliding and one-way gates in the single-file chute must be constructed so that the animals can see through them, otherwise the animals will balk. This is especially important at the junction between the single-file chute and the crowd pen. However, palpation gates for pregnancy checking or artificial insemination should be solid so that approaching animals do not see a person standing in the chute.

When a curved chute is built, it must be laid out properly so that it does not appear to be a dead end. A cow, sheep, or horse standing in the crowd pen must be able to see a minimum of two body lengths up the chute. Animals will balk if the chute is bent too sharply at the junction between the crowd pen and the single-file chute. This is one of the worst design mistakes. Figure 8.6 illustrates an efficient, curved facility that is easy to lay out. The lay out works really well for cattle and wild horses. The round crowd pen (tub) in this facility works efficiently for all species because animals moving through the tub think they are going back to where they came from. The entire facility consists of three half circles laid out along a layout line (Grandin, 1998b). Curved bugle-shaped layouts that work well with sheep are shown in Barber and Freeman (2000). Pigs will tend to jam in funnel-shaped crowd pens that work well for cattle and sheep. The entrance of the chute should have an abrupt entrance to prevent jamming (Hoenderken, 1976; Grandin, 1982, 1987). An offset equal to the width of one pig works well.

RESTRAINT PRINCIPLES FOR ANIMALS WITH A LARGE FLIGHT ZONE

Cattle or bison sometimes become severely stressed and agitated in a conventional squeeze chute. This is due to deep invasion of the animal's flight zone by the operator and other people that can be seen through the open barred sides. Agitation and struggling can be reduced by installing solid sides or rubber louvers on the open-barred sides (fig. 8.7). Six- to eight-inch (15 to 20 cm) wide louvers made from rubber conveyor belting can be installed on the drop down bars. The strips of belting are installed on a 45 degree angle. The bars can still be opened, but incoming animals cannot see out as they enter. People who handle bison and deer have used solid sides on squeeze chutes for many years. Try experimenting by covering up the sides of the squeeze chute with cardboard. The most important part to cover is the back half nearest the tailgate.

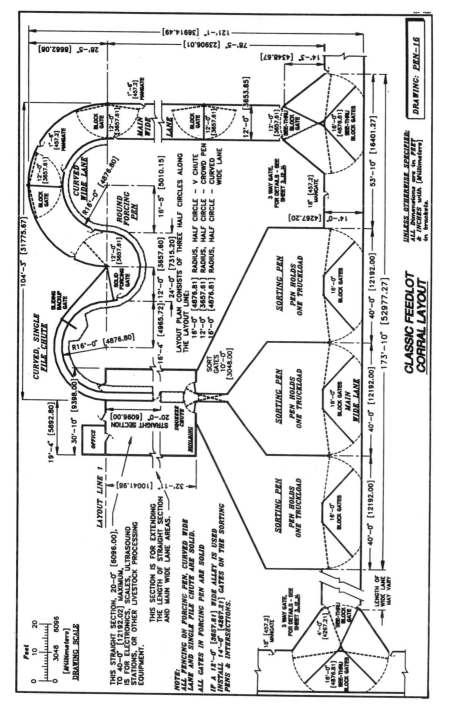

Figure 8.6. Corral system with a single-file chute, round crowd pen, and wide curved lane that are laid out in three half circles along a layout line. Curved facilities *must* be laid out correctly.

153

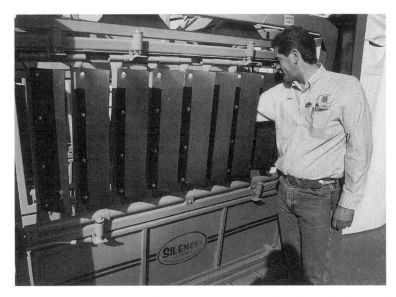

Figure 8.7.   Rubber louvers on the side of a squeeze chute prevent incoming cattle from seeing people. The louvers are on a 45°angle and they are attached to the drop down bars for easy access to the animal.

Bison squeeze chutes should have a solid gate located about 3 ft. to 4 ft. (1 m to 1.2 m) in front of the headgate. This gate prevents the animals from attempting to run through the headgate. A solid top is also recommended for bison and wild horses to prevent rearing. Even a piece of cardboard will work because it blocks vision. Many cattle sustain shoulder and neck injuries when they hit the headgate too hard. Cattle should go into and out of the squeeze chute at a walk. Solid sides will reduce lunging at the headgate and running. The animal lunges because it sees people through the open barred sides.

Observations of cattle handling at meat packing plants indicates that squeeze chutes on ranches and feedlots need to be modified. Blocking the animal's vision has a great calming effect. I spent 35 hours operating a restraining chute used for kosher slaughter. It consists of a box with completely solid sides and a small T-shaped opening in the front for the animal's head. When an animal enters the box it cannot see people. After it sticks its head through the front opening, a metal shield prevents it from seeing people. A light over the head hole entices the animal to stick its head through. Most cattle walk in quietly and seldom attempt to lunge at the head opening. The cattle at this packing plant were calmer than cattle entering a conventional squeeze chute with open bar sides.

Since the animals did not attempt to run through the chute, squeeze pressure could be applied slowly instead of suddenly. Slow steady motion had a calming effect. Sudden jerky motion or sudden bumping of the animal with the apparatus caused agitation and excitement. When the animal's vision was blocked by metal side panels, it would stand and allow its head and body to be positioned in the device. The cattle seldom resisted pressure from the apparatus if it was applied slowly and excessive pressure, which would cause pain and discomfort, was avoided. There is also the concept of optimum pressure. Sufficient pressure must be applied to make the animal "feel restrained" but excessive pressure, which would cause pain, must be avoided. Many people make the mistake of applying more pressure when an animal struggles. The animal will often stop struggling if the pressure is reduced slightly. Excessive pressure must be slowly eased off. A sudden release of the pressure will cause the animal to become excited.

Behavioral Principles of Restraint

Below is a list of the behavioral principles of low-stress restraint for grazing animals. Principles 1 and 2 apply to animals that are not completely tame and principles 3 through 7 apply to both tame and wild animals of all species.

1. *Block vision outside the facility* to prevent the animals from seeing people deep in their flight zone. Blindfolding or darkness will reduce stress. Both practical experience and research show that blocking vision has a calming effect on both mammals and poultry (Ewbank, 2000; Grandin, 1992, 2000a; Douglas, Darre, and Kinsman, 1984; Jones, Satterlee, and Cadd, 1998; Andrade et al., 2001; Joe Stookey, personal communication, 2002).

2. *Block vision of an escape route.* Animals will remain calmer if their vision is blocked until they are fully restrained and feel held in a restraint device (Grandin, 2000b, 1998c, 1991). Restraint devices for elk are equipped with curtains that block the animal's vision until the animal is fully restrained (Mathews, 2000). Cattle entering a restraining apparatus must see a lighted area or a small lighted window. They will not walk into a dark space.

3. *Slow steady pressure* applied by a restraint device is calming and sudden jerky motion by either equipment or people causes excitement and agitation (Grandin, 1992). The use of devices where the floor is suddenly dropped often causes fright. Their use is usually not recommended unless they are designed so that the animal's body does not suddenly fall.

4. *Optimum pressure.* A restraint device must apply sufficient pressure to provide the feeling of being held, but excessive pressure that causes pain must be avoided. Even pressure applied to the body has a relaxing effect (Grandin, Dodman, and Shuster, 1989)(fig. 8.8). Some pigs will go to sleep in a sling that fully supports them (Panepinto, 1983). The sling has openings for the legs and fully supports the body and head with even pressure. The device must be designed so that pressure is distributed over a wide enough body area to prevent pinching or pressure points. V-shaped restrainers that support the animal's body between two angled sides work well for sheep and fat pigs because the body is supported with even pressure (Regensburger, 1940). They work poorly for lean pigs with large hams because the restrainer pinches the hams and fails to support the shoulders. Lambooy (1986) observed that veal calves were not fully supported in a V restrainer. The double rail restrainer where the animal straddles two bars is more comfortable than a V restrainer for calves and cattle (Giger et al., 1977; Grandin, 1988).

For wild horses, elk, and deer, restraints are available that have heavy, thick foam padding that is covered with plastic. The thick foam prevents injuries and encases the animal with even pressure. If animals struggle or vocalize, the pressure may be too tight or

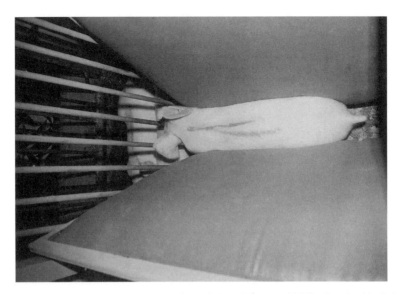

Figure 8.8.   Foam-padded V-shaped restrainer for a piglet. Piglets would fall asleep in this device when they had a herdmate beside them. The herdmate is located in front of the restrained pig. The two animals can touch each other.

the animal is being pinched or poked by a sharp edge. Excessive pressure from a restraint device will make cattle vocalize (Grandin, 1998a,b, 2000a). If animals vocalize or struggles in direct response to application of a restraint, there is likely to be a problem that needs to be corrected.

5. *A companion near them.* Animals will remain calmer during restraint if they have either a familiar person with them or a herdmate (fig. 8.8). Cattle and other grazing animals will stand more quietly and remain calmer if they can see another bovine within 3 ft. (1 m) of them, but they may lunge and become excited if they see herdmates many meters away. They become excited because they want to rejoin their herdmates.

6. *No fear of falling.* The restraint method must not trigger the righting reflex and fear of falling. This principle applies to both mechanical restraint devices and holding an animal in your hands. The animal's body must be supported. In devices where the animal is held with its feet off the ground, it must be held in an upright position with its body fully supported. Tilting chutes that lay an animal on its side must fully support the animal's body. Animals panic if they feel that they might fall.

Devices such as the Panepinto sling for pigs, the double rail, center-track conveyor restrainer, and V conveyor restrainers are designed to fully support the body. Westervelt et al. (1976) found that straddling a conveyor was a low-stress method of restraint. Animals will struggle if they feel off balance. More information on restraint device design can be found in Grandin, 1986; Panepinto, 1983; Mathews, 2000; Fowler, 1995; Grandin, 1988, 1991, 1992, 1994, 1995, 2000b; Haigh 1992, 1995, 1999; and Haigh and Hudson, 1993. Ramps and chutes leading into and out of any type of restraint device must be nonslip. Squeeze chutes with sides that squeeze evenly on both sides will keep the animal balanced.

The use of devices that invert animals onto their backs should be avoided. Full inversion is highly stressful for many types of animals (Dunn, 1990).

7. *Never leave an animal unattended* in a restraint device. Even a tame, trained animal may panic and injure itself if it is left alone.

Adjustment of Squeeze Chutes

The use of a complete squeeze chute is strongly recommended for animals that are not trained to head restraint. Restraint of the body will prevent the animal from fighting the headgate. For untrained extensively raised beef cattle, body restraint is less aversive than head restraint (Grandin, 1992). On hydraulic restraint devices, the pressure relief valve must be adjusted to prevent excessive squeeze pressure. The animal must be able to breath normally and show no signs of straining. Excessive pressure can cause severe injuries such as ruptured diaphragm or broken bones. If an animal strains or vocalizes (moos or bellows) when the valve lever is held down until the valve bypasses, the pressure setting is too high. Devices for restraining the head must be designed to avoid distress. If the animal struggles or vocalizes at the moment the device is applied, it will need to be redesigned or the pressure may have to be reduced.

To prevent choking in a headgate with curved stanchion bars (fig. 8.9), the squeeze sides must be adjusted so that the V shape of the sides prevents the animals from lying down (Grandin, 1980a). Pressure exerted by the headgate on the carotid arteries can kill the animal (White, 1961). If an animal collapses while held in a headgate, the headgate must be

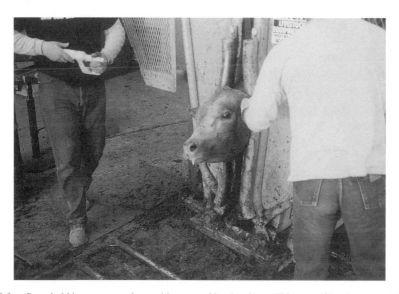

Figure 8.9.   Steer held in a squeeze chute with a curved bar headgate. This type of headgate provides good control of head movement and it must be used with a body squeeze to prevent the animal from lying down. If the animal lies down, it can choke. If a headgate is used with no body restraint, it should have straight vertical neck bars that allow the animal to safely lie down with no pressure on the underside of the neck. These principles apply to all species.

released immediately to avoid death. Some veterinarians prefer a chute that does not pinch the feet together at the bottom. If a squeeze chute with straight sides is used, it must be equipped with a straight bar stanchion headgate to prevent choking. An animal can safely lie down in a straight bar stanchion because no pressure is exerted on the underside of the neck. Care must be taken with self-catching headgates. Cattle can be injured if they run into the self-catcher at a high speed. Self-catchers are usually not recommended for wild horned cattle. It is also essential to adjust the self-catcher for the size of the cattle. NEVER, NEVER leave an animal unattended in any restraint device.

Severe injuries can occur if a self-catcher is adjusted too wide and the animal's shoulder passes part way through the closed gate. Latches and ratchet locks must be kept well maintained to prevent accidents to people. If a ratchet device becomes worn, replace it immediately. Friction-type latches must never be oiled. Oiling will destroy the ability of a friction latch to hold. On self-catching headgates, the mechanism must be kept maintained to prevent an animal from getting stuck part way through a closed gate.

Dark Box Chute and Dark Rooms

Cows and other animals can be easily restrained for artificial insemination (AI) or pregnancy testing in a dark box chute that has no headgate or squeeze (Parsons and Helphinstine, 1969; Canada Plan Service, 1984). This is an example of using behavior instead of force to restrain an animal. Even the wildest cow can be restrained with a minimum of excitement. Deer and elk are routinely handled in a darkened room. Deer that have a large flight zone in daylight can often be touched in a darkened room.

The dark box chute can be easily constructed from plywood or steel. It has solid sides, top, and front. When the cow is inside the box, she is inside a quiet, snug, dark enclosure. A chain or bar is latched behind her rump to keep her in. After insemination, the cow is released through a gate in either the front or the side of the dark box. If wild cows are being handled, an extra long, dark box can be constructed. A tame cow that is not in heat is used as a pacifier and is placed in the chute in front of the cow to be bred. Even a wild cow will stand quietly and place her head on the pacifier cow's rump. After breeding, the cow is allowed to exit through a side gate, while the pacifier cow remains in the chute.

AVOID AVERSIVE RESTRAINT METHODS

Animals that are being used for biomedical research or other research where they will be handled many times will be less stressed and easier to handle if they are trained to walk voluntarily into a restraint device. Feed rewards of the animal's favorite treat will make training easier. Training methods are covered in detail in Panepinto (1983); Grandin (1989); Grandin et al. (1995); Phillips et al. (1998); Hutson (1985); Ferguson and Rosales-Ruiz (2001); and Chilcott, Stubbs, and Ashley (2001). Painful restraint methods such as nose tongs should be avoided. Cattle that have been restrained with nose tongs become more and more difficult to restrain repeatedly. They also remember aversive experiences such as being accidentally banged on the head with the headgate of a squeeze chute

(Grandin et al., 1998b). The use of a halter is recommended. Practical experience has shown that cattle become easier and easier to restrain for blood testing from the jugular vein if a halter is used. Calves and polled cattle held in a headgate can be easily restrained for blood testing by a person pushing their heads over with his or her rear end. The person's rear covers the eyes and the animal will remain calmer. The animal will usually cooperate if steady pressure is applied and sudden jerky movement is avoided.

Electrical immobilization that paralyzes an animal must never be used as a substitute for well-designed restraint equipment. Scientific studies clearly show that electrical immobilization is highly aversive and detrimental to animal welfare (Pascoe, 1986; Grandin et al., 1986; Lambooy, 1985). Electrical immobilization with a small current should never be confused with electrical stunning that is used in slaughter plants. Electrical stunning uses a high-amperage current that induces instantaneous unconsciousness.

Nonslip Flooring

Low-stress animal handling is impossible if animals constantly slip on the floor (Grandin, 1983). Even slight slipping can make an animal become agitated and nervous. The two most common facility problems that make quiet handling difficult are slick floors and lighting problems that cause animals to balk. In many cases, older facilities that are not state of the art are often adequate provided that they are well maintained, have nonslip flooring, and do not have the lighting problems discussed previously.

Existing slick, concrete floors can be roughened with a concrete grooving machine. Grooves made by a concrete grooving machine are suitable for many different species. Rubber mats are available to provide nonslip footing in veterinary clinics, horse stocks, and feedlot cattle working facilities. In high-traffic areas in beef cattle facilities, a grating constructed from 1 in. diameter steel bars in 12 in. by 12 in. (30 cm by 30 cm) squares can be used. The bars must be welded flush so that all bars lie flat against the floor.

In new facilities, concrete should be deeply grooved for beef cattle. Make an 8 in. by 8 in. (20 cm by 20 cm) pattern of 1 in. deep V-shaped grooves (fig. 8.10). For dairy cattle, a less-rough pattern should be used because they are walking on the floor every day. A floor that is too rough can damage their feet.

LOADING RAMP DESIGN

A well-designed loading ramp has a level landing at the top (Grandin, 1990). This provides the animals with a level surface to walk on when they first get off the truck. This will help prevent falling on the ramp. The landing should be at least 5 ft. (1.5 m) wide for cattle for use on ranches and feedlots and at least 10 ft. (3 m) long in slaughter plants. Many animals are injured on ramps that are too steep. The slope of a permanently installed ramp for most species should not exceed 20 degrees and portable ramps should not exceed 25 degrees. On concrete ramps, stair steps are recommended because they are easier for animals to walk on when they become dirty or worn. The recommended dimensions for stair steps for cattle, horses, bison, and elk are a 31/2-in. (10 cm) rise and a 12-in. (30 cm) to 18-in. (45

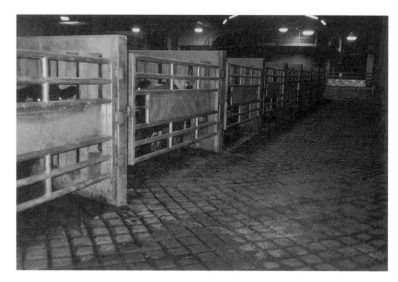

Figure 8.10.   Nonslip flooring for beef cattle. This flooring is suitable for use in working, sorting, and loading areas. In places where cattle walk every day, such as dairies, smaller grooves should be used to prevent hoof damage.

cm) tread length. If cleats are used, there should be 8 in. (20 cm) of space between the cleats. This provides space for the animal's foot to fit between the cleats without slipping.

Chutes for both loading and unloading should have solid sides to block the animal's vision. A ramp with solid outer sides and a "see through" center partition works well for pigs (fig. 8.11). Two pigs can walk up side by side and following behavior occurs because the

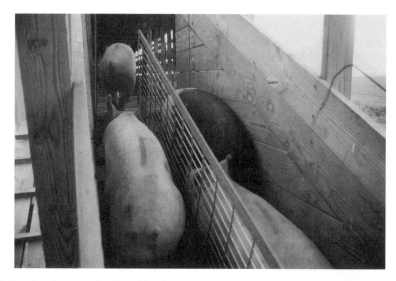

Figure 8.11.   Loading ramp for pigs with solid outer fence to block vision and an inner "see through" partition to promote following.

pigs can see each other through the divider. A loading chute for cattle, bison, or horses should be 30 in. (76 cm) wide and no wider. The largest bulls will fit through a 30 in. wide chute. Ramps designed with cattle specifications will work well for horses, bison, and other large animals.

Small animals such as weanling piglets will need small cleats that are spaced closer together (Phillips et al., 1989). This will prevent injuries to the dewclaws when the animal goes down the ramp. If the cleats are spaced too far apart, the animal will attempt to stop itself from slipping by using its dewclaws for brakes. Dewclaw injuries may occur when cleats are missing on a ramp. A basic principle of ramp design is that the steps or cleats should fit the stride length of the animal (Mayes, 1978). Larger animals need bigger cleats and wider spacing than small animals. Cleats should be sized and spaced so that an animal can easily place its foot between the cleats without slipping. If the cleats are too far apart, the animal's foot will slip between them, and, if they are too close together, the animal will slip because its foot will rest on top of the cleats instead of fitting between them.

CORRAL DESIGN

A corral constructed with round holding pens, diagonal sorting pens, and curved drive lanes will enable you to handle cattle more efficiently because there is a minimum of square corners for the cattle to bunch up in (Grandin, 2000b). The advantage of diagonal pens is that sharp 90-degree corners are eliminated. Yards with diagonal pens have good traffic flow because animals enter at one end and leave through the other. The principle of the corral layout in figure 8.6 is that the animals are gathered in either a big round pen or the lanes shown on this diagram and then directed to the curved lane for sorting and handling.

For holding less than 24 hours, gathering pen space can be figured at 20 sq. ft. (1.8 sq. m) per cow and 35 to 45 sq. ft. (3.3 to 4.2 sq. m) per cow and calf pair depending on calf size. Sorting pens should be designed to hold one truckload, which works out to 840 sq. ft. (78 sq. m). If cattle will be held overnight in a sorting pen, increase the size to 900 sq. ft. (84 sq. m). Figure 8.6 illustrates a three-way sorting gate in front of the squeeze chute for separating the cows that are pregnant from cows that are open or for sorting cattle by size. If the cattle are watered in the corrals, they will become accustomed to coming and going. When you need to catch an animal, you merely shut a trap gate and direct her up the curved reservoir lane to the chutes. This is an especially handy feature for AI. If more than one corral is built on the same ranch, they should both be laid out in the same direction. The mirror image of the designs will work.

The curved sorting reservoir terminates in a round crowding pen and curved single-file chute. The crowding gate has a ratchet latch that locks automatically as the gate is advanced behind the cattle. To load low stock trailers, open an 8-ft. (2.5 m) gate that is alongside the regular loading chute. This provides you with the advantage of the round crowding pen for stock trailers. More designs are in publications by Grandin (1997, 2000b).

Figure 8.6 illustrates a layout where cattle can be sorted many different ways after they leave the squeeze chute. Corral layouts with their capability will become more and more

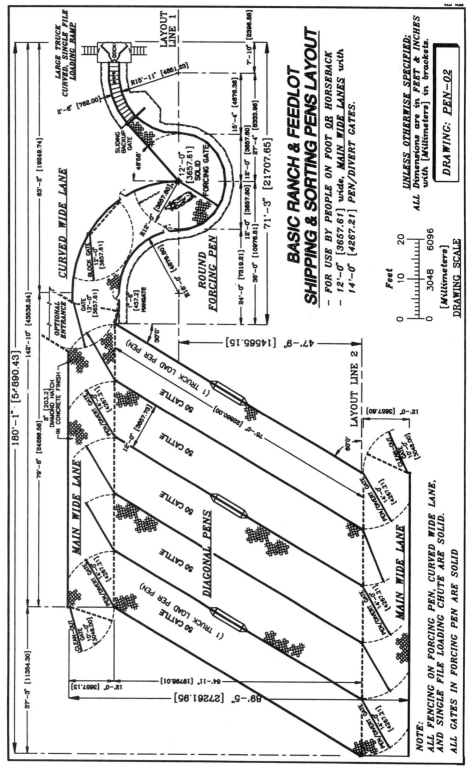

Figure 8.12.   Diagonal pens provide easy one-way traffic flow with no sharp corners for animals to bunch up in. Diagonal pens work well with many species of animals.

popular as more cattle have to be sorted to fit specific specifications. Cattle can be weighed, be examined with ultrasound, or have other evaluations in the squeeze chute and then be sorted into one of the pie-shaped pens. This type of layout will be needed when cattle are being individually identified with computerized systems.

Corral Construction Tips

Fences 5 ft. (1.5 m) high are usually sufficient for cattle such as Hereford and Angus. For Brahman cross and European Continental cattle, a 5 1/2-ft. to 6-ft. (1.6 m to 1.8 m) fence is recommended. Solid fencing should be used in the crowding pen, single-file chute, and loading chute. If your budget permits, solid fencing should be used in the curved reservoir lane. If solid fencing is too expensive, then a wide belly rail should be installed. This is especially important if the corral is constructed from thin rods. An 18 in. (45 cm) wide solid belly rail can also be installed on gates to prevent animals from hitting gates during sorting.

If a V-shaped chute is built, it should be 16 in. to 18 in. (41 cm to 45 cm) wide at the bottom and 32 in. to 36 in. (81 cm to 90 cm) wide at the top. The top measurement is taken at the 5 ft. (1.55 m) level. If the single-file chute has straight sides, it should be 26 in. (66 cm) wide for the cows and 18 in. to 20 in. (46 cm to 51 cm) wide for calves. When a funnel-type crowding pen is built, make one side straight and the other side on a 30 degree angle. This design will prevent bunching and jamming. The crowding pen should be 10 ft. to 12 ft. (3 m to 3.5 m) wide. The recommended radius for a round crowd pen is 12 ft. (3.5 m). Larger crowd pens are not recommended. The minimum radius is 10 ft. (3 m). Recommended cattle alley dimensions are 10 ft. (3 mm) for people on foot, 12 ft. (3.5 m) for people on foot and horses, and 14 ft. to 16 ft. (4.2 m to 4.8 m) for horses only.

In areas with solid fence, small man-gates must be installed so that people can get away from charging cattle. The best type of man-gate is an 18-in. (46 cm) wide, spring-loaded steel flap. The gate opens inward toward the cattle and is held shut by a spring. A person can quickly escape because there is no latch to fool with.

TROUBLESHOOTING HANDLING PROBLEMS

To solve a handling problem, one must determine the cause of the problem. Do you have a facility problem or a problem caused by the way people are handling the animals? Difficulties can arise from any one or more of the following factors:

1. Facility design problem such as a dead-ended chute (race).
2. Small distractions that cause balking, which can be easily corrected.
3. Too many animals placed in the crowd pen. Fill it half full.
4. Handlers who get the animals agitated, excited, and scared.
5. Animal temperament problem caused by flighty excitable genetics.
6. Problems with lighting and a chute entrance that is too dark.

You must determine whether you have a basic design problem, a small distraction that can easily be fixed, or an animal or handling technique problem.

REFERENCES

Amaral, A. 1977. Mustang life and legends of Nevada's wild horses. University of Nevada Press, Reno, NV.

Andrade, O., Orihuela, A., Solano, J. and Galina, C. S. 2001. Some effects of repeated handling and the use of a mask on stress responses in zebu cattle during restraint. Appl. Anim. Behav. Sci. 71:175–181.

Barber, A. and Freeman, R. B. 2000. Design of sheep yards and shearing sheds. In: Grandin, T. (Editor), Livestock handling and transport. 2nd ed. CAB International, Wallingford, Oxon, UK; 201–212.

Canada Plan Service. 1984. Herringbone AI Breeding Chute, Plan 1819 Agriculture Canada. Ottawa, Ontario, Canada.

Chilcott, R. P., Stubbs, B. and Ashley, Z. 2001. Habituating pigs for in pen non-invasive biophysical skin analysis. Lab Animal 35:230–235.

Douglas, A. C., Darre, M. D., and Kinsman, D. M. 1984. Sight restriction as a means of reducing stress during slaughter. In: Proceeding 30th European Meeting of Meat Researcher Workers, Bristol, UK; 10–11.

Dunn, C. S. 1990. Stress reactions of cattle undergoing ritual slaughter using two methods of restraint. Vet. Rec. 126:522–525.

Ewbank, R. 1968. The behavior of animals in restraint. In: Fox, M. W. (Editor), Abnormal behavior in animals. W.B. Saunders, Philadelphia, PA.

——. 2000. Handling cattle in intensive systems. In: Grandin, T. (Editor), Livestock handling and transport. CAB International, Wallingford, Oxon, UK, pp. 87–102.

Ferguson, D. L. and Rosales-Ruiz, J. 2001. Loading the problem loader: The effects of target training and shaping on trailer loading behaving horses. J. Applied Behavior Analysis 34:409–425.

Fowler, M. E. 1995. Restraint and handling of wild and domestic animals. 2nd ed. Iowa State University Press, Ames.

Giger, W., Prince, R. P., Westervelt, R. G., and Kinsman, D. M. 1977. Equipment for low stress animal slaughter. Transactions of the American Society of Agricultural Engineers 20:571–578.

Grandin, T. 1980a. Good restraining equipment is essential. Veterinary Medicine and Small Animal Clinician 75:1291–1296.

——1980b. Livestock behavior as related to handling facility design. International Journal of the Study of Animal Problems 1:33–52.

——. 1980c. Observations of cattle behavior applied to the design of cattle handling facilities. Applied Animal Ethology 6:19–31.

——. 1982. Pig behavior studies applied to slaughter plant design. Applied Animal Ethology 9:141–151.

——. 1983. Welfare requirements of handling facilities. In: Baxter, S. H., Baxter, M. R. and MacCormack, J. A. D. (Editors), Farm animal housing and welfare. Martinus Nijhoff, Boston, MA; 137–149.

——. 1986. Minimizing stress in pig handling. Lab Animal 15(3).

——. 1987. Animal handling. In: Price, E. O. (Editor), Farm animal behavior. Veterinary Clinics of North America, Food Animal Practice 3(2):323–338.

——. 1988. Double rail restrainer conveyor for livestock handling. J. of Ag. Eng. Res. 41:327–338.

——. 1989. Voluntary acceptance of restraint by sheep. Appl. Anim. Behav. Sci., 23:257–261.

——. 1990. Design of loading facilities and holding pens. Appl. Anim. Behav. Sci. , 28:187–201.

——. 1991. Double rail restrainer for handling beef cattle. Paper No. 91–5004, American Society of Agricultural Engineers, St. Joseph, Michigan.

——. 1992. Observations of cattle restraint device for stunning and slaughtering. Animal Welfare (Universities Federation for Animal Welfare, Potters Bar UK) 1:85–91.

——. 1994. Euthanasia and slaughter of livestock. J. Am Vet. Med. Assoc., 204:1354–1360.

——. 1995. Restraint of livestock. In: Proc. of the Animal Behavior and the Design of Livestock and Poultry Systems Intl. Conference. Northeast Regional Agricultural Engineering Service, Cooperative Ext., Cornell University, Ithaca, NY; 208–223.

——. 1996. Factors that impede animal movement at slaughter plants. J. Am. Vet. Met. Assoc. 209:757–759.

——. 1997. The design and construction of facilities for handling cattle. Livestock Production Sci. 49:103–119.

——. 1998a. The feasibility of using vocalization scoring as an indicator of poor welfare during slaughter. Appl. Anim. Behav. Sci. 56:121–128.

——. 1998b. Handling methods and facilities to reduce stress on cattle. In: Stokka, G. L. (Editor), Vet. Clinic of North America Food Animal Practice, 14:325–341.

——. 1998c. Solving livestock handling problems in slaughter plants. In: Gregory, N. G. (Editor), Animal welfare and meat science. CAB International, Wallingford, UK.

——. 2000a. Cattle vocalizations are associated with handling and equipment problems at beef slaughter plants. Appl. Anim. Behav. Sci. 71:191–201.

——. 2000b. Livestock handling and transport. CAB International, Wallingford, Oxon, UK.

——. 2003. Transferring results of behavioral research to industry to improve animal welfare on the farm, ranch and slaughter plant. Appl. Anim. Behav. Sci. 81:215–228.

Grandin, T., Curtis, S. E., Widowski, T. M. and Thurman, J. C. 1986. Electro-immobilization versus mechanical restraint in an avoid choice test. J. Anim. Sci. 62:1469–1480.

Grandin, T., Dodman, N. and Shuster, L. 1989. Effect of naltrexone on relaxation induced by flank pressure in pigs. Pharmocology, Biochemistry and Behavior, 33:839–842.

Grandin, T., Rooney, M. B., Phillips, M., Irlbeck, N. A. and Grafham, W. 1995. Conditioning of nyala (*Tragelaphu angasi*) to blood sampling in a crate using positive reinforcement. Zoo Biology 14:261–273.

Haigh, J. C. 1992. Requirements for managing farmed deer, In: Brown, R. D. (Editor), The biology of deer. Springer-Verlag, New York; 159–172.

——. 1995. A handling system for white-tailed deer (*Odocoileus virginianus*). J. of Zoo Wildlife Medicine 26(2):321–326.

——. 1999. The use of chutes for ungulate restraint. In: Fowler, M. E. and Miller, R. D. (Editors), Zoo and wildlife medicine. Current Therapy 4. W.B. Saunders, Philadelphia, PA; 657–662.

Haigh, J. C. and Hudson, R. J. 1993. Farming Wapiti and red deer. Mosby, Toronto; 67–98.

Hoenderken, R. 1976. Improved system for guiding pigs for slaughter to the restrainer. Die Fleischwirtschaft 56(6):838–839.

Hutson, G. D. 1980a. Sheep behavior and the design of sheep yards and shearing sheds. In: Wodzicka-Tomaszewska, M., Edey, T. N. and Lynch, J. J. (Editors). Behavior in relation to reproduction, management and welfare of farm animals. University of New England Publishing Unit, Armidol, NSW, Australia; 137–141.

——. 1980b. Visual field, restricted vision and sheep movement through laneways. Appl. Animal Ethology 6:175–187.

——. 1985. The influence of barley food rewards on sheep movement through handling systems. Appl. Anim. Behav. Sci. 14:263–273.

Jones, R. B., Satterlee, D. C. and Cadd, G. G. 1998. Struggling responses of broiler chickens shackled in groups on a moving line effect of light intensity, hoods and curtains. Appl. Animal Behavior Sci. 38:341–352.

Kilgour, R. 1971. Animal handling in works, pertinent behavior studies. In: Proceedings of the 13th Meat Industry Research Conference, Hamilton, New Zealand; 9–12.

Lambooy, E. 1985. Electro-anesthesia or electro-immobilization of calves, sheep and pigs with Feenix Stockstill. Vet. Quarterly 7:120–126.

——. 1986. Automatic electrical stunning of veal calves in a V-type restrainer. In: Proceedings, 32nd European Meeting of Meat Researcher Workers, Ghent Belgium, paper 2.2; 77–80.

Lehman, W. B. and Patterson, G. H. 1964. Depth perception in sheep: Effects of interrupting the mother neonate bond. Science 145:835–836.

Lynch, J. J. and Alexander, G. 1973. The pastoral industries of Australia. University Press, Sydney, Australia; 371–400.

Matthews, L. R. 2000. Deer handling and transport. In: Grandin, T. (Editor), Livestock handling and transport. 2nd ed. CAB International, Wallingford, Oxon, UK; 331–362.

Mayes, H. F. 1978. Design criteria for livestock loading chutes. Am. Soc. Ag. Engineers, Paper No. 78–6014, St. Joseph, MI.

Panepinto, L. M. 1983. A comfortable minimum stress method of restraint on Yucatan miniature swine. Lab Animal Sci. 33(1):95–97.

Parsons, R. A. and Helphinstine, W. M. 1969. Rambo AI breeding chute for beef cattle. One Sheet Answers, University of California Agricultural Extension Service, Davis, CA.

Pascoe, P. J. 1986. Humaneness of electrical immobilization unit for cattle. Am. J. Vet. Res. 10:2252–2256.

Phillips, M., Grandin, T., Graffam, W., Irlbeck, N. A. and Cambre, R. C. 1998. Crate conditioning of bongo (*Tragelephus eurycerus*) for veterinary and husbandry procedures. Zoo Biology 17:25–32.

Phillips, P. A., Thompson, B. K. and Fraser, D. 1989. The importance of cleat spacing in ramp design for young pigs. Canadian J. Anim. Sci. 69:483–486.

Regensburger, R. W. 1940. Hog stunning pen. U.S. Patent 2,185,949.

Rider, A., Butchbaker, A. F. and Harp S. 1974. Beef working, sorting and handling facilities. Am. Soc. Ag. Eng. Paper No. 74–4523, St. Joseph, MI.

Van Putten, G. and Elshof, W. J. 1978. Observations on the effect of transport on the well being and lean quality of slaughter pigs. Animal Regulation Studies 1:247–271.

Ward, F. 1958. Cowboy at work. Hasting Press, New York.

Westervelt, R. G., Kinsmon, D., Prince, R. P., and Giger, W. 1976. Physiological stress measurement during slaughter of calves and lambs. J. Anim. Sci. 42:831–834.

White, J. B. 1961. Letter to the editor. Vet. Res. 73:935.

Wyman, W. D. 1946. The wild horse of the west. Caxton Printers, Caldwell, ID.

9

Personnel Management in Agricultural Systems

Grahame Coleman

It is commonly held that some people are "naturals" in regard to their affinity for and ability to interact with farm animals. It might be because they are female or empathic or have a suitable personality or some special communication skills that allow them to be especially sensitive to the needs of animals. To regard some people as being dispositionally well suited to the care of animals is to beg the question of whether or not people can be taught to be good stockpeople. Clearly this has implications for the selection of stockpeople, on the one hand, and their training, on the other. Also, does a capacity to care for animals, in the pastoral sense, imply that people with such a capacity are best suited to manage farm animals? The role of technical knowledge and the kinds of people who are best able to acquire and utilize such knowledge are surely also key issues.

The aim of this chapter is to characterize the principal requirements for animal handlers; to relate these to human traits, acquired dispositions, attitudes, skills, and knowledge; and to identify the key imperatives for personnel management in livestock systems.

Job Requirements of Personnel in Livestock Systems

In general, farm personnel in animal agriculture are regarded as itinerant and unskilled workers. Farm managers are reluctant to invest too much effort in training stockpeople because of the high rate of turnover. The role of the stockperson, outlined in chapter 2, as the principal person responsible for the day-to-day welfare and productivity of the animals under his or her care has not received wide acknowledgment. However, recognition of this role of farm personnel in animal agriculture leads to the recognition of these personnel as important human resources that need to be selected, trained, and managed in a way similar to current practice in a wide range of white-collar industries. A duty statement for a modern stockperson from Hemsworth and Coleman (1998, 4) is:

- A good general knowledge of the nutritional, climatic, social and health requirements of the farm animal;
- Practical experience in the care and maintenance of the animal;
- Ability to quickly identify any departures in the behavior, health or performance of the animal and promptly provide or seek appropriate support to address these departures;
- Ability to work effectively independently and/or in teams, under general supervision, with daily responsibility for the care and maintenance of large numbers of animals.

As Hemsworth and Coleman have indicated, the stockperson is required to have

a basic knowledge of both the behavior of the animal and its nutritional, climatic, housing, health, social and sexual requirements together with a range of well developed
husbandry and management skills to effectively care and manage farm animals. For instance, farm personnel may have knowledge and skills in a number of diverse management and husbandry tasks such as estrus detection and mating assistance; semen
collection, semen preparation and artificial insemination; pregnancy diagnosis with
ultra-sonography; artificial rearing of early weaned animals; milk harvesting; controlling and monitoring of feed intake to optimize growth, body composition, milk production and reproductive performance; pasture management to optimize pasture
production; routine health checks; monitoring and adjusting climatic conditions in indoor units; administering antibiotics and vaccines; shearing and crutching of sheep;
teeth and tail clipping of pigs; castration of males; and effective and safe animal handling. These are skilled tasks and farm personnel are required to be competent in many
of these tasks. (p. 4)

The working environment in animal systems often places demands on personnel that
are not usually encountered in other workplaces. Those working outdoors may be exposed to extreme weather conditions, while those working both indoors and outdoors may
be exposed to wide variations in temperature, humidity, and levels of odor and dust. The
larger farm animals can also present a source of physical danger if managed carelessly or
improperly.

The job status of those working in animal systems is variable and generally not high.
Beynon (1991) reported that the families of pig stockpeople regarded employment in the
pig industry as having a low status. The poor image of farm personnel is often attributed
as a factor contributing to the problem of attracting people to and retaining staff in intensive animal systems. English et al. (1992) went so far as to suggest that farm personnel are
the world's most undervalued profession.

There is a clear need to identify the attributes that best allow a person to meet the job
requirements for a stockperson. These characteristics will be a combination of dispositions
(personality, empathy, etc.) and learned factors (skills, knowledge, etc.). In general, the
small amount of research that has been done on stockperson characteristics has adopted
one of two broad approaches. On the one hand, some studies have attempted to identify
the characteristics of stockpeople currently employed in agricultural systems on the assumption that there will be a match between the job requirements and the person. On the
other hand, a few studies have attempted to identify those characteristics that are associated with good performance stockpeople in agricultural systems. The implications that
may be drawn from these two kinds of studies are different. The fact that a stockperson is
employed in an agricultural system may be a result of a multitude of factors partly geographical and financial, and partly related to the characteristics of the person. Certainly, the
fact that a stockperson is currently employed in an agricultural industry does not imply that
the person is necessarily the best for the welfare or productivity of the animals under his
or her care. Those studies that explicitly relate personal characteristics to stockperson per-

formance are more likely to be useful in identifying appropriate training and, perhaps, selection strategies for stockpeople.

MEASURES OF PERFORMANCE

The principal prerequisites for good job performance are appropriate knowledge, skills, and abilities (KSAs). For example, in the pig industry, a stockperson working with the breeding herd must be skilled at estrus detection and at assisting matings, and if he or she does not have these skills, then production will be severely impaired. Less obvious, and also the subject of limited research, is the impact of stockperson skills in handling and interacting with intensively and extensively farmed animals. Research has shown that most stockpeople in the pig and dairy systems do not know, in detail, what aspects of handling that farm animals find aversive, despite the fact that it has been shown that aversive handling has negative consequences for the animal and its productivity and welfare (see chapter 2). The translation of skills and knowledge into appropriate animal management behavior is clearly an important aspect of stockperson performance. Equally, the extent to which a person is satisfied with the job and is prepared to remain in the job for a reasonable period of time is also important. Turnover is a major problem in many agricultural systems; in Australia, a turnover of 50 percent in six months among new pig farm personnel has been observed in our own research.

DETERMINANTS OF PERFORMANCE

There is a wide range of factors that influence an individual's performance in the workplace. Seabrook (1982) attempted to identify these in agricultural workers, but in the absence of any empirical data was able to identify some generic factors only. There is a need for greater specificity in identifying the characteristics relevant to stockperson performance. First, there are characteristics of the individual. On the one hand, a range of dispositional factors—that is, relatively stable characteristics of the person that initiate and mediate or moderate behavior—provides a basic framework within which the individual interacts with his or her environment. On the other hand, there is a range of learned factors, including not only skills and knowledge but also learned motivations, which affect behavior. Second, there is a range of environmental factors that provide physical constraints within which the person works. And finally, there is a range of demographic factors such as family size, distance from work, and so on.

Dispositional Characteristics

The principal dispositional characteristic that is invoked to account for a range of human behaviors is personality. Although there is some disagreement among psychologists, it is reasonably well accepted that a personality trait is a relatively enduring characteristic that exerts a general effect on that person's behavior and that we cannot observe directly but can infer from the person's behavior. Gordon Allport defined personality as "the dynamic organization within the individual of those psychophysical systems that determine his unique adjustments to his environment"(Allport, 1937, p. 48).

Today most researchers agree that personality can be characterized in terms of five dimensions (the so-called big five): (1) extraversion/introversion, (2) emotional stability, (3) agreeableness, (4) conscientiousness, and (5) intellect (Costa and McCrae, 1992). Extraversion is associated with sociability, assertiveness, and an outgoing nature. Emotional stability refers to a trait similar to Eysenck's (1966) neuroticism and includes such things as anxiety, embarrassment, and insecurity. Agreeableness is associated with cooperation, good nature, and tolerance. Conscientiousness is characterized by dependability, hard work, and perseverance. Intellect includes being imaginative, cultured, and original (Barrick and Mount, 1991). These personality factors appear to be useful in matching people to some kinds of jobs. Barrick and Mount found that conscientiousness predicted job success across a range of job categories and was the most significant personality characteristic associated with sales performance. There was also a less-strong relationship between extraversion and sales performance. Another measure of personality type, Briggs Type Indicator (MBTI), identifies the basic preferences of people in regard to how they use their perceptions and judgment and, therefore, how they differ in their reactions, values, motivations, skills, and interests. The MBTI has four bipolar dimensions: extraversion-introversion, thinking judgment-feeling judgment, sensing perception-intuitive perception, and judgment-perception.

In agricultural systems, there is little evidence relating personality directly to good work performance. Seabrook (1972a,b) reported that the stockperson's personality was related to behavior of the cows and milk yield of the herd. He found that high milk yield was associated with herds in which the stockpeople were introverted and confident and where the cows were most willing to enter the milking shed and were less restless in the presence of the stockperson. In general, self-confidence was associated with moderate to high yield regardless of degree of introversion. In an unpublished study, Beveridge (1996) investigated the relationship between personality types as measured by the MBTI and dairy stockperson behavior toward cows. The most common personality type among dairy stockpeople was the introverted-sensing-thinking-judgment type. There was a negative relationship between judgment-perception scores and negative behavior toward cows. Thinking-feeling scores tended to be correlated positively with positive and mildly aversive behaviors and negatively with clearly aversive behaviors. The MBTI correlated more strongly with measures of stockperson attitude but showed no correlations with milk yield. In a recent study by Waiblinger, Menke, and Coleman (2002), stockperson personal characteristics, based on the measures used by Seabrook, also did not correlate significantly with milk yield, but did correlate with the attitudes of stockpeople. Agreeableness correlated negatively with positive attitude toward awareness of cows and positively with positive attitude toward contact with cows while caring for them. Agreeableness also correlated with several stockperson behavior variables: negatively with percentage of neutral behaviors, positively with absolute number and percentage of positive behaviors, and tended to correlate negatively with the percentage of negative behaviors.

Significant relationships have been found in the pig industry between personality types of stockpeople and productivity in farrowing units. Seabrook (1996) reported that pig performance, measured by litter size, was associated with carers with confident personalities, emotional stability, independent personality, rational behavior, and low aggression. Ravel et al. (1996), using an established but currently less-frequently used test, the 16 PF, found that self-discipline was a trait that appeared to be important at all farms studied; high insecurity and low sensitivity were associated with piglet survival at independent owner-operated farms; while stockpeople that were highly reserved and bold, suspicious, tense, and changeable were associated with higher piglet mortality at large integrated farms.

It is difficult to extract a pattern from these varied results. The fact that several researchers, in different contexts and using different measures of personality, have been able to find direct or indirect relationships between carer personality and production outcomes does suggest that personality may well be a relevant factor in animal systems. The perennial problem of different measures of personality with variable validity coupled with a variety of outcome measures serves to obscure the picture. Also, the fact that the dependent variables often are farm outcomes rather than the performance of individual stockpeople means that, because many factors can intervene between stockperson characteristics and the productivity and welfare of the animals under his or her care, it may be difficult to determine the causal sequence between stockperson characteristics and productivity.

Apart from personality measures, it may be the case that degree of empathy predisposes people to be good stockpeople. Certainly, the idea that stockpeople will perform best if they have good insight into the emotional responses of the animals under their care has strong intuitive appeal and is consistent with Hemsworth and Coleman's (1998) findings that stockperson behavior is an important determinant of farm animal productivity. Empathy can be described as the capacity to put oneself in the place of another. It has two basic components, an attributional and an experiential element. These elements may take the form of vicarious experience of another's emotions or it may simply be a capacity for role taking. Chlopan et al. (1985) have concluded that the most appropriate way of considering empathy is to regard it as being multifaceted and containing both role-taking and vicarious experience components. While empathy is a dispositional characteristic, unlike personality, there is some argument about whether empathy is innate or learned. In a recent review, Duan and Hill (1996) distinguished between a trait approach, which is widely adopted by psychotherapists and others, and a situation-specific social learning approach, which is amenable to training.

In the agricultural literature, the term *empathy* has been used to describe the bond that exists between humans and animals under their care (English et al., 1992). In fact, an empathic bond may exist between stockpeople and their animals; however, empathy does not refer to the bond itself, which may have its origins in a number of factors of which empathy is one. Empathy refers to the way in which stockpeople may feel a bond with their animals because of being able to put themselves in the animal's position or to understand the way in which the animals are reacting.

Only limited empirical data from agriculture are available. Beveridge (1996) found that empathy toward animals was positively associated with positive attitudes toward interacting with cows and positive beliefs about cows but not directly with stockperson behavior toward cows. Coleman , Hemsworth, and Hay (1998) found that empathy toward animals was associated with positive beliefs about pigs and about handling pigs. These two findings suggest that empathy may be a factor underlying the development of positive attitudes toward pigs. This will be discussed in more detail below. However, in a recent study, Coleman (2001) found that empathy was associated with positive behavior toward pigs and a high level of intention to remain working in the pig industry. This study is discussed in some detail below.

As has been discussed in chapter 2 and reviewed extensively by Hemsworth and Coleman (1998), attitudes toward farm animals and toward working with farm animals have been associated with stockperson behavior toward animals, and stockperson behavior has affected fear levels and subsequent behavior in farm animals. More recent work (e.g., Lensink, Boissy, and Veissier, 2000; Waiblinger et al., 2002) has provided additional support for this. Attitudes are learned dispositions, which are often invoked both in everyday use as well as in research to explain behavior. In particular, Ajzen and Fishbein (1980) have proposed that the immediate cause of behavior is attitude, specifically attitude toward the behavior in question. The key to their theory is the idea that specifically targeted attitudes dispose individuals to specific behaviors. The antecedents of those attitudes begin with a range of demographic, personality, and other variables leading to a range of beliefs about the situation, which in turn lead to behavioral attitudes. Many of the empirical results showing that attitudes are good predictors of stockperson performance across a range of agricultural systems have been given in chapter 2.

Data from the studies by Beveridge (1996), Coleman et al. (1998), and Waiblinger et al. (2002) as well as those reviewed in chapter 2 provide evidence in support of the proposed relationship between personality variables and attitudes, on the one hand, and between attitudes and stockperson behavior, on the other. These results are consistent with the Ajzen and Fishbein (1980) approach, which suggests that this characteristic may influence the development of attitudes but not directly affect behavior.

The extent to which a person applies himself or herself to a task will depend, in part, on the extent to which the person "wishes" to achieve the task. In other words, a good stockperson is one who is motivated to apply skills and knowledge to the management of the animals under his or her care. What this means, of course, is that the person must be motivated. In general, it is accepted that motivation alone is insufficient for good work performance; if a person does not have the knowledge, skills, or opportunity to perform a job, then motivation will not make any difference. However, if a person does have the knowledge, skills, and opportunity to perform the task, what is the role of motivation in professional stockperson behavior?

There is little systematic study of the effect of motivation on stockperson performance. However, a study carried out in India (Singh, 1983) showed that productivity, as measured by progressive farm behavior, was associated with career interest, upward striving, attitude toward making money on the farm, intelligence, tolerance for work pressure, and punctuality. This suggests that motivational factors, such as upward striving and need to make money, can contribute to productivity on a farm.

Environmental Variables

There is no direct evidence relating environmental variables with work performance in agricultural industries. However, the relevance of the work environment to worker performance has come under some scrutiny recently. Ashforth and Kreiner (1999) have argued that "dirty work" does not necessarily lead to low worker self-esteem associated with the stigma of working in such an industry. The argument is that where there is a strong occupational work-group culture, workers may see themselves as belonging to an important group. They also argue, however, that if the work environment involves physical isolation or high turnover, then self-esteem may well be adversely affected by the work environment. Data from two separate studies in Australia indicate that a typical turnover rate in the pig industry is on the order of 50 percent over a six-month period. This suggests that there is a high risk of morale problems among the workers in agricultural systems, particularly the pig industry, and that strategies to improve job satisfaction may be highly desirable.

Demographic Variables

One of the principal demographic variables that is mentioned regularly in discussions about animal stockpeople is gender. Given the social and biological role that women occupy in caring, nursing, and, still predominately, raising children, there is the assumption that there is a perhaps biological or learned ability for women to care for their animals sensitively. These assumptions merit some consideration. Girls have been found to have stronger bonds with pets in some studies (Kidd and Kidd, 1990; Triebenbacher, 1998; Vidovic, Stetic, and Bratco, 1999) but not in others (Melson and Fogel, 1988; Stevens, 1990). Leaving aside the inconsistency in the results, it may be the case that boys are less willing to reveal emotional attachments than are girls. There is also the possibility that boys and girls may use different language to express emotions or even to construe their interactions with animals differently. There are limited available data relating to stockpeople in agricultural systems. Lensink et al. (2000) found that being female was associated with more positive contact with veal calves than being male. Also, the study by Coleman (2001) found that gender was a predictor of some aspects of work performance. This will be discussed in more detail below.

There appear to be no data on stockperson performance in any workplace relating to age, family characteristics, health status, or education. To the extent that most of the skills required to care for animals are not intellectually demanding but require conscientiousness, persistence, and some sensitivity, then it is not surprising that many of these variables have not been shown to be related to stockperson performance. Even the kinds of judgment that are required to appropriately care for animals are similar to those that are part of everyday life skills and are utilized in making a range of domestic and social decisions.

AN INTEGRATED STUDY OF STOCKPERSON PERFORMANCE

Coleman (2001) recently reported the results of a preliminary study that is currently undergoing further validation. However, because the study provides an integrated evaluation of many of the variables so far discussed, it will be reported in some detail. A total of 144 inexperienced stockpeople participated in a study in which stockpeople, at commencement of employment, completed a set of computerized questionnaires, which included measures of personality, motivation, turnover potential, performance potential, attitudes, and empathy toward pigs. Those stockpeople who remained at the piggery for six months completed a second set of computerized questionnaires, which included measures of work performance. At this time, direct supervisors were also asked to assess job performance in terms of animal handling, conscientiousness, and other skills, and independent observers also assessed animal handling, work ethic, and technical knowledge.

Stockperson performance was assessed using ratings of stockperson behavior toward their pigs, technical knowledge, conscientiousness, satisfaction, and intention to leave the job soon (intention to turnover) (table 9.1). Stockperson behavior toward their pigs, technical knowledge, and work ethic were directly assessed by an independent observer. A supervisor report of satisfaction and conscientiousness was used to measure these aspects of stockperson performance. Intention to turnover was assessed using the Michigan Organizational Assessment Questionnaire (Cammann et al., 1979).

Females were rated as more conscientious by their supervisors, and were independently rated as having greater technical knowledge and a better work ethic compared to males. The self-reported PDI-EI Performance measure (Personnel Decisions, Inc., 1996) was significantly correlated with all three measures of independently observed performance. A person scoring high on this measure is likely to adhere to rules, show stability of behavior, take care while performing tasks, and take responsibility. On the other hand, the PDI-EI

Table 9.1.   Predictors of Pig Stockperson Performance

| | Stockperson performance variable[2] | | | | | |
| | Supervisor ratings | | Independent observer ratings | | | Stockperson |
Predicator variable[1]	Conscientiousness	Satisfaction	Technical knowledge	Behavior toward pigs	Work ethic	Intention to turnover
Sex	0.29*	0.10	0.45**	−0.03	0.29*	−0.06
PDI performance	0.32*	0.39**	0.27	0.29*	0.22	−0.35**
PDI tenure	0.03	0.18	0.13	0.15	0.05	−0.28*
Positive attitude	0.27*	0.26	0.23	0.23	0.11	−0.37**
Empathy affect	0.11	0.12	0.27	0.37**	0.19	−0.41**
Empathy attribution	0.13	0.05	0.33*	0.30*	0.17	−0.39**

Source: From Coleman (2001).

$*p < .05$, $**p < .01$; n = 50–64.

[1]Predictor variables are as follows: Sex: 1 = male, 2 = female; Experience: years experience working with pigs; PDI performance: expected job performance; PDI tenure: likelihood of remaining in a job for at least 3 months; Positive attitude: positive attitude toward pigs; Empathy affect: concern about animals' feelings; Empathy attribution: belief that animals are like humans.

[2]Stockperson performance variables are as follows: Conscientiousness: how conscientious supervisors judge stockpeople to be; Satisfaction: how satisfied supervisors judge stockpeople to be; Technical knowledge: independent observer's rating of stockperson's technical knowledge; Work ethic: independent observer's rating of stockperson's work ethic; Behavior toward pigs: independent observer's rating of stockperson's handling of pigs; Intention to turnover: likelihood of seeking a new job in the next year.

Tenure measure correlated with intention to remain in employment over the next year. A positive attitude toward the characteristics of pigs correlated significantly with conscientiousness and intention to remain in the job. Finally, empathy toward animals correlated with technical knowledge, behavior toward pigs, and intention to remain in the job. Another finding was that 50 percent of new stockpeople left their jobs within six months of employment.

One of the important features of this study is that all the measures of stockperson characteristics were taken in an initial interview and the performance measures six months later. Therefore, these measures of stockperson performance have the potential to be used to identify potentially good stockpeople.

As is always the case in research, this study leaves some tantalizing questions. Why do women appear to perform better than men? Is it because they self-select in animal care jobs? Do (male) raters rate females higher in gender-stereotyped areas of behavior? Are females better stockpeople and are they more conscientious? Notably, being female was not associated with better observed behavior toward pigs.

Although a "big five" measure of personality was used in this study, no consistent relationships between personality and stockperson performance were observed. However, neuroticism was associated with observer rating of work ethic ($r = 0.39$, $p < .01$) and a trait unique to the Kline and Lapham (1991a, 1991b) Professional Personality Questionnaire, tendermindedness, was related to intention to turnover ($p = 0.28$, $p < .05$).

SELECTION AND TRAINING OF STOCKPEOPLE

Most of the studies that have examined the role of personality, empathy, and attitudes in the performance of stockpeople have concentrated on behavior toward the animals under their care. There is a good reason for this. As Hemsworth has pointed out in chapter 2, very strong evidence has accumulated to show that the behavior of stockpeople toward their animals has a major impact on both the welfare and the productivity of the animals. To the extent that the dispositional factors so far discussed affect the behavior of stockpeople toward their animals, either directly or indirectly through behavior-specific attitudes, they should be targeted in selection and training of stockpeople. While it is well accepted that personality is not susceptible to change and therefore cannot be targeted through training, it may be a useful measure for screening purposes as an adjunct to the identification of other characteristics that may be relevant to stockperson performance.

Apart from the few instances involving personality, none of the factors associated with stockperson performance in the agricultural research literature were innate dispositions but were characteristics formed by psychosocial development. It is unclear whether any of the factors identified by Seabrook (1972a,b) represent innate human traits, and the work by Ravel et al. (1996) stands as the one instance where an established measure of personality has been used and where there is a relationship with animal production, but no indication of stockperson behavior. This leads to the conclusion that there are two broad strategies that may be adopted in managing stockpeople in agricultural systems. To the extent that innate characteristics are relevant to stockperson performance, it may be appropriate to use, for example, personality attributes as a basis for stockperson selection. However, there are several considerations that argue against this approach. First, it has yet to be established which, if any, personality characteristics are generically important for stockperson performance. Second, and perhaps more important, it remains to be determined whether personality is a direct determinant of stockperson performance or whether certain kinds of people gravitate toward work with animals in agricultural systems or whether personality factors tend to affect the development of attitude and behavior. Certainly, this moderating role of personality in stockperson behavior is consistent with the approach of Ajzen and Fishbein (1980) described above, in which personality influences the development of attitudes, but it is the attitudes that are the proximal causes of behavior. Depending on the causal status of personality, training may well be a more appropriate approach than simply selection on the basis of personality attributes. However, before this can be done with any confidence, systematic research that uses well-established, current, and well-validated measures of personality and that targets a range of performance measures needs to be carried out.

Empathy and attitudes are susceptible to change and, therefore, selection processes that identify deficits in these areas can be used, not so much as an employment tool but as a means for identifying areas that should be targeted through training. Such a strategy has the added advantage that evidence from the organizational psychology literature indicates that training programs improve worker job satisfaction and job retention.

While it is clear that appropriate training that targets attitudes and behavior can improve stockperson behavior and, subsequently, pig reproductive performance (Hemsworth and Coleman, 1998), it is also important to identify those characteristics that identify potentially good stockpeople when they have little experience working with pigs. Attitudes are unreliable predictors of behavior when they are not associated with relevant experience (Ajzen, 1988). Therefore, it is important to persist with investigations into dispositional factors that are not dependent upon specific animal-care experience. The recent study by Coleman (2001) gives some indication that personal attributes, such as empathy and attitudes toward animals and toward aspects of work, may well be useful in identifying inexperienced people who are likely to be good stockpeople.

There are several practical impediments to using selection strategies in agricultural systems even if certain individuals are better suited to work with farm animals. Many agricultural facilities are located in rural areas often not near large population centers. As a consequence, there is limited availability of a wide pool from which to select stockpeople. Further, people from urban areas with limited experience in working with animals or in "dirty" environments may not be inclined to apply to work in farm animal systems. Therefore, it is important to optimally train and, having trained, to retain those workers who are attracted to farm animal work.

RETENTION OF STAFF IN AGRICULTURAL SYSTEMS

Steel, Griffeth, and Hom (2002) recently reviewed quit-rate statistics in the United States. Across all companies, national average turnover rate is about 15 percent per year. In the manufacturing sector, turnover rates are a little higher at 15 to 25 percent. Data for farm workers are not reported, however, our own data from Australia (Coleman, 2001) indicate turnover rates among new pig stockpeople of around 50 percent over a six-month period, and anecdotal reports from the United States show similar figures. It is difficult to place a monetary cost on turnover, but Steel et al. report that the average cost per employee is of the order of ten thousand dollars (US) when averaged across all industries and across all employee categories.

Steel et al. (2002), based on an integration of turnover frameworks, concluded that employee expectations regarding their jobs and employee morale contribute substantially to employees intention to stay in the job and hence retention. As indicated earlier, Beynon (1991) reported that employment in the pig industry has a low status and that this poor image contributes to the problem of attracting and retaining stockpeople in intensive animal systems. However, Ashforth and Kreiner (1999) have argued that "dirty work" does not necessarily lead to low worker self-esteem associated with the stigma of working in such an industry. The argument is that where there is a strong occupational work-group culture, workers may see themselves as belonging to an important group. They also argue, however, that if the work environment involves physical isolation or high turnover, then self-esteem may well be adversely affected by the work environment. Therefore, strategies that target employee morale by increasing job satisfaction and by ensuring that employee expectations are met are important for the agricultural industries, just as they are in other industries. Strategies that have been employed to improve retention include appropriate selection techniques, realistic induction training, and job enrichment programs (Steel et al., 2002).

Variables relevant to selection of stockpeople in agricultural systems have already been discussed. Steel et al. (2002) caution that selection strategies based on demographic variables in particular and, perhaps, other personal characteristics may constitute discrimination and therefore be at least undesirable and possibly illegal. Nevertheless, variables such as the PDI performance and tenure as well as measures of attitude may be regarded as strategies for identifying individuals suitable to the stockpeople. Of course, such measures should never be used in isolation but should form part of a selection strategy that involves interview and evaluation of the motivations, past experience, and skills of the applicant.

There appears to be no research on the value of appropriate induction strategies for stockpeople. Anecdotally, it appears that induction programs are widely used and that new stockpeople are often given initial video and face-to-face introductions to the job followed by some weeks of on-the-job training. English (2002) reported improved pig production following the introduction of staff induction procedures and training, which he attributed to improved knowledge, understanding, and skills; improved team work; increased motivation; and job satisfaction. He did not report any changes in job retention. Steel et al. (2002) suggested that an appropriate strategy to improve retention may be to present new stockpeople with realistic previews of the job as a way of preparing the applicant for the less-pleasant aspects of the job situation. This has the effect of lowering stockperson expectations, which may improve retention rates.

Both overall job satisfaction and organizational commitment are good predictors of turnover (Griffeth, Hom, and Gaertner, 2000). In addition, Hull and Tyagi (1996) found that dairy plant managers adopted a principally authoritarian management style and had employees with low job satisfaction and weak motivation. Therefore, techniques designed to improve stockperson job satisfaction should be employed in agricultural systems. Again, there are few data to demonstrate the effectiveness of such strategies for stockpeople.

Coleman et al. (1998) found clear relationships between pig stockperson attitudes and job-related subscales. In particular, the willingness of stockpersons to attend training sessions on their own time was correlated with positive attitudes toward pigs and working with pigs. Job enjoyment and opinions about working conditions showed a similar relationship with attitudes. There is also anecdotal evidence to suggest that dairy stockpeople may benefit from training programs directed toward handling in other ways. In a more recent study, Coleman et al. (2000) found that six months after the completion of a similar training program, the retention rate for pig stockpeople who had participated in the training program was 61 percent compared to the rate for those who had not participated of 47 percent. Hemsworth et al. (2002) found that dairy farmers who had undertaken a program similar to the pig handling program subsequently reported a much improved working environment. There were fewer periods of cow restlessness, the farmers themselves felt calmer and more relaxed, and there were fewer days when things seemed to go consistently wrong. Taken together, these studies suggest that training programs that target improved animal handling by stockpeople may have the secondary outcome of improving job satisfaction and retention rates.

CONCLUSION

It is time to return to the questions raised at the beginning of this chapter. Is it the case that some people are "naturals" in their ability to work with farm animals? Are empathy and concern for welfare the principal requirements for stockpeople? The evidence reviewed here certainly suggests that there are a number of dispositional characteristics that make individuals suitable to be stockpeople in agricultural systems. There is evidence to suggest that positive attitudes toward animals and toward working with animals as well as empathy are good predictors of subsequent behavior toward those animals. Further, there are good data to show that stockperson handling of animals affects stress and fear levels in those animals and subsequently their productivity. Also a measure of attitude toward work, the PDI performance score is a good predictor of stockperson performance in all areas— work ethic, behavior toward the animals under his or her care, technical knowledge, and preference to stay in the job. However, none of these variables could reasonably be described as innate. Appropriate training and experience can be used to target each of these areas with the likely consequence that stockperson performance will improve. While there is some evidence to suggest that personality traits may be associated with people choosing agricultural systems as areas of employment, evidence to suggest that personality predicts those individuals who are likely to be good animal handlers has yet to be uncovered. The general organizational psychology literature suggests that conscientiousness is a personality attribute associated with good work performance, but this relates to overall job commitment and is not specifically related to handling animals. The answer to the original question, therefore, must be that stockpeople are made not born. While sensitivity to the animals under their care is an important attribute for stockpeople, so are good technical knowledge and a general conscientiousness in the workplace. All of these should be the targets of strategies to recruit and train stockpeople in agricultural systems.

Personnel management in agriculture needs to match other industries. It appears that recruitment, performance, and turnover of stockpeople in agricultural systems are in a kind of recursive loop. An apparent unwillingness to invest in validated selection and training strategies leads to the employment of stockpeople who may not be ideally suited to animal care and who do not receive the opportunity to develop the attributes appropriate to the job. Equally important, the absence of a corporate policy that identifies stockpeople as key agricultural workers who should be the beneficiaries of programs to improve skills and motivation must reduce the status of workers in agricultural systems.

Employers in agricultural systems need to engage in practices that will improve the status of the industry, improve productivity, improve marketability of jobs in agricultural systems, and accommodate the fact that the potential pool of employees may be limited by geography and job image. A balanced approach will take advantage of people who are highly motivated, have dispositions and styles good for handling animals, and are amenable to appropriate training. By means of appropriate skills training, animal management training, and exercises to improve communication and group cohesion, management will have the opportunity to attract and retain the best possible staff and, in so doing, improve all aspects of the intensive animal farming sector.

REFERENCES

Ajzen, I. (1988). *Attitudes, personality, and behaviour*. Milton Keynes: Open University Press.

Ajzen, I., and Fishbein, M. (1980). *Understanding attitudes and predicting social behaviour*. Englewood Cliffs, NJ: Prentice-Hall Inc.

Allport, G. W. (1937). *Personality: A psychological interpretation*. New York: Holt and Company.

Ashforth, B. E., and Kreiner, G. E. (1999). "How can you do it?" Dirty work and the challenge of constructing a positive identity. *Academy of Management Review* (3), 413–434.

Barrick, M. P., and Mount, M. (1991). The big five personality dimensions and job performance: A meta-analysis. *Personnel Psychology*, 44, 1–26.

Beveridge, L. M. (1996). Studies on the influence of human characteristics and training on stockperson work performance and farm animal behaviour. Unpublished Ph.D. thesis, University of Aberdeen.

Beynon, N. M. (1991). Analysis of stockmanship. *Pig Veterinary Journal*, 26, 67–77.

Cammann, C., Fichmann, M., Jenkins, D., and Klesh, J. (1979). *The Michigan organisational assessment questionnaire*. Ann Arbor: University of Michigan.

Chlopan, B. E., McCain, M. L., Carbonell, J. L., and Hagen, R. (1985). Empathy: Review of available measures. *Journal of Personality and Social Psychology*, 48(3), 635–653.

Coleman, G. J. (2001). Selection of stockpeople to improve productivity. Paper presented at the 4th Industrial and Organisational Psychology Conference, Sydney, NSW.

Coleman, G. J., Hemsworth, P. H., and Hay, M. (1998). Predicting stockperson behaviours towards pigs from attitudinal and job related variables and empathy. *Applied Animal Behaviour Science*, 58(1), 63–75.

Coleman, G. J., Hemsworth, P. H., Hay, M., and Cox, M. (2000). Modifying stockperson attitudes and behaviour towards pigs at a large commercial farm. *Applied Animal Behaviour Science*, 66(1–2), 11–20.

Costa, P. T. and McCrae, R. R. (1992). The five-factor model of personality and its relevance to personality disorders. *Journal of Personality Disorders*, 6, 343–359.

Duan, C. and Hill, C. E. (1996). The current state of empathy research. *Journal of Counselling Psychology*, 43, 261–274.

English, P. (2002). Staff induction procedures and training. *Pig Progress*, 18, 28–29.

English, P., Burgess, G., Segundo, R. and Dunne, J. (1992). *Stockmanship: Improving the care of the pig and other livestock*. Farming Press Books, Ipswich, UK.

Eysenck, H. J. (1966). *Dimensions of personality*. Routledge and Kegan Paul Ltd., London

Griffeth, R. W., Hom, P. W. and Gaertner, S. (2000). A meta-analysis of antecedents and correlates of employee turnover: Update, moderator tests, and research implications for the next millennium. *Journal of Management*, 26, 463–488.

Hemsworth, P. H. and Coleman, G. J. (1998). *Human-livestock interactions: The stockperson and the productivity and welfare of intensively-farmed animals*. CAB International, Oxon UK.

Hemsworth, P. H., Coleman, G. J., Barnett, J. L., Borg, S. and Dowling, S. (2002). The effects of cognitive behavioural intervention on the attitude and behaviour of stockpersons and the behaviour and productivity of commercial dairy cows. *Journal of Animal Science*, 80, 68–78.

Hull, M. B. and Tyagi, K. C. (1996). Motivational styles, goal orientation and job satisfaction in dairy plants. *Indian Journal of Dairy Science,* 47, 385–391.

Kidd, A. H. and Kidd, R. M. (1990). The social and environmental influences on children's attitudes toward pets. *Psychological Reports*, 67, 807–818.

Kline, P. and Lapham, S. (1991a). The validity of the PPQ: A study of its factor structure and relationship to the EPQ. *Personality and Individual Differences*, 6, 631–635.

——. (1991b). The validity of the V scale of the PPQ. *Personality and Individual Differences*, 6, 637–641.

Lensink, J., Boissy, A. and Veissier, I. (2000). The relationship between farmers' attitude and behaviour towards calves, and productivity of veal units. *Annales de Zootechnie*, 49, 313–327.

Melson, G. F. and Fogel, A. (1988). The development of nurturance in young children. *Young Children. National Association for the Education of Young Children, US*, 43(3), 57–65.

PDI Employment Inventory. (1996). Personnel Decisions Inc., Minneapolis, MN.

Ravel, A., D'Allaire, S., Bigras-Poulin, M. and Ward, R. (1996). Influence of management, housing and personality of the stockperson on preweaning performances on independent and integrated swine farms in Quebec. *Preventive Veterinary Medicine*, 29, 37–57

Seabrook, M. (1996). The role of the human factor in increasing performance and profitability in pig production. Filozzo Rhone Poulenc Conference, Moderna, Italy, 2–13.

Seabrook, M. F. (1972a). A study on the influence of the cowman's personality and job satisfaction on milk yield of dairy cows. Joint Conference of the British Society for Agriculture Labour Science and the Ergonomics Research Society, National College of Agricultural Engineering, UK, September, 1972.

——. (1972b). A study to determine the influence of the herdsmen's personality on milk yield. *Journal of Agriculture Labour Science*, 1, 45–59.

——. (1982). Motivation and performance. *Ergonomics*, 25, 65–72.

Singh, S. (1983). Effect of motivation, values, cognitive factors and child rearing among Punjab farmers. *Journal of Social Psychology*, 120, 273–278.

Steel, R. P., Griffeth, R. W. and Hom, P. W. (2002). Practical retention policy for the practical manager. *Academy of Management Executive*, 16, 149–181.

Stevens, L. (1990). Attachment to pets among eight graders. *Anthrozoos*, 3, 177–183.

Triebenbacher, S. L. (1998). The relationship between attachment to companion animals and self-esteem: a developmental perspective. In C. C. Wilson and D. C. Turner (Eds.), *Companion animals in human health* (pp. 135–148). London, UK: Sage Publications, Inc.

Vidovic, V. V., Stetic, V. V. and Bratco, D. (1999). Pet ownership, type of pet and socioemotional development of school children. *Anthrozoos,* 12, 211–217.

Waiblinger S., Menke C. and Coleman G. (2002). The relationship between attitudes, personal characteristics and behaviour of stockpeople and subsequent behaviour and production of dairy cows. *Applied Animal Behaviour Science.* 79(3), 195–219.

II

Practical Applications

10

Production Practices and Well-Being: Beef Cattle

Joseph M. Stookey and Jon M. Watts

This chapter discusses the impact of various management practices on the well-being of beef cattle. It focuses specifically on the routine painful procedures commonly applied to beef cattle: dehorning, branding, and castration. However, painful treatments are not the only issues threatening beef cattle welfare. Because of their particular relevance to this industry, we also discuss the impact of abrupt artificial weaning and the buller steer syndrome that occurs in large feedlot pens.

For some procedures, a multitude of instruments or techniques can be used to obtain the same outcome (to remove horns, for example). We believe that where choices exist, there is an obligation to identify and adopt the most welfare-friendly option. In several cases, we propose that the industry abandon some traditional practices. We do this at the risk of being criticized for advocating what may appear to some producers to be a less-practical alternative.

Many current practices have evolved without accounting for the pain delivered by the procedure, thereby creating much of the welfare controversy that exists today for the beef industry. When these were first carried out, and throughout much of their history, anesthetics and analgesics were not available. Furthermore, opinions on the sentience of animals and the significance of their suffering were mainly the province of philosophers. Now that alternatives are available, even imperfect ones, it is appropriate that we try to direct the future evolution of livestock management in a manner more sympathetic to the needs of the animal. In general, practices that we know cause pain are indefensible if performed with no attempt to minimize or mitigate it.

Livestock industries today face many controversial issues, such as biosecurity, food safety, environmental stewardship, and animal welfare. Each one of these issues deserves the industry's attention, and each one can be solved by the same basic approach. Only high intention, sincere effort, intelligent direction, and skillful execution will yield progress on these issues. The problems will not go away on their own or be solved by accident. This chapter provides some insight on alternatives that may help improve the well-being of beef cattle.

THE EFFECTS OF AGE ON THE IMPACT OF A PROCEDURE

A common theme that resurfaces within each discussion about routine procedures is whether the age of the animal impacts upon the degree of suffering. We are certain that it does, but we believe this for reasons that are not entirely related to pain perception. The

185

Canadian veterinary profession recommends that castration and dehorning of cattle be performed in the first week of life (CVMA, 2003). However, the beef industry has yet to conform to a standard age at which these procedures are actually carried out. Branding, where practiced, is sometimes done repeatedly with changing ownership of an animal. The swine, poultry, and dairy industries usually castrate, debeak, tail dock, and so forth at a very early age. A major practical advantage to doing these tasks early is that the young animals are easier to restrain. This is arguably of benefit to the animal as well as the producer in that the task can be done more quickly and surely, minimizing handling stress.

From an animal's perspective though, this is probably not the most relevant factor. It is likely that there are both advantages and disadvantages to performing a procedure at a given age, depending on the task and the manner in which it is carried out. It was believed at one time that the ability to feel pain is absent in young animals, or poorly developed compared with their older counterparts. Recent research has shown that this is incorrect; in fact the opposite may be true. The perception of pain at a young age is now well documented (Anand and Scalzo, 2000; Ruda et al., 2000). The studies show not only that neonates do feel pain, but also that young animals may develop increased pain sensitivity following repeated painful experiences as a neonate. This, however, should not be taken to mean that doing the procedures later is preferable. Rather, it implies that the obligation to mitigate pain through the use of anesthetics and analgesics applies as much, or more, to young as to older animals. The great advantage to the animal of doing these tasks early is that it recovers sooner from the physical injury. Very young animals show quicker wound healing and experience fewer complications. Thus, the total amount of suffering from the time of the procedure until the wound heals is likely to be less if it is done at a young age. It is mainly for this reason that we agree that castration and dehorning should be done within seven days of birth.

The potential effects of these procedures on an animal's welfare are not limited to the pain of the procedure itself and the risk of subsequent infection. There may also be long-term negative psychological consequences of an unpleasant treatment. Memory of the painful procedure and its associated stimuli may contribute to fear of, and aversion to, certain people, places, sounds of equipment, and so on. This could lead to greater distress upon subsequent handling. One piece of evidence that is missing is whether age impacts upon the memory of painful procedures. Humans usually do not recall as adults the pain associated with surgical procedures, such as circumcision, that are often performed on infants, in some cultures without anesthesia. It may be that by performing the procedures early, we minimize the long-term psychological impact on the animal. We know that the pain system is stimulated by early experiences and that receptors and axons change as a result of early painful experiences (Anand and Scalzo, 2000). So, in a sense the body "remembers," but it is uncertain if the painful experience is remembered in a cognitive sense. If the ability to remember painful experiences is underdeveloped in neonates compared to older animals, as is true for some cognitive skills, then the scale might be further tipped in favor of completing necessary chores at an early age.

BRANDING

Cattle were branded in ancient Egypt as early as 2700 B.C.E. Today in many countries, branding continues to be a useful, though obviously painful, means to establish proof of ownership.

Since 1982, the United Kingdom has prohibited hot-iron branding (MAFF, 1992). In contrast, under some state regulations, as in New Mexico, a person who owns cattle *must* brand them (NMSA, 1978) using either hot-iron or freeze-branding techniques. Unbranded livestock, except calves running with branded cows, are subject to seizure by the authorities. Purchased livestock must be rebranded by the new owner within 30 days (NMSA 1978).

Branding comes at a cost to the animal, but also to the industry. The June 1996 Canadian Beef Audit reported that 37 percent of the cattle at the slaughter plants in Canada were branded, 6 percent of these cattle had multiple brands (Schwartzkopf-Genswein, 2000). Cows had the largest number of brands (51 percent) and multiple brands (19 percent). While branding may be a deterrent to cattle theft, ironically branding was estimated in 1993 to result in an average loss between $9.00 and $13.00 US per hide (USDA, 1993) and more recently estimated to cost the Canadian beef industry $3.57 per head or $9.5 million Cdn per year due to hide damage (Schwartzkopf-Genswein, 2000).

Branding may contribute to a loss of consumer support for the industry. Applebee's International, a restaurant chain in North America, announced in 2001 that it would require suppliers to adhere to standards, including a suggestion that animals not be branded. This company has since decided to review its policy after industry complaints, but Applebee's interest in this area is indicative of the dissatisfaction that restaurants and groceries have about the branding of cattle.

Is branding necessary? If branding causes pain to the animal, reduces hide prices, and also causes customer dissatisfaction, then why continue the practice? It should be possible in some settings, say at commercial feedlots, to provide sufficient security, penning, and ear tagging to eliminate the need for branding. Unfortunately, there are many locations where security is an issue, and there are few alternatives other than branding that offer absolute proof of ownership in cases of owner disputes. As a result, some lending institutions in North America require that the animals be permanently identified with a visible brand to ensure that cash receipts from the sale of the animal are returned to the rightful owner or lender. Another contributing factor to the widespread use of branding, such as in western Canada, is the practice of communal grazing. The commingling of cattle from various owners and subsequent owner disputes has inevitably led community pasture associations to require that animals be branded prior to entry.

Is it possible to create a permanent visible mark without branding? If compounds could be found that cause permanent visible marks without painful application, side effects, or residues in cattle, then perhaps branding could be replaced. We have investigated this possibility using depigmenting compounds and have successfully identified numerous compounds that have a depigmenting effect when applied on cattle. Unfortunately, we have found no compound that produced a permanent visible mark that survived after shedding and regrowth of the hair (Schwartzkopf et al., 1994).

Unfortunately, ear tags and electronic identification systems have often fallen short in terms of permanence and costs compared to branding in extensive operations. However, identification techniques that seemed impossible or expensive just a few years ago are likely to become the norm in the future. Currently, the European Union (EU) and the United Kingdom (UK) both have mandatory animal identification regulations in place, and

Canada has initiated a national identification system that requires all cattle to carry an individual bar-coded ear tag at the time of sale. Other countries are certain to follow this lead. Branding may become obsolete simply because individual animal identification systems with trace-back capabilities are being viewed as essential for disease control, food safety, and country-of-origin food labeling. One futuristic identification technique that is tamper proof and animal welfare friendly is retinal imaging (Golden and Shadduck, 2000). This technology is being specifically adapted for use in livestock and makes use of each animal's individual uniqueness in the pattern of blood vessels at the back of their eyes. The blood vessel pattern can be viewed through the pupil with a scanner and digitally recorded. Much like a fingerprint database for humans, a retinal image database could be kept for cattle. The Optibrand system can even combine the animal's retinal image data with encrypted global positioning system (GPS) information that is virtually impossible to falsify. Such a system would enable food producers, retailers, and governments to rapidly, accurately, and inexpensively track an animal's identity, ownership, and movements. However, until such technology is accepted, branding despite its drawbacks still offers the best proof of ownership in many locations throughout the world.

One alternative to hot-iron branding is freeze branding, which uses liquid nitrogen to supercool the branding irons. Upon application of the irons, the melanocytes within the hair follicles are permanently destroyed resulting in the growth of white hairs. Freeze branding was promoted in the 1960s as the "painless alternative" to hot-iron branding. However, research has shown that both branding methods cause physiological and behavioral responses indicative of pain (Lay et al., 1992a). It has not been simple to determine which procedure is the least painful. Lay and coworkers (1992a) gained some confidence that hot-iron branding was more painful when they used tame dairy cows in their comparison. However, the differences between the two treatments were not as clear when cattle were not habituated to handling (Lay et al., 1992b). Cortisol responses in branded and control animals were similar, suggesting that a large proportion of the hormonal response was a consequence of the handling and restraint required to perform branding. Another study (Schwartzkopf, Stookey, and Welford, 1997b) showed that the aversion or reluctance to reenter the branding area was no different for the next four days after the procedure for branded animals compared to controls that had simply been restrained in the same location. However, Schwartzkopf and coworkers (1997b) demonstrated a clear distinction between hot-iron and freeze branding by quantifying behavioral responses at the time of branding. By using strain gauges attached to the head gate, we detected significant increases in the exertion force against the head gate during hot-iron branding compared to freeze branding and controls. We also found that hot-iron branded cattle vocalize more at the time of branding, and their calls have a higher fundamental frequency compared to freeze-branded animals (Watts and Stookey, 1999). It now seems clear that hot-iron branding *is* more painful than freeze branding. There are drawbacks to freeze branding, however. These include the increase in time required to brand the animal, the high cost of liquid nitrogen, and the ineffectiveness of a freeze brand on white or light colored cattle.

One point to keep in mind is that though branding is certainly painful, the effects on the animal appear to be relatively short-lived. Surprisingly, there is no noticeable setback in weight gain or health following branding (Schwartzkopf et al., 1997a). This is in contrast to other painful or stressful procedures, such as castration, dehorning, transportation, or weaning, which always cause a setback. From a welfare perspective, branding may represent a very small negative blip in an animal's lifetime of experiences. Nevertheless, given the options, we believe the beef industry should disallow multiple branding, restrict the use of branding to cattle on extensive pasture situations, use freeze branding whenever the color of the cattle allows for it, and work toward a satisfactory alternative to, and the eventual abolition of, hot-iron branding.

DEHORNING

The ancestors of domestic cattle evolved horns under natural selection because they conferred a survival or reproductive advantage upon the possessor. Historically, they may even have been selected for artificially in the development of certain breeds, partly for their aesthetic qualities and partly in association with desirable production traits. In contemporary beef production, it is difficult to see any advantage arising from the possession of horns. Indeed, their only function outside of the showring seems to be as weapons. Horns are used by cattle in competitive encounters with their conspecifics and against people in offensive or protective situations. Leaving horns on beef cattle makes these encounters potentially more dangerous, both to people and to other cattle. Furthermore, injury arising from the use of horns as weapons leads to additional suffering for the animals and to economic losses for the producer.

When horns are left on feedlot cattle, the amount of bruised trim from the carcasses has been reported to be twice the amount measured from equivalent hornless groups (Meischke, Ramsay, and Shaw, 1974; Grandin, 1980). The Canadian Beef Quality Audit 1998–1999 has estimated that bruising costs the industry over $4 million Cdn a year, though the percentage of bruising attributable to horns remains unknown. One way to avoid bruising from cattle with horns is to remove them. Ideally this would be done as early as possible. If not dehorned until arrival at a feedlot, cattle can experience a setback in average daily gain that can be detected for up to 106 days (Goonewardene and Hand, 1991), evidence of the long-term effects of the pain and suffering that the dehorning procedure inflicts upon cattle of this age.

The Horned Cattle Purchase Act introduced in 1939 in Saskatchewan, Canada, required that a penalty of $2 Cdn be charged to the seller at the time of sale for all horned animals. This program was designed to encourage cow-calf producers to dehorn their calves prior to sale. In 2002, the act was amended and the fee was hiked to $10. This is a useful strategy other authorities might consider to encourage earlier dehorning of cattle.

Dehorning cattle prior to arrival at the feedlot, say at three months of age, does not eliminate the pain of the procedure, however (Sylvester et al., 1998). Dehorning cattle shortly after birth, using caustic paste or hot iron, has also been shown to be painful (Morisse, Cotte, and Huonnic, 1995). The use of local anesthetics administered prior to dehorning in calves has been shown to reduce the behaviors associated with the immediate pain response (Morisse et al., 1995; Sylvester et al., 1998), but this is not common practice within the beef industry. Even when local anesthetics are administered prior to dehorning, their effectiveness in blocking pain is limited to a few hours after dehorning. Cortisol levels rise after the effect of the local anesthetic wears off (Petrie et al., 1996), evidence that postoperative pain persists for a considerable time after the procedure. Since the beef industry rarely uses local anesthetics for dehorning, it seems unlikely that it would embrace the use of long-acting analgesics in combination with local anesthetics, which would be needed to control both postoperative and immediate pain responses (McMeekan et al., 1998, 1999; Faulkner and Weary, 2000). In the UK, dehorning of cattle is a veterinary procedure regulated under the Protection of Animals (Anaesthetics) Acts 1954, 1964, and Amendment Order 1982 (MAFF, 1992).

The North American beef industry is reluctant to use analgesics for dehorning of young calves because of the additional time and costs associated with the blocking procedure. Skilled operators can restrain and dehorn a calf faster than is required for injections of local anesthetics to be administered and to take effect. Those opposed to using analgesics would argue that the additional stress caused by an increase in restraint time may offset the benefits of pain control. There is no evidence to support or refute such claims, and more research is needed to determine the relationships between fear, pain, restraint time, and stress. The increased economic cost of pain relief comes primarily from the fees of the veterinarian, who is licensed to dispense controlled drugs; the drugs themselves are relatively inexpensive. One way to reduce this cost would be to offer a certification program that specifically trains and allows producers to possess anesthetics and analgesics and administer them to the animals prior to dehorning. A similar compromise has been reached between elk producers and the Alberta Veterinary Association to assist elk producers in removing velvet antler using anesthetics.

A logical alternative to dehorning, and one that is welfare and industry friendly, would be to use polled bulls to sire calves that do not need dehorning. This is especially attractive given a growing body of evidence that polled beef sires are the equal of their horned counterparts in every measure of productivity (e.g., Stookey and Goonewardene, 1996). Horns are inherited as an autosomal recessive gene, polledness being dominant (Long and Gregory, 1978). In one breeding season, a producer could take a herd of horned cows and breed them to a polled bull (homozygous for the polled condition) and produce an entire calf crop of polled calves.

Unfortunately, there are still pockets of resistance due to the belief that polled bulls are inferior. Comparing traits from bulls at test stations in Alberta and Saskatchewan from 1985 to 1993, Stookey and Goonewardene (1996) detected no differences between horned and polled bulls in Herefords (n = 1,860) or Charolais (n = 578) in average daily gain, adjusted yearling weight, backfat thickness, or scrotal circumference. In another study, polled German Simmental cattle were no different from their horned counterparts in growth, carcass yield, carcass composition, health, and reproductive performance (Lange, 1989). Horned and polled crossbred lines from various beef breeds were no different in live weight, fertility, and mortality rates (Frisch et al., 1980). Recent comparisons of three beef synthetic lines found no differences between horned and polled cattle in weight at birth, weaning weight, preweaning and postweaning average daily gain, carcass weight, and carcass characteristics (Goonewardene et al., 1999a) nor were there differences in reproductive traits such as pregnancy rates, dystocia scores, cow weights, and cow condition scores (Goonewardene et al., 1999b).

It already appears that the use of polled beef bulls may be increasing. One reason for this is that some of the polled breeds are valued for their calving ease, color, or carcass traits. Also, the exotic beef breeds in North America that were bred up from foundation stock, including the Limousin, Simmental, and Charolais breeds, are reporting a gradual increase in the numbers of polled animals. It is interesting to note that some breeders in North America have begun exporting semen and animals with the polled condition back to their country of origin, where polled animals are not readily available.

Horned-Hereford breeders seem to be the exception to the trend and are maintaining a strong registry and a resistance to change to polled breeding. In fact, the horned-Hereford breeders have used the horns as indicators or "advertisements" of their tradition and their selection for specific traits in an attempt to distance themselves from polled Herefords. Many horned-Hereford breeders would resist switching to polled bulls simply to address the welfare issue of dehorning, because at the same time they would have to give up tradition, possible clientele, and years of selection following specific lines. Nevertheless, the practice of dehorning will continue to be a welfare issue as long as beef calves are being sired by horned bulls and as long as they are being dehorned without pain control.

CASTRATION

As with dehorning, there has been no lack of imagination in devising methods to castrate cattle. In the case of castration, however, it may be harder to convince the industry to do the job in a particular way, at a certain age, solely on animal welfare grounds. This is because, while horns on cattle offer no benefit whatsoever to the producer, the possession of testicles, up to a point, can be advantageous. Growth rate and average daily gain is higher in bull calves than it is in steers (table 10.1), at least if the steers are not implanted. The feed efficiency of bulls is higher, the carcass is leaner, and the dressing percentage is greater.

Is castration of male beef calves really necessary? Writing for the Universities Federation for Animal Welfare, in the United Kingdom, John Webster (1999) argues that if bulls can reach slaughter weight by 18 months of age, the answer is no. In the UK and throughout the European Union, the use of hormone growth promoters has been banned since 1988. Intact males should therefore have a worthwhile advantage in growth rate over unimplanted steers. With some imagination and appropriate management, it should be possible to reduce or eliminate the need to castrate in North America, too. As long as bulls are slaughtered at a reasonable age, taste panels are apparently unable to discriminate between their meat and the meat of steers (Rollin, 1995). The practice of castration is part of the tradition of the industry for one good reason. Steers are easier to handle. A greater emphasis on selection for temperament together with improvements in handling management could greatly reduce aggression in bulls and help to overcome stress-induced problems such as dark cutting as well. Replacing the anabolic effects of testicles with artificial growth implants probably contributes to the incidence of buller steer syndrome. This welfare problem, and indeed the costs of implanting, would also be reduced if there were a greater acceptance of the advantages of raising bulls.

There are, however, serious disadvantages to raising intact bulls (table 10.1). Bulls are more aggressive than steers. They are also more difficult to handle (Hinch and Lynch, 1987). They are potentially more destructive of equipment and more likely to injure each other. In addition, people are more at risk of injury when working with bulls. If bulls are regrouped before slaughter, they are more likely to show dark cutting. The hide from bulls tends to be harder to remove. The meat is actually leaner than steer meat but, in some taste tests, consumers have rated bull meat as less palatable. Aware of these negative traits, packers discount bulls. Overall, if one disregards the welfare issues, there are many compelling disadvantages in raising and marketing intact males. This helps explain why castration is a routine procedure in the beef industry.

Method of Castration

A range of devices is available including Burdizzo, Newberry knife, elastrator, emasculator, and the humble pocketknife. These are variously intended to sever, crush, or constrict blood flow. Although all are undoubtedly painful in varying degrees, there has been considerable debate as to which is the least painful castration procedure. Some researchers have argued that rubber rings are more painful than surgical castration (Shutt et al., 1988). However, Zobell and coworkers (1993) have shown the setback in older animals was greater following surgical castration compared to animals castrated with the bloodless elastrator. Results from a study of our own on castration of older bulls (unpublished data)

Table 10.1.   Advantages and Disadvantages of Raising Intact Bulls Versus Steers

Advantages of raising bulls	Disadvantages of raising bulls
Growth (compared to nonimplanted steers)	Increased aggressive manner
• 17% higher ADG	More difficult to handle
• 13% higher feed efficiency	Receive discounted prices
Carcass traits	Carcass traits
• leaner meat (35% less fat)	• 73% increase in dark cutters*
• 0.2% higher dressing percent	• hide is harder to remove
	• lower consumer acceptance
	• less tender, less marbling
	• lower quality grade
	• darker meat

Source: Adapted from Seideman et al. (1982).
*The 73% increase in dark cutters occurs if bulls are recently mixed prior to slaughter.

were equivocal. Pain responses at the time of castration were more pronounced in animals surgically castrated with a Newberry knife than with rubber rings. But the rubber bands caused a delay in wound healing, suggesting prolonged discomfort, compared with the knife. Another study (Fisher et al., 1996) concluded that surgical castration was more stressful than the Burdizzo method, but that local anaesthetic was less effective for Burdizzo castration. Taking into account immediate and longer-term effects of these traditional castration techniques, it is not clear that one method is less costly to the well-being of the animal.

Age at Castration

It is clear to us that the welfare of male calves is better if they are castrated at the right time than if a particular tool is used to remove the testicles. All the evidence we have suggests that younger is better, and within a few days of birth is best of all. Bagley et al. (1989) found that intact bull calves gained 5 percent faster from birth to weaning compared to steers castrated at birth, but implanted steer calves gained 4 percent faster than control steers. They concluded that there is no benefit in delaying castration. Baker, Strickland, and Vann (2000) found no differences in average daily gain, weaning weight, or weight per day of age between calves castrated and implanted shortly after birth and at 150 days and intact controls. Bull calves could be routinely castrated at birth and implanted, which would result in nearly equal gains compared to bulls. The main advantage of castrating at birth would be that the healing process is so much quicker in younger animals (Johnstone, 1944).

Perhaps because implantation appears necessary if very young steers are to equal the growth rates of bull calves, some producers hold the view that late-age castration is desirable for reasons of productivity. Devices are available that are intended for castration of older bulls, weighing 750 pounds or more, using the rubber band method. The benefits of delayed castration are questionable, however. Recently, Gazzola et al. (2002) concluded that there was no commercially useful increase in growth rate with castration as late as 16 months. The rubber band devices are being marketed as a low-stress method for castration compared with traditional techniques. This is a disingenuous claim, in our view, because from the point of view of minimizing stress, animals in this size/age range should not be castrated at all. Moreover, it is not clear that this method is in all respects superior to surgical castration. For example, Fisher et al. (2001) found that cattle banded at 9 and 14 months of age showed less acute behavioral reactions immediately after castration than surgically castrated animals of the same age. Unfortunately, the 14-month-old banded cattle developed persistent wounds above the bands, which lasted up to several weeks after the scrotums fell off. The banded cattle also grew more slowly than the surgical group in the 56 days following treatment. Similarly, Knight et al. (2000) found that cattle castrated by banding at 14 months grew slower over the first 35 days postcastration compared with surgically castrated animals, and showed lower live weights after 122 days. Whether delayed castration offers any significant benefit in growth compared with implanting steers is uncertain. Regardless of the technique used, delayed castration should be deplored on welfare grounds.

Immunological Castration

Research in the last decade has raised the possibility that functional castration could be achieved practicably, without the pain and setback associated with conventional methods. Immunological castration attempts to vaccinate the animal against its own hormones. The gonadotropin-releasing hormone (GnRH) from the hypothalamus is a small messenger made up of only a few proteins. This hormone travels to the pituitary and activates a cascade of events that ultimately leads to sexual maturity and fertility. If an animal could be vaccinated against its own GnRH, the animal would launch an immune response against itself and produce antibodies that intercept the GnRH message, preventing it from arriving at the pituitary. In theory, you could castrate the animal through injections or vaccinations. Such a procedure would eliminate most concerns about the painfulness of castration. Studies to date have shown that vaccination against GnRH reduces testicular growth (Adams et al., 1996) and bull-like behavior (Jago et al., 1997, 1999) while possibly improving meat quality (Jago et al., 1999). The research in this area is promising, but the technique has not evolved to the point where it is straightforward and reliable enough for the needs of the industry.

Our conviction is that, from a welfare perspective, male cattle should be castrated early, if they are to be castrated at all. Ideally, this should be done before one week of age. The age at castration is much more important than the method used. Routine castration of mature cattle should not be done but, if it is necessary to castrate an isolated older individual, this should be performed as a veterinary procedure with local anesthesia and analgesics.

WEANING

Artificially weaning cows and calves by abrupt separation is perhaps the greatest psychological stressor imposed on beef cattle during their lifetime. The changes in behavior, such as increased vocalizations, decreased feeding, decreased time spent lying, and increased walking, persist for three to five days after separation. Inevitably there is a setback in weight gain for abruptly weaned beef calves during the first week after separation and often an increase in morbidity, even if the food and surroundings are familiar.

However, there are very good management, nutritional, and economic reasons why producers would want to impose an artificial weaning date upon cows and calves, despite the apparently negative impact upon the animals. Adult cattle have lower nutritional requirements compared to calves and feed sources can be more efficiently used if adults and young cattle are fed separately. In addition, body condition scores for lactating females drop during prolonged lactations, especially if nutrients or forages are limited or of poor quality. By imposing an artificial weaning date, producers are shifting the balance of responsibility for raising the calf away from the mother and onto themselves, in an attempt to maximize the cow's future production.

Under natural weaning conditions, animals rarely show overt signs of distress. Young mammals and adults appear programmed to accept the natural weaning process; yet when it is abruptly thrust upon them through our management practices, both cows and calves display severe signs of distress. This suggests that some component of traditional weaning imposes undue stress upon our cattle.

If left to nature, the weaning process in beef cattle would follow the milk production curve of the cow, peaking around 90 days postpartum and then declining gradually. Natural weaning in zebu cattle (*Bos indicus*) was reported to take about two weeks and occurred, on average, at 11.3 months of age for bull calves and 8.8 months of age for female offspring (Reinhardt and Reinhardt, 1981). There is never complete and abrupt abandonment of the calf by the cow. Instead, they maintain a lifelong relationship of social contact and companionship even after the birth of successive sibling calves (Reinhardt, 2002).

In many countries, the beef industry is segregated into cow–calf producers, backgrounders, and finishers; thus, cattle may change owners, locations, and groups one or more times prior to reaching slaughter weight. Many calves are taken from the cows directly to the auction market. These calves experience all of the stressors associated with weaning within a few days (table 10.2). There is good evidence that multiple concurrent stressors have a greater impact upon an animal than if the animal experiences one stressor at a time (McFarlane et al., 1989; Curtis, Johnson, and McFarlane, 1990; Hyun et al., 1998).

Age at Weaning

Weaning is artificially imposed at a time that reduces the normal lactation by two to four months. However, Reinhardt and Reinhardt (1981) showed that the natural age at weaning of cattle has tremendous variation. It is likely that natural weaning age in cattle is dependent on the dam's milk production rather than age, as it is in sheep (Arnold, Wallace, and Maller, 1979). The variation that some producers observe from year to year in the amount

Table 10.2.   List of Potential Stressors Associated with Traditional Weaning in Beef Cattle

---

Age at weaning is younger than natural age.
New social environment:
   absence of adults
   mixing of unfamiliar animals
   formation of new social hierarchy
Physical separation of mother and calf
Premature end of lactation (even though milk still available)
Transportation
New location
New diet

---

of calling between cows and calves after weaning is likely the result of year-to-year variation in forage, milk supply, pregnancy status, and how close to a natural weaning age the calves were at the time of separation. The age at which we artificially impose weaning is probably not, in itself, a stressor.

New Social Environment, Absence of Adults

In contrast to the calves' previous social conditions, a pen of newly weaned calves will typically be without any adult animals. Prior to weaning, calves are in constant contact with their dams who provide them with protection, as well as lead them to forage and water (Fraser and Broom, 1990). Newly weaned calves are reported to have low feed intake for the first two weeks following their arrival at the feedlot (Cole and Hutcheson, 1988; Fluharty, Loerch, and Smith, 1994). In red deer, the presence of an adult has been shown to reduce weaning stress and the fear response (Pollard, Littlejohn, and Suttie, 1992).

Several researchers have asked whether the presence of unfamiliar adult "trainer" cows in a feedlot would facilitate the introduction of newly weaned calves. Loerch and Fluharty (2000) found a slight benefit in performance and a lower morbidity in two out of three trials. However, Gibb et al. (2000) reported lower rates of gain for calves housed with trainer cows and no difference in health or immune function. Our conclusion is that there are no proven significant benefits from this procedure.

Presence of Familiar Adults

We conducted a small pilot study with eight crossbred cow-calf pairs to determine if cows and calves that were familiar herd mates would benefit from each other's presence following abrupt separation when calves averaged six months of age. The eight pairs were a subset of a larger herd that had been together since calving. For two days prior to weaning and four days after weaning we observed the pairs during daylight hours. On the day of weaning we divided the group into two nonadjacent pens, so that each contained four cows and four calves, but none of the cows were penned with their own calves.

Before separation, we did not observe cross suckling or attempts by the calves to nurse from any cow other than their mother. Similarly, no cows were seen to groom a calf other than their own. They did not vocalize except when supplemental feed was being delivered by tractor and wagon.

During the days following weaning, both cows and calves behaved in a manner that we would call "typical" for newly weaned cows and calves. The rate of vocalizing was exceptionally high for the first two days following separation and gradually declined. There was a significant reduction in the time spent eating and ruminating. To our surprise, the cows were not observed to lie down during the first 12 hours following weaning and their time spent ruminating was reduced by 75 percent.

We observed only two tentative and unsuccessful attempts by calves to nurse from cows after the separation. It seemed obvious to us that the cows and calves were only interested in reuniting with their partners. There was no redirected maternal care despite the fact that udders were engorged and there were bawling calves present from their own herd. Likewise, calves did not appear "calm" despite the presence of familiar cows.

Fence-Line Weaning

Weaning by separating mothers and offspring into adjacent pens so that some social contact is possible has been shown to be of some benefit in horses (McCall, Potter, and Kreider, 1985). Fence-line weaning has also been shown to reduce behavioral indicators of stress in elk (Haigh et al., 1997) and beef calves (Stookey et al., 1997). In our studies, we found fence-line weaned calves consistently walked less and lay more than remotely separated cows and calves. Fence-line weaned calves gained more during the first week after weaning, but there were no long-term benefits on growth rate. More recent work has shown that fence-line weaned calves gained more the first week following weaning and were still heavier than traditionally weaned calves after ten weeks (Price, 2002). Statistically, we can detect some advantages to fence-line weaning, but they are not obvious to the casual observer. Given a choice between remotely separating cows and calves or using fence-line weaning, we recommend producers allow fence-line contact following weaning.

Two-Step Weaning

Recently, the doctoral research of Derek Haley has shown that by weaning in two stages, first by taking away the milk and second by separating the pair several days later, the entire weaning process can be made significantly less stressful (Haley, Stookey, and Bailey, 2002). In these studies, nursing was prohibited by a plastic antisucking device, which hung from the calf's nose and prevented calves from getting the teat into their mouths (fig. 10.1).

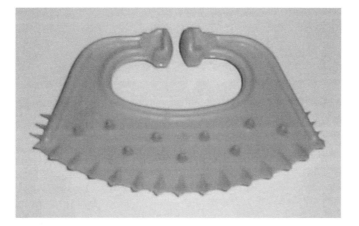

Figure 10.1.   The plastic antisucking device used to terminate nursing. The device acts as a physical barrier preventing calves from getting the cow's teat into their mouths.

One of many trials, used 12 beef cow-calf pairs and randomly assigned pairs to a control (abrupt-weaning treatment) or to the two-step weaning procedure. Nursing was prevented for four days prior to separation for the two-step calves. Prior to imposing the treatments, baseline information about the nursing and general behavior patterns of the cow-calf pairs was collected for four days. We then observed the animals during the four-day period while nursing was prevented for the two-step weaning group and while control groups were allowed to nurse. Finally, we observed cows and calves for the four days following their separation. All antisucking devices were removed on the day of separation. During the baseline period, vocalizations by both cows (fig. 10.2) and calves (fig. 10.3) were extremely rare. The only behavioral change associated with preventing nursing, during the next four days, was a slight increase in the amount of vocalizing (cows = 24 vocalizations/day; calves = 6 vocalizations/day). On the four days after cows and calves were separated, two-step cows vocalized 80 percent less than the control cows weaned the traditional way. For calves, the difference was even more remarkable; treated calves vocalized 95 percent less than traditionally weaned calves, calling at the same rate they did during baseline observations.

Two-step cows and calves spent more time eating, compared to controls and two-step calves spent roughly 50 percent less time walking than the abruptly weaned calves after separation.

We conducted another trial to determine the relative distance that calves walked before and following separation, using electronic pedometers. Half of the calves were randomly assigned to the control (abrupt separation) and the other half were weaned following the two-step procedure.

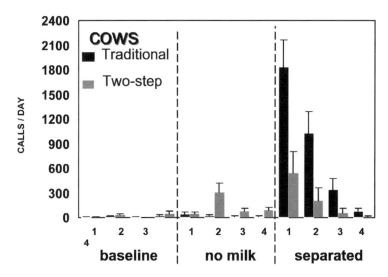

Figure 10.2.   The vocalizations per day by cows weaned by abrupt separation and by the two-step method during three distinct periods of time.

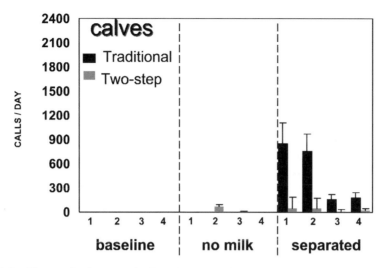

Figure 10.3.   The vocalizations per day by calves weaned by abrupt separation and by the two-step method during three distinct periods of time.

Applying the same average stride length to all steps (75 cm), we found that controls walked nearly three times farther than two-step calves during the first two days after separation (40 vs 15 km; $P < 0.05$). Two-step weaning drastically reduces the behavioral indicators of stress associated with the traditional abrupt method of weaning. Our conclusion is that simultaneously removing the mother and the milk, as is done in traditional weaning, causes a far greater behavioral response than if the two events occur at separate times (Haley et al., 2001). In retrospect, it appears that the two-step weaning procedure mimics the natural weaning process and as a result reduces many of the behavioral signs of stress associated with weaning. Based on these behavioral responses, two-step weaning represents the latest and best alternative to traditional weaning.

HOUSING STEERS IN FEEDLOTS AND THE BULLER STEER SYNDROME

The buller steer syndrome is a behavioral problem among feedlot steers, characterized by the repeated mounting of a steer (referred to as the buller) by a group of steers (known as the riders) who persistently follow and perform the mounting behavior. We believe this is partially the result of management decisions that place animals at higher risks. The behavior of buller steers in feedlot pens has recently been investigated by Jean Clavelle. In one observational study, bullers received on average 61 mounts per hour (range 43–114 mounts/hour) (Clavelle, 2002a). Exposed to such harassment, a buller steer becomes exhausted, often shows loss of hair, swelling and trauma on the rump and tail head, and in extreme cases can suffer broken bones or may even die from injuries. The syndrome is an obvious welfare issue. Proper management of cases requires prompt isolation and removal of the buller to a separate hospital or sick pen where bulling usually subsides.

The annual incidence of buller steers within the feedlot industry is reported to fall between 2 and 4 percent, but the incidence per pen can be quite variable ranging from 0.0 percent to 11.2 percent per pen (Taylor et al., 1997). Numerous causative factors have been implicated as contributing to the incidence, including the use of anabolic agents, improper implantation, reimplantation or double dosing, changes in weather and seasonal factors, excessive mud or dusty pen conditions, entry weights, disease, group size, improper or late castration, feeding management, transportation, handling, mixing, dipping, and aggressive social dominance behavior. Of these factors, entry weights, weather, and seasonal factors have not withstood scientific scrutiny and should be dropped from the list of causative factors (Irvin et al., 1979). The perceived seasonal effects are more likely related to the increase in bullers observed immediately after feedlot entry, which tends to be seasonal (Taylor et al., 1997).

There is very strong evidence that the use of anabolic agents contributes to the development of bullers (Irvin et al., 1979). Historically, the incidence of buller steers was low (1.5 percent) back in 1968–1970, when the agent used as a growth promotant was diethylstilbestrol (DES) at the 10 mg level in the feed. In 1971, DES was increased to the 20 mg level and the incidence of buller steers edged upward (2.09 percent). A further jump to 2.8 percent was noted in 1972 when the industry switched to anabolic hormone implants. It was up to 3.67 percent by 1974 (Pierson et al., 1976). Even higher incidences of buller steers have been reported with the use of the stronger implant combinations of trenbolone acetate and estradiol. It is uncertain if the use of growth promotants in nursing calves (which is increasing) is further compounding the incidence of bullers in the feedlot. The common practice is to implant all animals upon entry into the feedlot, disregarding the possibility that incoming cattle may already be implanted. That may be a mistake in terms of buller activity.

One difficulty in implicating implants as the main culprit is that during the time implants were increasing in popularity and potency, the number of cattle in feedlots nearly doubled. The number of animals per pen was also increasing as the incidence of bullers was rising. One study has shown a correlation between the number of steers in the pen and the incidence of bullers; for every ten head increase per pen, the buller incidence increases 0.015 percent (Brower and Kiracofe, 1978).

The buller steer syndrome may also be partially related to the establishment of social hierarchies among unfamiliar animals and may develop through the normal mounting behavior that accompanies aggressive behavior. This theory helps explain the increase in bullers that occurs shortly after entry into the feedlot and the resurgence of bullers following regrouping. It also explains why the incidence is lower in pens that are made up of a single group as opposed to pens assembled from multiple groups.

What has recently become clear is that the standard description, which states that a buller steer voluntarily stands to be mounted (Blackshaw, Blackshaw, and McGlone, 1997), is probably wrong for the majority of bullers. Instead, buller steers try to avoid mounts and take advantage of corners, water troughs, dirt mound and feed bunks to help fend off riders (Clavelle, 2002b). In her observational studies, Clavelle (2002a) has also discovered that some buller steers miss detection by feedlot personnel but are able to recover and avoid further abuse on their own. The implications from these recent findings are that physical structures or barriers might be designed to offer protection for steers. Research is needed to investigate this possibility, and engineers should begin thinking of pen designs that facilitate manure handling, animal handling, *and* mounting protection. In addition, pen size should not exceed two hundred steers per pen (Blackshaw et al., 1997). One of us (JMW) has hypothesized that the proportion of bullers might represent merely the most extreme manifestation of a larger welfare problem, chronic social stress in very large groups. However, evidence for or against this idea has yet to be gathered. Finally, the role of implants in the incidence of bullers is too overwhelming to ignore. The buller steer issue is indeed an animal welfare issue and contributing factors must be identified and corrected. If specific implant protocols are contributing to the problem, they should be adjusted, and pharmaceutical companies must play a role in helping to address animal welfare issues that they may have helped create.

CONCLUSIONS

Several common production practices in the beef industry have inherent negative consequences for the well-being of the animals. These procedures can cause pain and physical injury and also psychological distress. Where their use is mandated in current production systems, caretakers should attempt to reduce to a minimum their impact on the animal. We are certainly able to make recommendations to improve welfare based on science and sound logic. However, few improvements in animal welfare will come about without producers accepting that some costs might be incurred. One exception is dehorning, which could practically be abolished in the beef industry if there were sufficient will among breeders to do it, simply through the use of polled sires. Painful procedures in general should be done as early as possible in an animal's life. This promotes more rapid healing and may not have such prolonged psychological consequences. Production systems should be modified as necessary to reduce stresses on the animals. Important in this regard is consideration of the normal behavior and social system of cattle. For example, the stress of artificial weaning could be considerably reduced through the use of a two-stage weaning technique, which is closer to the way cattle wean themselves under natural conditions. The buller steer syndrome is seen in feedlots where groups of steers, all of a similar age range, are penned together in very large numbers. While it may be helpful to provide antimounting structures in the pen or to tinker with implanting protocols, one solution we know will practically eliminate the syndrome, though not without some cost, is simply to avoid penning feedlot steers together in such large groups.

REFERENCES

Adams, T. E., Daley, C. A., Adams, B. M., Sakurai, H. 1996. Testes function and feedlot performance of bulls actively immunized against gonadotropin-releasing hormone: effect of age at immunization. J. Anim. Sci. 74, 950–954.

Anand, K. J., Scalzo, F. M. 2000. Can adverse neonatal experiences alter brain development and subsequent behavior? Biol. Neonate. 77, 69–82.

Arnold, G. W., Wallace, S. R., Maller, R. A. 1979. Some factors involved in the natural weaning processes in sheep. Appl. Anim. Behav. Sci. 5, 43–50.

Bagley, C. P., Morrison, D. G., Feazel, J. I., Saxton, A. M. 1989. Growth and sexual characteristics of suckling beef calves as influenced by age at castration and growth implants. J. Anim. Sci. 67, 1258–1264.

Baker, J. F., Strickland, J. E., Vann, R. C. 2000. Effect of castration on weight gain of beef calves. Bovine Practitioner 34, 124–126.

Blackshaw, J. K., Blackshaw, A. W., McGlone, J. J. 1997. Buller steer syndrome review. App. Anim. Behav. Sci. 54, 97–108.

Brower, G. R., Kiracofe, G. H. 1978. Factors associated with the buller-steer syndrome. J. Anim. Sci. 46, 26–31.

Clavelle, J. L. 2002a. A description of mount behaviour during the buller steer syndrome in a western Canadian feedlot. Proceedings of 5th North American Regional Meeting of the ISAE. Quebec City, Canada. July 20–21, p 9.

——. 2002b. The buller steer syndrome. MS Thesis. Department of Large Animal Clinical Sciences, University of Saskatchewan, pp 54–97.

Cole, N. A., Hutcheson, D. P. 1988. Influence of protein concentration in prefast and postfast diets on feed intake of steers and nitrogen and phosphorus metabolism of lambs. J. Anim. Sci. 66, 1764–1777.

Curtis, S. E., Johnson, R. W., McFarlane, J. M. 1990. Multiple stressors affect chick performance additively. Poul. Digest 49, 36–37.

CVMA. 2003. Animal welfare position statements of the Canadian Veterinary Medicial Association. Castration/tail docking/dehorning of farm animals C36893 http://www.cvma-acmv.org/welfare.asp.

Faulkner, P. M., Weary, D. M. 2000. Reducing pain after dehorning in dairy calves. J. Dairy Sci. 83, 2037–2041.

Fisher, A. D., Crowe, M. A., Alonso de la Varga, M. E., Enright, W. J. 1996. Effect of castration method and the provision of local anesthesia on plasma cortisol, scrotal circumference, growth, and feed intake of bull calves. J. Anim. Sci. 74, 2336–2343.

Fisher, A. D., Knight, T. W., Cosgrove, G. P., Death, A. F., Anderson, C. B., Duganzich, D. M., Matthews, L. R. 2001. Effects of surgical or banding castration on stress responses and behaviour of bulls. Aust. Vet. J. 79, 279–284.

Fraser, A. F., Broom, D. M. 1990. Farm animal behavior and welfare (3rd Ed.). Bailliere Tindal, London.

Frisch, J. E., Nishimura, H., Cousins, K. J., Turner, G. H. 1980. The inheritance and effect on production of polledness in four crossbred lines of beef cattle. Anim. Prod. 31, 119–126.

Fluharty, F. L., Loerch, S. C., Smith, F. E. 1994. Effects of energy density and protein source on diet digestibility and performance of calves after arrival at the feedlot. J. Anim. Sci. 72, 1616–1622.

Gazzola, C., Jeffery, M. R., White, D. H., Hill, R. A., Reid, D. J. 2002. Effect of delayed castration on the growth rate, behaviour and serum insulin-like growth factor–concentration of beef cattle on tropical pasture. Anim. Sci. 75, 41–47.

Gibb, D. J., Schwartzkopf-Genswein, K. S., Stookey, J. M., McKinnon, J. J., Godson, D. L., Wiedmeier, R. D., McAllister, T. A. 2000. Effect of a trainer cow on health, behavior and performance of newly weaned beef cattle. J. Anim. Sci. 78, 1716–1725.

Golden, B. L., Shadduck, J. A. 2000. The role of retinal imaging in source verification. Robert E. Taylor Beef Symposium, Fort Collins, CO, 12–13 December. http://ansci.colostate.edu/ran/beef/blg002.html.

Goonewardene, L. A., Hand, R. K. 1991. Studies on dehorning steers in Alberta feedlots. Can. J. Amin. Sci. 71, 1249–1252.

Goonewardene, L. A., Pang, H., Berg, R. T., Price, M. A. 1999b. A comparison of reproductive and growth traits of horned and polled cattle in three synthetic beef lines. Can. J. Anim. Sci. 79, 123–127.

Goonewardene, L. A., Price, M. A., Liu, M. F., Berg, R. T., Erichsen, C. M. 1999a. A study of growth and carcass traits in dehorned and polled composite bulls. Can. J. Anim. Sci. 79, 383–385.

Grandin, T. 1980. Bruises and carcass damage. Int. J. Stud. Anim. Prob. 1, 121–137.

Haigh, J. C., Stookey, J. M., Bowman, P., Waltz, C. 1997. A comparison of weaning techniques in farmed wapiti (*Cervus elaphus*). Anim. Welfare 6, 255–264.

Haley, D. B., Stookey, J. M., Bailey, D. W. 2002. A procedure to reduce the stress of weaning on beef cattle: On-farm trials of two-step weaning. Proceedings of the 5th North American Regional Meeting of the ISAE. Quebec City, Canada July 20–21, p 8.

Haley, D. B., Stookey, J. M., Clavelle, J. L., Watts, J. M. 2001. The simultaneous loss of milk and maternal contact compounds the distress at weaning in beef calves. Proceedings of the 35th International Congress of the ISAE. Davis, CA, August 4–9, p 41.

Hinch, G. N., Lynch, J. J. 1987. A note on the effect of castration on the ease of movement and handling of young cattle in yards. Anim. Prod. 45, 317–320.

Hyun, Y., Ellis, M., Riskowski, G., Johnson, R. W. 1998. Growth performance of pigs subjected to multiple concurrent environmental stressors. J. Anim. Sci. 76, 721–727.

Irvin, M. R., Melendy, D. R., Amoss, M. S., Hutcheson, D.P. 1979. Roles of predisposing factors and gonadal hormones in the buller syndrome of feedlot steers. J. Amer. Vet. Med. Assoc. 174, 367–370.

Jago, J. G., Cox, N. R., Bass, J. J., Mathews, L. R. 1997. The effect of prepubertal immunization against gonadotropin-releasing hormone on the development of sexual and social behaviour in bulls. J. Anim. Sci. 75, 2609–2619.

Jago, J. G., Matthews, L. R., Trigg, T. E., Dobbie, P., Bass, J. J. 1999. The effect of immunocastration 7 weeks before slaughter on the behaviour, growth and meat quality of post-pubertal bulls. Anim. Sci. 68, 163–171.

Johnstone, I. L. 1944. The tailing of lambs: the relative importance of normal station procedures. Australian Vet. J. 20, 286–291.

Knight, T. W., Cosgrove, G. P., Death, A. F., Anderson, C. B., Fisher, A. D. 2000. Effect of method of castrating bulls on their growth and liveweight. NZ J. Agric. Res. 43, 187–192.

Lange, H. 1989. Investigations on polledness and head conformations. Thesis, Ludwig-Mazimilians-Universat Muchen, Federal Republic of Germany.

Lay, D. C., Friend, T. H., Bowers, C. L. Grissom, K. K., Jenkins, O. C. 1992a. A comparative physiological and behavioral study of freeze and hot-iron branding using dairy cows. J. Anim. Sci. 70,. 1121–1125.

Lay, D. C., Friend, T. H., Randel, R. D., Bowers, C. L., Grissom, K. K., Jenkins, O. C. 1992b. Behavioral and physiological effects of freeze or hot-iron branding on crossbred cattle. J. Anim. Sci. 70, 330–336.

Loerch, S. C., Fluharty, F. L. 2000. Use of trainer animals to improve performance and health of newly arrived feedlot calves. J. Anim. Sci. 78, 539–545.

Long, C. R., Gregory, K. E. 1978. Inheritance of the horned, scurred and polled condition in cattle. J. Herid. 69, 395–400.

MAFF. 1992. Summary of the law relating to farm animal welfare. Ministry of Agriculture, Fisheries and Food PB 0493, MAFF Publications, London, pp 9–24.

McCall, C. A., Potter, G. D., Kreider, J. L. 1985. Locomoter, vocal and other behavioural responses to varying methods of weaning foals. Appl. Anim. Behav. Sci. 14, 27–35.

McFarlane, J. M., Curtis, S. E., Shanks, R. D., Carmer, S. G. 1989. Multiple concurrent stressors in chicks. 1. Effect on weight gain, feed intake and behavior. Poul. Sci. 68, 501–509.

McMeekan, C. M., Mellor, D. J., Stafford, K. J., Bruce, R. A., Ward, R. N., Gregory, N. G. 1998. Effects of local anaesthesia of 4 to 8 hours' duration on the acute cortisol response to scoop dehorning in calves. Aust. Vet. J. 76, 281–285.

McMeekan, C. M., Stafford, K. J., Mellor, D. J., Bruce, R. A., Ward, R. N., Gregory, N. G. 1999. Effects of local anaesthetic and a non-steroidal anti-inflammatory analgesic on the behavioural responses of calves to dehorning. NZ Vet. J. 47, 92–96.

Meischke, H. R. C., Ramsay, W. R., Shaw, F. D. 1974. The effect of horns on bruising cattle. Aust. Vet. J. 50, 432–434.

Morisse, J. P., Cotte, J. P., Huonnic, D. 1995. Effect of dehorning on behaviour and plasma cortisol responses in young calves. Appl. Anim. Behav. Sci. 43, 239–247.

NMSA. 1978. New Mexico Statutes CHAPTER 77. Livestock Code ARTICLE 9. Brands, Ownership, Transportation and Sale of Animals sect. 3 Necessity of brand; rebranding required; exceptions. http://www.law.utexas.edu/dawson/brands/NM_BRAND.HTM.

Petrie, N. J., Mellor, D. J., Stafford, K. J., Bruce, R. A., Ward, R. N. 1996. Cortisol responses of calves to two methods of disbudding used with and without local anaesthetic. NZ Vet. J. 44, 9–14.

Pierson, R. E., Jensen, R., Braddy, P. M., Horton, D. P., Christie, R. M. 1976. Bulling among yearling feedlot steers. J. Amer. Vet. Med. Assoc. 169, 521–523.

Pollard, J. C., Littlejohn, R. P., Suttie, J. M. 1992. Behaviour and weight change of red deer calves during different weaning procedures. Appl. Anim. Behav. Sci. 35, 23–33.

Price, E. O., 2002. Fenceline weaning of beef calves. http://danrrec.ucdavis.edu/sierra_foothill/sfrec _2002_fenceline_weaning.pdf.

Reinhardt, V. 2002. Artificial weaning of calves: benefits and costs. J. Appl. Anim. Welfare Sci. 5, 251–255; and http://www.awionline.org/Lab_animals/biblio/jaaws7.html.

Reinhardt, V., Reinhardt, A. 1981. Natural sucking performance and age of weaning in zebu cattle (*Bos indicus*). J. Agr. Sci., 96, 309–312.

Rollin, B. E. 1995. Farm animal welfare. Iowa State University Press, Ames, p 63.

Ruda, M. A., Ling, Q. D., Hohmann, A. G., Peng, Y. B., Tachibana, T. 2000. Altered nociceptive neuronal circuits after neonatal peripheral inflammation. Science. 289, 628–631.

Schwartzkopf, K. S., Stookey, J. M., Hull, P. R., Clark, E. G. 1994. Screening of depigmenting compounds for the development of an alternate method of branding beef cattle. J. Anim. Sci. 72, 1393–1398.

Schwartzkopf, K. S., Stookey, J. M., Janzen, E. D., McKinnon, J. 1997a. Effects of branding on weight gain, antibiotic treatment rates and subsequent handling ease in feedlot cattle. Can. J. Anim. Sci. 77, 361–367.

Schwartzkopf, K. S., Stookey, J. M., Welford, R. 1997b. Behavior of cattle during hot-iron and freeze branding and the effects on subsequent handling ease. J. Anim. Sci. 75, 2064–2072.

Schwartzkopf-Genswein, K. 2000. Quality Assurance Practices—Branding. http://www.agric.gov.ab .ca/livestock/beef/qa/branding.html.

Seideman, S. C., Cross, H. R., Oltjen, R. R., Schanbacher, B. D. 1982. Utilization of the intact male for red meat production: A review. J. Anim. Sci. 55, 826–840.

Shutt, D. A., Fell, L. R., Connell, R. Bell, A. K. 1988. Stress responses in lambs docked and castrated surgically or by the application of rubber rings. Aust. Vet. J. 65, 5–7.

Stookey, J. M., Goonewardene, L. A. 1996. Comparison of production traits and welfare implications between horned and polled beef bulls. Can. J. Anim. Sci. 76, 1–5.

Stookey, J. M., Schwartskopf-Genswein, K. S., Waltz, C. S., Watts, J. M. 1997. Effects of remote and contact weaning on behaviour and weight gain of beef calves. J. Anim. Sci. 75 (Suppl. 1), 157.

Sylvester, S. P., Mellor, D. J., Stafford, K. J., Bruce, R. A., Ward, R. N. 1998. Acute cortisol responses of calves to scoop dehorning using local anaesthesia and/or cautery of the wound. Aust. Vet. J. 76, 118–122.

Taylor, L. F., Booker, C. W., Jim, G. K., Guichon, P. T. 1997. Sickness, mortality and the buller steer syndrome in a western Canadian feedlot. Aust. Vet. J. 75, 732–736.

United States Department of Agriculture (USDA). 1993. Branding practices in beef cow/calf herds. Http://www.aphis.usda.gov/vs/ceah/cahm/Beef_Cow-Calf/chapa/chapbrnd.pdf

Watts, J. M., Stookey, J. M. 1999. Effects of restraint and branding on rates and acoustic parameters of vocalization in beef cattle. Appl. Anim. Behav. Sci. Amsterdam; New York: Elsevier, 1984-. Feb 15, 1999, v 62 (2/3), pp 125–135.

Webster, A. J. F. 1999. Beef cattle and veal calves. In Ewbank, R., Kim-Madslien, F., Hart, C. B. Management and welfare of farm animals: The UFAW farm handbook. Universities Federation for Animal Welfare: Wheathampstead, UK, pp 49–82.

Zobell, D. R., Goonewardene, L. A., Ziegler, K. 1993. Evaluation of the bloodless castration procedure for feedlot bulls. Can. J. Anim. Sci. 73, 967–970.

11

Animal Well-Being in the U.S. Dairy Industry

Franklyn B. Garry

INTRODUCTION

A reasonable discussion of the well-being of dairy animals relies heavily on an understanding of the structure and function of dairy production systems. The dairy industry in the United States has undergone dramatic changes over the last 40 to 50 years, and these changes are ongoing. The impetus for change is mostly provided by economic factors, plus the availability of new technology. As with other livestock production areas, changes are reflected in increased production per animal, increased total production, and decreased input of human labor per animal or per pound of production. Many features of these changing production systems have the potential to positively or negatively impact animal welfare, such as housing, nutrition and feeding systems, animal handling, and disease control programs.

Some discussions of animal welfare in livestock production environments focus on a few specific practices or details of animal management that some people have considered abhorrent (e.g., debeaking of poultry, use of gestation crates for sows, downer cow management in the slaughter industry). These isolated aspects of livestock production become the lightning rods for those trying to change industry practices. Unlike the pork and poultry industries, the dairy industry has received little such attention and very few practices have achieved widespread notoriety as indicative of dairy animal suffering. This is a very good time for the dairy industry to take stock of some of the impacts that production practices can have on animal welfare with an eye toward continual improvement of animal well-being. It is reasonable to presume that future dairy industry changes, predicated primarily on the improvement of animal welfare rather than primarily on the improvement of economic efficiency, could profoundly benefit both the animals and the industry.

The following discussion of animal well-being in the dairy industry will first review some of the fundamental changes in dairy production systems that have occurred over the last several decades. Based on this overview, we will then consider specific features of animal well-being as they relate to current management practices.

CHANGING FEATURES OF U.S. DAIRY PRODUCTION

A common vision of dairy farming for much of the public is the image of a small herd of dairy cows grazing in a pasture and periodically being called to the barn for milking. This

207

image is accurate as a snapshot of dairying on a nice summer day on some dairies in the traditional dairy regions of the country. However, it provides only a glimpse of the full picture, which would include details of how the cows are housed in bad (winter) weather, how they are fed when pasture forage is not available, what other activities the dairy producer is doing besides milking cows, and what kind of housing and management is provided for youngstock. Furthermore, that common image is in sharp contrast to that of a dairy with a thousand or more cows, housed in large, open, dirt lots in the western United States' arid lands, and fed mixed and processed silage and grain exclusively from a feedbunk. Dairy animal management is continuing to undergo dramatic change, and both of these snapshot views are accurate for some settings, illustrating that animals in the industry experience a diverse range of environments and management practices.

Some statistics can help to demonstrate the magnitude of change that has occurred in the U.S. dairy industry over the last 50 years. In 1950, there were approximately 22 million dairy cows, producing 5,300 lb of milk per year, for a total of 117 billion lb of total U.S. milk. By the year 2000, there were only 9.2 million cows, averaging 18,200 lb of milk, for a total of 167 billion total lb. That is, fewer than half as many cows are producing 3.4 times as much milk per cow, and 50 percent more total production. In 1950, the U.S. Census of Agriculture reported that there were approximately 5.4 million farms in the United States, of which 3.7 million had milk cows; thus, 68.3 percent of farms had some milk cows. In 1997, these numbers had changed to 1.9 million farms and 116,874 had milk cows, so that only 6.1 percent of farms had milk cows. Thus, we have reduced the number of farms with milk cows to 0.3 percent of the number 50 years earlier. Average number of milk cows per farm in 1950 was 6 head, and 98.3 percent of operations had less than 30 cows. In the year 2000, cows per operation had increased to 88 head, and 29.6 percent of operations had fewer than 30 head, while 20 percent had greater than 100 head. Although there were still numerous small farms in the year 2000, only 1.8 percent of all milk cows were on farms with less than 30 head and 36 percent of all U.S. milk cows were on farms with more than 500 head. Thus, the dairy farms are, on average, very much larger, and the trend is clearly for the disappearance of small farms.

The geographic location of milk production in the United States has also changed. While milk is produced in all 50 states, the magnitude of production is very different between various states and regions. The top ten dairy-producing states provide 70 percent of all milk production, and the top five states account for 53 percent of the total. The top five milk-producing states in 2000 were the same as those in 1975: California, Wisconsin, New York, Pennsylvania, and Minnesota, though the order of ranking was different. The traditional dairy states have been northeast, Great Lakes, and Corn Belt states, plus Texas and California. Since 1975, however, there has been a profound shift in the location of dairy production. California is now the leading dairy state. From 1975 to 2000, it has increased total production by nearly threefold (10.8 billion lb to 32.2 billion lb), now producing almost 50 percent more milk than the next highest state, Wisconsin (23.2 billion lb). In the same time frame, Idaho increased production from 1.6 to 7.2 billion lb, and New Mexico from 366 million to 5.2 billion lb, and now both states are in the top ten for total production. Arizona increased from 840 million to 3.0 billion lb, and Colorado increased from 845 million to 1.9 billion lb of total milk during the years from 1975 to 2000.

These statistics demonstrate very profound trends in the changing dairy industry. Consistently, there has been increased production from fewer total cows, more production per cow, many more cows per herd, with many fewer herds, and dramatically increased milk production in some nontraditional dairy states in the western United States with arid climates. More detail concerning these features of the dairy industry can be found in a recent USDA report from which these numbers were obtained (Blayney, 2002). It seems important to emphasize that while these trends have radically changed the face of the dairy industry, the industry is not adequately characterized by focusing only on the large operations. That the average herd size is still 88 cows is an illustration of the fact that there are still many small traditional dairy farms. It is more accurate to view U.S. dairies as being tremendously diverse, with some small farms at one end of a spectrum, and very large farms at the other.

These statistics, in themselves, do not tell us anything about dairy animal well-being. For this magnitude of change to occur in such a short time period, however, powerful and persistent forces had to be at work. These forces, and their consequences can profoundly affect animal well-being, both directly and indirectly. Although we cannot fully analyze all of the complexities of the dairy industry in this chapter, it is worth considering the nature of some of these forces, and how they ultimately affect animals.

FORCES THAT CHANGE THE U.S. DAIRY INDUSTRY

Like most livestock products, milk sold by a producer is primarily marketed as a raw commodity. Other entities besides the producer then process the product and eventually reap the benefits of retail sale. There are exceptions to this, in the form of "producer-processors" who take milk from production through to retail sale, sometimes including home delivery, but these are a relatively small number of producers. Generally, the producer, like the producer of other commodities, has very little control of the price paid for the raw product. However, milk is a very perishable commodity that must be kept highly sanitary and processed and sold promptly. In the early 1930s, when milk prices dropped dramatically due to poor ability of consumers to pay, there was little coordination of milk marketing systems and danger that major disruptions of milk supply would develop. The federal government intervened in the name of public interest, fair marketing, and provision of a stable supply of this highly perishable product. The result, over many years of modification, is an extremely complex milk marketing system that attempts to maintain consistent pricing of milk across regions of the country based on complex formulas regarding milk composition, supply, demand, transportation, and end use. More details on milk marketing and pricing can be found in a recent book (Bailey, 1997).

Very significant results of the way milk is priced for producers are that they cannot control their price, and that milk prices tend to hover near the actual cost of producing the milk. For example, the actual sale price of milk to producers in 2000 approximated what it was in 1980, about $10 per hundred pounds. Facing this situation, it is clear to most producers that the way to profit from their business is to continually seek means to keep their cost of production as low as possible. It is a common mantra for commodity livestock producers that if you can't control the price you receive then you need to control the cost you invest. This is the mindset of most successful dairy producers, and several consistent trends result. It is increasingly the case that the most important skills a producer needs in order to continue dairying are business skills, rather than animal handling and husbandry skills.

Referring back to the statistics above, it is apparent that in times gone by, many dairies were a component of a diversified farming operation. Dairy producers have traditionally looked at dairy farming as a way of life, an avocation that provides a good environment for the family, where cows and cow care are central elements of family activity. There appears to be a progressive shift toward dairy production as a highly specialized business, designed and operated to generate income, more than a shared family activity. Producers who fail to adjust to this economically driven change will eventually go out of business if they fail to generate sufficient income. Increasing numbers of dairies are solely dedicated to milking many dairy cows on a relatively small piece of property, where all other aspects of the entire process are hired out, such as feed production. It is appropriate to say that dairying is becoming increasingly "industrialized." In order to operate as a successful business, there is great pressure to minimize human labor input, make decisions based on economic efficiency, find ways to decrease overhead costs, and maximize production at any given cost level. These are examples of the thought process that drives producers to increase herd size as a means to take advantage of the economies of scale and move dairying as a business to regions in the country where overhead costs, such as housing structures and feed costs, are lowest. These factors are not inherently good or bad, and they do not automatically produce poor animal welfare. Rather, they supercede animal welfare concerns in terms of their importance in decision making. Fortunately for the animals, many management changes that improve productivity also are beneficial to the animals in some way, but this is not always the case.

Another factor in the changing face of dairy production is the ongoing development of new technology. This factor facilitates the "industrialization" of production methods. New technologies have radically improved forage and grain production, harvest, storage, and feeding methods. Similarly, milk harvest, cooling, storage, and transportation methods have been dramatically altered over the last half-century. Computerization is under continual improvement for monitoring and measuring techniques, animal tracking and identification, and animal production and management procedures. Some results of these technological advances are revolutionary changes in animal nutrition, animal breeding and selection processes, housing, and waste management systems. These promote and facilitate the trend toward larger and more industrialized farms and a move away from pasture-based grazing systems toward confinement feeding systems. The effects on animals can be seen as highly beneficial in some cases, for example, the fact that nutritional deficiency is unusual in modern dairy cattle, but again, the total effect on animal welfare is more complex. The developments in technology may improve industrial efficiency, and may enhance a producer's opportunity to make money in the business, but could be neutral or even detrimental to animal well-being. In such cases, the technology will still be adopted for the sake of improving profitability, and negative consequences for the animals then become items that need to be "managed."

Dairying has traditionally been a family-based, rather than corporate, enterprise. Despite the changes highlighted to this point, the industry has retained this characteristic. Although there are several different business organizations that are used, such as partnerships and family corporations, less than 1 percent of all dairies are run by nonfamily corporations. Thus, on dairies of all sizes, the overwhelming majority of decisions are made by individuals or families, not by corporate boards. This is extremely important, because the industry is steeped in a tradition of caring for animals, and today's dairy owners/operators generally come from a dairy background that emphasizes good animal husbandry. Many dairies maintain purebred animals, even when their primary income is from commercial sale of milk, reflecting that even commercial producers still see cattle as individually important members of the farm operation. There are long-standing principles regarding animal well-being that are held as ideals by many, and perhaps most, dairy producers. These include the notion that you have to care for the animals if you expect them to care for you, and that animals should be properly handled, fed, and housed.

Although some dairy producers would argue that their industry is not subsidized, in fact there are very substantial public policies that directly or indirectly influence dairy production, even when these policies are not overt subsidies. In fact, the U.S. dairy industry is considered one of the most heavily subsidized agricultural enterprises in the country (OECD, 2002). Some of the public interventions include dairy price supports and government purchase of surplus dairy products, which influence milk prices and are a part of the effort to maintain fairly stable dairy product supply. There are also import quotas and tariffs that modify competition from other world dairy sources. As mentioned above, milk pricing is a very complex phenomenon, and could not be properly analyzed in this chapter. It could be argued that the system works to the public benefit by supplying an abundant and relatively constant supply of dairy products, but it is also appropriate to note that an effect of the milk-pricing and supply-demand market system is a relatively low milk price paid to producers compared to the cost of production, and a modest oversupply of dairy products. This continues to hold producers in a position where economic efficiency of production is a driving force in producer decision making. Beyond the price of milk, other government policy influences are also prominent in dairying. Grain prices are dramatically affected by government policy, and inexpensive cattle-feed grains are the norm. Federal development of water resources has had a profound impact on agriculture in the western states. Despite its relative scarcity, water is available at low cost for agricultural use. This has stimulated the growing of forages on western lands at low cost and with extremely high cattle-feed value. This fact, plus the availability of water for intensive livestock production, accounts for much of the development of the dairy industry on arid lands in the western United States. The western climate allows animals to be maintained without extensive housing costs, as are found in the wetter and colder traditional dairy states, and this combination of factors decreases the cost of dairy production in a region where it would be impossible without the historic government program intervention.

OVERVIEW OF DAIRY ANIMAL WELL-BEING

From the description of the dairy industry above, it should be clear that dairy production in the United States has changed dramatically over the last several decades. These changes impact dairy animals in profound ways, with mixed effects on their well-being. It is relatively easy to identify one or another specific aspect of dairy animal care that can be taken out of context and used to demonstrate either improvement or deterioration of animal well-being. Such approaches are often used by industry antagonists, or industry supporters, when two sides take issue in an argument. The remainder of this chapter attempts to examine a number of issues with an eye toward identifying areas where a focus on animal management and well-being could benefit animals and the dairy industry together.

In general, dairies have not experienced the type of extreme criticism that has been focused on the swine or poultry industries. This is probably attributable to multiple factors that work in favor of animal welfare even during a process of industrialization. Dairy producers have traditionally had a strong animal welfare ethic and, as mentioned above, most dairies are still operated by individuals or families who maintain this approach. It is characteristic of producers to hold both the herd, and individuals within the herd, in high esteem, to take pride in their animals and to pride themselves on the care of their animals. Furthermore, each individual animal typically has a substantial monetary value. These factors militate against any tendency to view animals as cogs in the production cycle or as production machines, as may more easily occur with low individual animal value, corporate ownership, and situations where the decision-makers are remote from the animals. In general, it is fair to say that dairy animals are well cared for in the modern dairy industry. Typical dairy husbandry provides good nutrition, circumstances that promote animal interaction and normal expression of individual and herd behavior, space and opportunity to get exercise, and protection against adverse weather conditions. There are exceptions to these generalizations. Numerous animal welfare concerns exist in the industry, but they tend to be complexities of the balance between an excessive focus on economics and production efficiency rather than an expression of disregard for, or diminution of the importance of the animals themselves.

There is clearly pressure on producers to increase production efficiency and total production as the means to improve their business and maintain their livelihood. In such an environment, animal welfare may be important to the producer, but it is not the motivation for change. Rather, economics and growth drive change, while animal welfare is an important, but secondary, consideration. Additionally, as the enterprise grows it may no longer be the producer or the family members who provide primary animal care. It is very easy for the producers to believe that animals are faring better than is truly the case, if they are without an appropriate training process for employees, specific guidelines for animal handling and welfare, a monitoring system for assessing these features, or a decision-making system that adjusts to specific individual animal needs. Very few dairies, as they get very large, make the time investment to specifically focus on animal welfare and the employee training and monitoring required for enhancement of animal welfare. In this situation, individual animals can fall outside the average for the herd and go unnoticed. For example, an animal with a debilitating disease may suffer for a considerable time before being euthanized, even though the producer would not conceive of letting the animal suffer if it had been noticed earlier. In other words, when production systems get very large, it is easier to say that each individual is valued than it is to take action based on that principle.

New feed preparation technologies, advances in measurement of feed characteristics, better understanding of animal nutritional needs, and computer-based management systems have provided the ability to revolutionize dairy nutrition programs. Similarly, technologies that measure and monitor animal production performance provide opportunities to fine-tune animal health and management programs. Although many people like to idealize "life on a small farm in times gone by," the management of such systems is often haphazard and based on poor information. Animal welfare in such production systems can be highly variable, and is less dependent on the size of the operation than the skills and focus of the manager. Cattle in those systems may be pampered and exquisitely managed, or alternatively may suffer from poor nutritional and health management. Producers on small, diversified farming operations may pay attention to animal needs only when they are not attending to the other farm problems. By contrast, large specialized dairies that purchase feed and only run a dairy business that harvests milk from cows can afford the time to focus specifically on things that influence the cows. Most modern large dairies can capitalize on economies of scale to afford the new technologies that promote tremendous improvements in animal production. This would seem to be great groundwork for improving overall animal well-being, and indeed some would claim that this feature characterizes the modern, intensively managed large dairy. Unfortunately, the push to increase production brings other liabilities, such as diseases of nutritional excess, metabolic and digestive disorders associated with feeding errors, and disorders in some individuals who do not tolerate well those management factors that promote extremely high production in the majority of their herdmates. These problems are known as "production diseases" because they rarely occur in animals that are not managed to perform at extremely high production levels.

To be realistic, it seems foolish to look at old-style and small-scale dairy production systems and suggest that they provided ideal animal welfare. Clearly, some managers and some settings provided good animal welfare with grazing systems, exercise, and low stress. Other circumstances in a similar time, style, and place could provide squalor, starvation, poor housing, and exposure to the elements, due to monetary constraints, lack of information, or lack of resources. In similar fashion, the modern, large-scale, intensified dairy systems have the potential to provide for excellent animal welfare, but may produce new disease problems, inadequate attention to individual animal problems, and improper training for employees to recognize and manage animal problems.

DOES HIGH PRODUCTIVITY EQUATE WITH GOOD ANIMAL WELFARE?

A common contention among defenders of industrializing animal management systems is that increased animal productivity is synonymous with improved animal well-being. This argument holds that the animals in a highly productive system must be faring well or they would not be producing so well. There is logic to this suggestion. It is true, for example, that a healthy, well-fed dairy animal will grow and produce better than her counterpart afflicted with disease and poor nutrition. Proponents of a particular animal-management system or of a particular performance-enhancing technique, when challenged about the effects of that technique on the animals, will commonly point to herd productivity as proof that the effects must be positive and that animal welfare is good. Taken to its logical conclusion, we should then believe that animals in the modern dairy industry must be vastly better off than they were 50 years ago, because production averages during that time have more than tripled.

Unfortunately, this is a flawed argument. Herd productivity is not an ideal surrogate measure for good animal welfare. There are several reasons that cows today produce more milk than cows did in previous years, and they do not necessarily equate with animal well-being. The two most important causes of increased production are (1) genetic changes due to selection of breeding stock for high productivity, and (2) improvements in animal nutrition and feeding systems. Neither of these changes can be assumed to unfailingly result in animal welfare improvement. In fact, these changes put the animals at increased risk of health problems under certain circumstances. For example, cows with genetic potential for extremely high milk production are prone to metabolic diseases that can be very debilitating, and even life-threatening, if feeding programs do not meet their high nutritional needs. For another example, which will be explored further below, cows on diets that promote extremely high production are at increased risk to suffer from gastrointestinal ailments induced by the ration. Under optimal conditions, the genetically selected and well-fed cow may indeed experience good health, high productivity, and optimal well-being. But a modern dairy cow can also produce more milk than her counterpart of 20 years ago and suffer numerous insults to her overall well-being that were far less common on dairies two or three decades ago.

Another flaw in the argument that high productivity equals good welfare is that herd productivity is calculated as an average. Similar to any other numerical average, herd productivity numbers do not tell the story of each individual in the herd. For virtually all populations, only a certain number of animals are close to the average, while others can deviate quite far from the average and are not adequately characterized by the number. In typical populations, the average animal may be producing quite well but a percentage of animals is producing quite poorly. To follow the logic of the concept that productivity equals welfare, then these animals are suffering. Alternatively, if they are not suffering, then productivity alone is not a good measure of welfare.

On the other hand, having argued that high productivity is not equivalent with animal well-being, the two are associated and productivity is a relevant evaluation that can help assess animal welfare. Physiological responses to stress and adverse circumstances can indeed limit production performance. One of the primary indicators that something has gone wrong in any livestock operation, including dairies, is a reduction in animal performance. It is worth noting that some of the improvements in animal nutrition that result in increased production have indeed reduced the types of animal suffering that occur with poor nutrition and nutritional deficiencies. Animal scientists, nutritionists, and dairy producers have substantially improved nutritional programs for postweaned youngstock, for example. Overt nutritional deficiency disorders are quite uncommon on modern dairies, and can often be promptly diagnosed and corrected when they do occur. An improved understanding of the nutritional needs of these growing animals has resulted in remarkable improvements in growth rates and decreased disease rates. Not all well-fed animals are, by default, also experiencing optimal well-being, but it seems fair to say that, all other management features being equal, a healthy, growing, well-nourished young animal, as typified in many modern dairies, is better off than its less well-fed counterpart in management systems of the past.

It is also worth commenting here on the common notion that "old-style dairies" were somehow far superior, from an animal welfare point of view, to the modern "industrialized" dairy. Although I have argued above that high productivity does not equate with optimal welfare, the trend toward industrialization in the dairy industry, which is closely linked with increased productivity, often provides benefits to the animals that accrue from the push to increase production. It is a pleasant thought that cows on pasture, maintained as part of a diversified family farm, were animals in an optimal environment. The reality is, however, that diversified farms that produce milk as only one of several components of the operation have the liability that they cannot afford to attend to the animals as their only priority. For example, a farm that produces multiple species of animals and harvests its own feedstuffs has greater needs for different housing and storage facilities, plus an array of machinery, than does a dairy that raises and feeds only dairy animals and purchases all feeds. An aspect of the management changes that increase milk production is an increased focus on the management of the cattle as the highest priority (i.e., specialization within the industry). As anyone who has worked with small, diversified farms can attest, management time and money can get spread very thin, and some things will receive attention due to urgency while other things suffer from lack of attention. Only a limited amount of operating money and effort is spent on the animals in such a setting because many other demands, such as planting crops, harvesting, facility maintenance, and machinery repair also require investment of time and money. It is common on such operations that animals occasionally, or even routinely, suffer from neglect of basic essentials, such as appropriate feed, suitable housing, and removal of manure. The trend to specialize farms for milk production, and to industrialize the process, can reduce the likelihood of such neglect as part of the means to increase animal productivity. While a blanket statement that high productivity equals good welfare is not accurate, it is reasonable to argue that many of the features of management systems that promote high productivity do improve some aspects of animal care. The subjects to be discussed below provide specific areas of concern that contravene this argument and that need to be addressed by the dairy industry.

ENVIRONMENTAL STRESS

Stressful events are not unique to domesticated production animals and, over the course of evolution, all species have developed adaptive responses to stressors. Stresses become problematic when they are excessive in duration or magnitude, such that they overwhelm these protective mechanisms. There are numerous stressors that dairy cattle encounter in the course of life in any production setting. Some stressors may be considered somewhat of a fact of life, such as adverse animal interactions in a population setting, or the physiological stresses of late pregnancy. While it is unrealistic to view almost any particular stressor as completely avoidable, it is quite realistic to manage most stressors so that they are not frequent, prolonged, or grossly detrimental to the animals. Several of the subsequent topics focus on particular stresses that dairy animals frequently or consistently encounter in certain management settings. This topic of environmental stress includes the physical stresses associated with climate and housing conditions of dairy cows.

The predominant dairy breed in the United States is the Holstein Friesian. These animals originate from northern Europe, and are well adapted to temperate climate. The other common dairy breeds originate from the British Isles and Western Europe and are also adapted to cooler temperate conditions. In the United States, these animals tend to fare well in the northern states with cold winters and moderate summer temperatures. The traditional housing management system for such cattle includes access to pasture during the warm seasons when grass is available and confinement in barns during the winter. Winter confinement serves both to centralize the animals for feeding when pasture is unavailable, and to protect the cattle from the most adverse weather conditions. Even without such protection, however, dairy cattle are fairly resistant to cold conditions. Adult cattle generate very substantial heat both by metabolism and from rumen fermentation. For adult animals, the lower critical temperature (the point at which additional metabolic activity is needed to maintain body temperature) is estimated between -20 and $-35°C$ (-5 to $-35°F$). For baby calves, the tolerance to cold is much less, and lower critical temperatures are estimated as $+10°C$ ($50°F$) for newborns, to $0°C$ ($30°F$) for one-month-old calves. These estimates are based on assumptions of no wind, moderate humidity, a dry hair coat, and moderate body condition. In wet or windy weather, or for lean animals or a wet hair coat, the effects of cold will be much more profound. With modest measures to ensure protection from adverse conditions, dairy cattle are quite tolerant of cold, and winter weather has not typically been seen as a major problem. There are exceptions to this generalization, the most common of which are young calves without adequate feed supply to meet metabolic demands in the cold, or growing heifers that are not afforded the expense of enclosed housing during extreme bouts of weather (Chase, 2003).

The preceding comments might be taken to suggest that old-style dairies in northern U.S. regions do not present environmental stress problems for the cattle. Indeed, this is the dairy management setting that seems to be idealized by many in the public at large as the way dairies ought to be. A more balanced view of this issue suggests that winter housing in barns may not be as idyllic as it seems. Because buildings are a major expense, most confined dairy barns provide limited space and close quarters for the cattle. Adequate ventilation is difficult to achieve in such buildings. The result in many cases can be significant animal congestion, limited exercise for prolonged periods of time, injuries caused by confinement in small stalls, and air quality problems that predispose to infectious respiratory disease. One of the housing-design changes over the last several decades is the development of free-stall barns, which are large, relatively open structures with alleyways, feeding, and resting areas. In free-stall barns, cows are not restrained, allowing them to move where they wish and rest in any stall they wish. These structures are relatively efficient in use of space, but provide shelter against the elements, excellent freedom of animal movement, and usually very good ventilation. Since they are a major expense, these structures typically accompany significant herd expansion and are associated with the trend to industrialize dairy production. Additionally, herds housed in free-stall barns are often restricted from grazing because it can be more efficient to raise and harvest forage to feed in the barn than to harvest pasture by grazing. Some may argue that this housing and feeding change negatively affects the cows since grazing is a normal activity that is curtailed or eliminated. One could alternatively argue that free-stall housing can represent a major improvement in animal care since the cows are well fed, well sheltered from adverse weather, and provided with a well-ventilated environment and freedom of movement.

Dairy industry growth in the arid West has proceeded with remarkable vigor, such that numerous states have more than tripled their dairy production over the last 25 years. The multiple reasons for this growth include favorable land prices, mild winters that allow minimal investment in animal housing costs, availability of forages with high feeding value due to extensive irrigation, and resultant low costs of production. Average herd sizes in the western states are very large compared to those in the central and northeastern United States. Along with the movement of dairy animals to these regions have come very significant problems with heat stress. The effects of heat stress are profound on these animals that are well adapted to cold conditions. High relative humidity exacerbates the impact of ambient temperature, and therefore the potential for heat stress is more closely related to a temperature-humidity index than to environmental temperature alone. Heat stress may be the single biggest animal-welfare challenge facing these western dairies. Similar or greater heat-stress problems occur in the humid southern and central states. Affected cows show increased core body temperature, altered respiration, abnormal gastrointestinal function, increased water loss, reduced feed intake, reduced and altered milk production, delivery of low-birth-weight calves, reduced reproductive performance, and other negative effects. In severe cases, animals can die of heat stress. The problem can also occur in northern areas of the country, but generally is less common and less profound. In the western and southern states, heat-stress conditions can persist unabated for months at a time (Staples and Thatcher, 2003).

It is not news to dairy producers that heat has profound negative effects on their cattle. Virtually all of the dairy-trade periodicals contain frequent articles about the problem and new ideas on how to manage it. There are several striking and sobering aspects of the response the dairy industry has had to this problem. The movement of the industry to areas where heat stress is common is not being made for the benefit of the animals, but for purely economic/cost of production reasons. The overwhelming majority of literature that focuses on heat stress details the effects of the phenomenon on production parameters, with scarcely a mention of the fundamental animal suffering that takes place while production is declining. Thus, heat stress is seen almost exclusively as an economic/production problem, rather than as the animal welfare issue that it really is. These trends in the response of producers to the well-being of their animals are very different from the traditional ethics of animal care that have been standard in the industry. There are means to reduce the impact of heat on the cattle, including modified shelters, fans that move large volumes of air around the cattle, water-spraying misters, and alterations in diet. These mitigations are broadly applied, and it would be inaccurate to imply that the problem is not taken seriously. Heat stress is the common focus of considerable research and management effort.

This problem and the discussions of its magnitude and management stand out as the type of issues that arise in dairy animal welfare, resulting directly from the economic forces that drive change in the industry. Heat stress is seen as an issue that has to be managed, with minimal thought given to geographic location as a means to minimize the problem, that is, manage cows in a friendlier environment.

COW COMFORT, EXERCISE, AND HOUSING DESIGN

Housing and handling facilities have a profound impact on animal well-being. There are numerous dimensions to the cow's physical environment beyond weather conditions. At a minimum, these would include good air and water quality, space to move and express normal behaviors, surfaces that provide good footing, areas to lie and rest, adequate eating areas to promote good feed access, and restraint and holding facilities that minimize the likelihood of injury. One of the reasons for the appeal of the scenario of small herds on pasture is that it appears to provide all of these environmental benefits. As mentioned previously, the pasture-based management setting can also have significant compromises in its provisions for animal welfare, given that winter housing may be far less idyllic. Furthermore, weather and specific geographic features of the local landscape may also compromise welfare of pastured animals. The trends toward specialization and industrialization of dairy activities, and the growth of larger herds with novel housing needs, have focused attention on some of the specific details of dairy cow housing requirements. The very substantial capital investments that are made in dairy housing and handling facilities have forced these changes and promoted the science of understanding cow comfort. This is an ongoing process, and facility design is not a perfected area of agricultural engineering, but tremendous progress has been made.

Producers, veterinarians, and design consultants have learned to ask some of the relevant questions about cow environment and behavior that have been ignored out of ignorance in the past. How much slope and what texture should footing surfaces have to promote drainage, provide good traction for cow locomotion, maintain normal hoof health, and avoid injury? What bedding materials and what bedding maintenance are optimal to keep cows comfortable? What stall and stall divider designs and dimensions provide the optimal environment for cows to lie down and rise again comfortably with minimal risk of injury, minimal manure contamination, and optimum udder health? What amount of time should cows spend lying down and ruminating versus eating or exercising? What restraint chutes and alleyway designs promote the best access to the cows for treatment and the least likelihood of cow injury? What handling techniques should be taught and promoted to farm workers and animal handlers? Recent publications (e.g., Northeast Regional Agricultural Engineering Service, 1995) are beginning to more definitively address the facility design features that improve the cow's environment. Other publications (Berry, 2001; Kahler and Zielinski, 2001) use the term *cow comfort* to define this area of animal welfare concern and link it closely with cow productivity. Lay journals written for dairy producers frequently present ideas and suggestions to assist in evaluation and promotion of cow comfort as a critical issue in dairy management. Increasingly, facilities have been designed and/or remodeled with the best interests of the cows as the top priority.

Because knowledge in the area of dairy facility design is still far from ideally developed, different consultants and contractors provide different and often divergent recommendations. Thus, many facilities are inadequately designed or built. Many operators are still in need of education about cow comfort assessment and the maintenance of appropriate housing and facilities. Many cows in dairy production systems live in environments that are far from ideal and suffer discomfort, injuries, or ill health as a result. While significant progress in the design of cow facilities has been made, there is still much room for improvement. Nevertheless, the issue of cow comfort may be the single most compelling example of a scenario where focus on animal welfare is the best approach to improving dairy production. It has been repeatedly shown, both in anecdotal reports and in scientific evaluations, that cows maintained in an environment that promotes animal well-being are more productive, and the farms are more profitable. This particular area of concern supports the rationale that placing animal-care priorities on par with economic efficiency priorities is beneficial to both the animals and the production system. Because most dairy producers are predisposed to favor ideas and investments that benefit their animals, as long as they do not conflict with economic priorities, the notion of building facilities that improve cow welfare is generally met with enthusiasm. As new knowledge and means to attain this goal are developed, they will almost certainly be widely adopted.

PRODUCTION DISEASES

The term *production disease* refers to conditions that occur infrequently or not at all in animals that are not pushed to achieve high performance, but that increase in frequency in high-production settings. There are several production diseases of dairy cattle that will be discussed here, each representing a significant negative impact to animal welfare. Further information about these diseases can be sought from a recent text (Smith, 2002). Some problems, such as mastitis and other infectious diseases have higher prevalence in the modern dairy industry than 40 or 50 years ago. The increased occurrence rates of such infectious problems may be influenced by the promotion of production, but are substantially affected by housing and environment and so they are not categorized here as production disease and are considered separately.

Subacute Rumen Acidosis and Laminitis

Cows that produce the vast quantities of milk that typify modern dairy production (many herds produce an average of eight to ten gallons of milk per cow per day) require intense nutritional support. Methods to provide these nutrients to dairy cattle have been developed over the last several decades, revolutionizing the field of dairy nutrition. Processed feeds with high energy density are commonly used, and these promote very high rates of rumen fermentation. When the feeding program is well tuned to the needs and physiological limits of the cow and her rumen, she can derive the necessary nutrients and maintain optimal

health. Unfortunately, the balance between sufficient energy supply and excessive generation of rumen acids can be fairly tenuous, and subacute ruminal acidosis (SARA) is common in cows on most dairies with high average production. Typically, this is a subclinical
problem, so the cow does not manifest overt illness, although that too can occur. Cows
with mild or moderate reduction of feed intake due to this form of indigestion can develop
chronic and recurrent metabolic problems. Many cows with SARA show minimal disease
signs at the time of the rumen problem, but alterations in blood flow to the feet and alterations in hoof growth occur as a result. This related problem is known as subclinical
laminitis, although clinical and severely painful acute laminitis occurs in some cattle.
Weeks to months after the onset of laminitis, affected cows frequently develop severe
lameness associated with one or more sole or hoof wall diseases that are sequellae to the
hoof-horn insult. These noninfectious foot diseases represent approximately half of all foot
lameness in dairy cows. A recent national survey of the U.S. dairy industry estimated that
lameness occurred in 17 percent of all dairy cattle during the 12 months preceding the
study. Lameness is one of the top two or three animal health concerns in dairy cattle, and
it clearly represents a very substantial animal welfare concern (NAHMS, 1996; NAHMS,
1997b).

Other features of animal management also contribute to the occurrence of laminitis.
Foot trauma contributes to the problem, often associated with excessive time spent standing on concrete or reduced time spent lying down. These factors can be managed with appropriate housing and stall design. Inappropriate design of feedbunks, crowding of pens,
and animal interactions that prevent feedbunk access also contribute by promoting infrequent feeding and overconsumption of feed when feed access does occur. Again, these
problems can be managed to minimize laminitis, if they are monitored and observed. The
two most important management techniques used to control laminitis and its severe clinical effects are nutritional modification to minimize SARA, and foot trimming to minimize
the effects of abnormal hoof growth. Virtually all high-producing dairies have cows affected with this problem. It appears the problem can be managed to decrease its impact,
but it has become accepted as a feature of dairy production that cannot be completely prevented. The bottom line is that laminitis is a disease that presents a major dairy-animal
welfare concern, and that clearly results from the drive to increase milk production (Greenough and Weaver, 1997).

Metabolic Disease

Cattle can develop several metabolic problems that are relatively unique to ruminant
species (uncommon in other animals) and that become increasingly problematic in animals
bred and managed for very high production. The most characteristic of these are hypocalcemia (milk fever), ketosis, fat cow disease, and fatty liver disease. Hypocalcemia occurs
when the demand for calcium in milk exceeds the ability of the cow to supply it from bone
reserves or from dietary intake. Ketosis and abnormal fat metabolism problems are sequellae of the unique fat metabolism of ruminants.

Milk fever has historically been a major metabolic problem of dairy animals. It most commonly occurs at the time or shortly after the onset of lactation when the rapid increase in calcium excretion in milk exceeds the cow's ability to mobilize sufficient supply, resulting in reduced blood calcium levels. The problem manifests as profound weakness and recumbency. It can lead to death in severe cases, but it is usually observed and treated before that outcome. The disease responds very favorably to treatment. Unfortunately, because cows are large animals, they can also suffer severe muscle damage when they are involuntarily recumbent, and downer cows are a major potential complication of the disease. For many years this disease occurred at a fairly consistent frequency (5 percent to 10 percent of dairy cows) across the dairy industry because increased understanding of the problem and improved detection and treatment were offset by increased milk production levels and increased cow susceptibility. However, recent development of preventive measures that entail modification of dietary mineral intake have dramatically reduced the occurrence of this disease in well-managed herds. This particular problem, though included as a production disease with some very debilitating effects, can actually provide a good success story for the dairy industry.

Ketosis is a disease condition characterized by abnormally high circulating levels of ketones, which are partially oxidized fatty acids. Affected animals show poor appetite, general malaise, and weight loss. Ruminants rely on fat metabolism to supply the majority of their energy needs, and a low level of ketone production and utilization is normal. However, when dietary energy intake is lower than energy demand—a circumstance called "negative energy balance"—cattle utilize stored fats very extensively and may produce ketones in excess of utilization, resulting in disease. Dairy cattle genetically selected for very high milk yield experience rapid increases in milk production early in lactation and commonly experience negative energy balance. Therefore, ketosis has become a very common disease in dairy cows. The problem may occur in 3 percent to 20 percent of cows in a herd at a given point in time, with outbreaks occurring when feeding errors or other problems limit cows' ability to consume sufficient feed. Like the other production diseases, this problem can be managed, and indeed it is the focus of considerable management effort. But also characteristic is that it cannot be eliminated in high-producing herds and remains a significant cause of animal suffering in many herds. Two related diseases are fatty liver disease and fat cow syndrome. Fatty liver disease is a condition characterized by chronic, persistent ketosis that does not respond well to common treatment methods. Essentially, fatty liver disease is a severe and chronic form of ketosis, with much the same predispositions but more severe additional complications that seem to result from the accumulation of excessive fat in the liver. Fat cow syndrome is a yet more extreme disease related to abnormal fat metabolism. This occurs in obese cattle near the time of parturition. It can occur in outbreaks, affecting multiple animals, in herds that have mismanaged feeding regimens such that cows consume excessive energy during late lactation when energy demand is low. The negative energy balance in these obese animals can be extreme because they cannot consume sufficient feed, and additionally they have extensive fat deposition in multiple organ tissues. Their metabolic crisis is very severe, and affected cows typically become recumbent and die. The disease was most common 10 to 20 years ago as the ability to deliver very-high-energy feeds improved, but producers did not yet understand how to manage energy delivery and cow weight management. Fortunately, the occurrence of this problem is now unusual in well-managed herds.

Abomasal Displacement

The abomasum is the gastric secretory compartment of the complex ruminant stomach system. It functions approximately similarly to the stomach of monogastric species. Feedstuffs that have undergone fermentation in the forestomach compartments pass into this compartment before passing into the intestines. Prior to the 1970s, disease of this stomach compartment was extremely infrequent. As feeding systems were altered to promote increased energy delivery and increased milk production, a disease called abomasal displacement was increasingly frequently recognized. The problem occurs when gas accumulates in this compartment, making it buoyant so that it floats upward in the abdomen either to the right or left side, where it can be identified by simple physical examination techniques. Unfortunately, the displaced location is not compatible with normal function. Affected animals develop decreased appetite, malaise, metabolic problems, body fluid disturbances, and further disruption of gastrointestinal function. The cause is multifactorial, including several physiological or feed-related factors that result in increased gas production and/or decreased abomasal motility. Under some management conditions, the problem can occur as outbreaks, or can be endemic, such that it affects 10 percent to 20 percent of cows in a herd over a year's time. This problem is so characteristic of feeding problems that can occur when feeding is targeted toward high milk production, that many dairies use the disease as an indicator to fine-tune their management. Thus, some producers monitor this disease and accept that their strategy and implementation are sound if abomasal displacement occurrence rates are below 3 to 5 percent per year. Some people have come to accept that this problem is a cost of high production, and they do not envision complete prevention.

Numerous other problems might be considered under this heading, but those discussed here are notable both for their frequency of occurrence and their clear link with genetic selection and dairy management that emphasize very high milk production. Although all of these problems can occur occasionally in cattle managed for lower production levels, or can result by accident or gross mismanagement, they are so closely tied to production performance that they are almost accepted as part of normal dairying by many in the industry. These production diseases represent an example where management focused to maximize animal well-being, rather than to maximize production, could provide benefit to animals and producer alike. Cows affected by these problems not only suffer, but also represent a real financial and production liability. It is not realistic to expect zero occurrences under any management strategy, since these are biological problems that cannot be absolutely controlled. However, it is realistic to manage with a target of no endemic or routine occurrence, given that maximal production is not the only indicator of success. Unfortunately, the economic forces affecting the dairy industry and described above make this option a very difficult choice for a modern producer who expects the operation to succeed. It is plausible that managing toward eliminating these production diseases could be economically rewarding, since the costs of disease treatment, reduced performance of sick cows, and increased loss or culling of cows could offset some revenue loss due to decreased total milk production. For many producers, the choice is to balance between the risks of too little production and too high disease occurrence, and accept that a certain proportion of animals will suffer with these diseases.

DOWNER COW PROBLEMS

The term *downer cow* refers to animals that are recumbent and unable to rise. The circumstances that predispose to these problems include inadequately balanced diets that induce metabolic disease, or housing and flooring conditions that promote poor footing and promote injury. Once a cow becomes involuntarily recumbent, a vicious cycle of additional problems can occur as a result of ongoing muscle injury. Mature dairy cattle typically weigh between 1,200 and 1,600 lb. If they are recumbent and unable to move their body mass, the limbs and tissues on which they are lying are rapidly injured by bruising and decreased blood flow to the tissues, complicating the original problem that made them recumbent. As a result, it is common for an animal to be down due to one specific problem, but then fail to rise even if that problem is addressed. For example, hypocalcemia will produce muscle weakness and recumbency, but the cow may develop hind limb injuries during the problem and fail to rise even after the hypocalcemia is corrected with appropriate therapy.

Downer cow problems have achieved considerable notoriety in some settings, particularly when they occur in animals penned prior to slaughter or at sale barns. In many such cases, the cause of the problem in the individual animal was weakness or debility, which was the reason the animal was sent to sale or slaughter and was also the cause of the final downer event. In other words, many of these cases represent very poor judgment by the original owner, who has chosen to defer an animal health problem to another buyer or to eliminate the problem by slaughter. Most such cases clearly should have been dealt with on the original farm, either with treatment or euthanasia.

On dairies, these downer cow cases cannot be completely avoided. Some are due to unforeseeable, or unpreventable circumstances. Sooner or later all cattle owners have animals that become downers. Except on a case-by-case basis it is difficult to generalize what the most appropriate disposition of such animals may be. Clearly these situations warrant a thorough examination of the animal to determine the cause of the problem. In many cases, appropriate care, with the right housing, will allow affected animals to regain normal health and return to productivity. Alternatively, euthanasia is often an appropriate choice when it is clear that the prognosis for recovery is poor and prolonged recumbency represents needless suffering. On most dairies, downers do not represent a significant animal welfare dilemma. It is so clear to any producer that the condition has occurred and that this condition represents a major problem for the individual animal in addition to a major economic loss, that such occurrences are typically dealt with very expediently. While it could be argued that bad decisions may be made concerning the care and/or disposition of some affected animals, I believe this is infrequent. Furthermore, if there are specific predisposing circumstances that lead to frequent occurrence of downers, these are typically dealt with effectively because any other course is a plan for financial ruin.

INFECTIOUS DISEASE PROBLEMS

There are numerous infectious diseases of concern to dairy operations that represent challenges to animal well-being. Information from the National Animal Health Monitoring System Dairy '96 Study (NAHMS, 1996; NAHMS, 1997b) demonstrates that infectious diseases represent a tremendous area of concern in dairy animals. Clinical mastitis occurs in 13.4 percent of all dairy cows, respiratory problems in 2.5 percent, and diarrhea in 3.4 percent. Approximately 50 percent of the dairy cow lameness reported in the Dairy '96 survey was apparently infectious in nature (NAHMS, 1997b). In dairy calves, scours, diarrhea, and respiratory problems are responsible for 85 percent of all calf deaths from birth to weaning, and death rates of calves through that age range averaged 10 percent to 13 percent in the NAHMS survey. It is common for 35 percent to 50 percent of dairy calves to become ill and require medical attention between birth and weaning (approximately eight weeks of age). These estimates of average disease incidence provide only one side of the infectious disease picture. Even more troublesome than ongoing disease losses is the development of explosive new infectious problems. Despite the lower profile infectious diseases may have assumed in some discussions of herd health and productivity, infectious agents are still as important as ever and perhaps even more problematic as animal density and herd size increase.

Increased dairy size and concentration of many animals in a single location are factors that promote the transfer of contagious infections. Rapidly increasing the size of herds requires considerable trade and traffic of animals between herds and areas of the country, facilitating spread of pathogens. A look at the findings from the NAHMS Dairy '96 Study puts in perspective the opportunities for disease spread with animal movement. Between 45 percent and 80 percent of dairies of different herd sizes brought cattle onto their operation within the year preceding the study. Of the purchased and introduced animals, fewer than 25 percent were quarantined and even fewer were adequately tested for infectious diseases. These statistics alone emphasize the high risk of infectious disease introduction in most dairies. Between 20 percent and 50 percent of dairies fail to require common vaccinations before introducing new cattle into their herds. Thirty to 80 percent of dairies fail to require milk somatic cell counts (an indicator of udder infection) and 60 percent to 90 percent of dairies fail to request milk culture before introducing new animals into the herd. Although the circumstances that occur with herd expansion can promote spread of infectious disease, this does not explain all of the infectious disease challenge faced by the modern dairy industry. Small farms included in the NAHMS survey had similar or higher rates of infectious disease occurrence as the larger farms. It appears that some diseases such as salmonellosis may be more common in large herds, while other problems such as contagious mastitis are more common in the smaller herds. It is inaccurate to say that large herd size promotes disease in general. It is more accurate to say that as herds consolidate, we are missing opportunities to minimize and limit disease occurrence and spread.

Unfortunately, the trend toward increased herd size, animal density, and animal trade is not paralleled by increased awareness of effective disease control measures. It seems that confidence in technological advances as the means to solve problems extends to the area of infectious disease control. Vaccination has apparently become the most widely used tool for prevention of infectious disease. It is promoted and incorporated into almost all disease prevention programs for individuals and herds. Progress in vaccine production technology is the focus of major corporate ventures and is widely publicized in lay and professional publications. The emphasis on vaccination is so pervasive that many have come to rely on vaccination as the primary means of infectious disease control. Unfortunately, the protection against infection or disease afforded by most vaccines is not nearly as thorough as most producers or their veterinarians would like to believe. The interaction between disease agent and host is extremely complex and different from disease to disease. Thus, it is textbook knowledge that vaccines are more commonly useful in modifying disease manifestations than in actually preventing infection or disease. The development of new antimicrobial agents has also been useful for controlling infectious disease problems when they do occur. Remarkable new drugs have been periodically developed over the course of the last several decades. Producers and veterinarians have been lulled into a false sense of security that antibiotics can effectively cure infected animals. But again that faith is typically extended beyond what is realistic. Antibiotics have essentially no benefit in combating viral diseases and very limited efficacy in treating many bacterial diseases, such as those where the pathogen is resistant to the drug or is located in a body region that the drug does not penetrate.

There are numerous management procedures that can be implemented to decrease animal exposure to infectious agents but that have not been widely adopted in modern dairy management. These procedures may be called biosecurity or biocontainment practices, and include separation of different animal groups, prevention of contact between healthy and sick animals, cleaning and hygiene procedures, minimizing manure contamination of premises or feed, and so on. Looking more specifically at calf management, for example, some infectious diseases are spread from dams to newborns, and the time of separation of the calf from the cow can have an impact on the transmission of these diseases. In the NAHMS survey, only 13 percent of operations separated newborn calves from the dams within 1 hour of birth. Twenty-five percent of operations separated the calves beyond 12 hours after birth. Fifteen percent of operations allowed calves to stay with their dams more than 24 hours. Thirty percent of operations failed to wash teats and udders before colostrum was collected for administration to the calves. Approximately 55 percent of operations used the calving area as a hospital area for sick cows. Fecal contamination is a common means for spread of many enteric infections. Developing more fully integrated approaches to infectious disease control could have a profound impact on dairy animal welfare.

CALF MANAGEMENT PRACTICES

Calf-rearing practices in the modern dairy industry present some very real problems regarding animal welfare. As described above, an excessive number of dairy calves die from infectious diseases (estimated 10 percent to 13 percent between birth and weaning), but this figure does not reflect the entire story. In a later section, we will discuss some issues regarding calf delivery (birthing) and associated disease and death losses. In this section, we will focus on some other calf-care issues.

Orphan Rearing and Early Weaning

Some people have voiced concerns about the fact that dairy calves are orphaned at birth or soon after, that is, the cow and calf are separated after birth and the calf is raised separately while the dam enters the milking herd. It is true that this separation is not natural, and the idea of the cow-calf pair bonding and remaining together is appealing as a closer reflection of natural maternity. Indeed, that model is the mainstay of beef herd production where the principle product is the growing calf. In the dairy industry, where the product is milk, there are obvious problems with such an approach. The economic argument is that it is preferable to sell the milk and to rear calves using less-valuable commodities, such as non-saleable milk or milk replacer. There are multiple features to the process of rearing dairy calves as orphans. One is the decision to wean earlier than normal, that is, at six to eight weeks rather than six to eight months. This is both economical and conducive to good growth. Calves left to their own dietary preferences would continue to suckle milk for many months. In natural settings, this could extend to approximately a year, until the dam produces the next offspring. The calf's preference does not represent a physiologic necessity, however. With proper feed availability, calves can adequately digest solid feeds by six to eight weeks of age such that they will grow as well or better if weaned to a completely solid diet at that time. While it is certainly true that beef calves are not typically weaned until well beyond two months of age, they also are not typically provided the additional nutrition that dairy calves receive in the weaning process. It is interesting that such management decisions are viewed negatively by some of the public, when similar decisions regarding human child weaning and nutrition are commonplace and unquestioned by most, that is, human babies are rarely allowed to nurse until the mother ceases lactation or the child voluntarily declines nursing.

There is more than the economics of milk disposition at the heart of this dairy management decision. In addition to the reasons to wean calves early, there are reasons to separate the pair shortly after birth. Dairy cattle are handled directly by humans on a daily basis, and orphan-rearing a calf bonds it to humans from the beginning of its life, facilitating subsequent animal management. It also seems apparent that early separation of the pair is less stressful than separation after significant bonding has taken place. As with other species, the neonate appears to bond with whoever supplies its needs, even if the individual is a different species. If humans intervene before the calf has bonded to the dam, there is little evidence of stress or concern on the part of the baby calf. Likewise, it seems much more stressful to the dam to remove a calf after the pair has closely bonded over time than to circumvent considerable interaction by removing the calf shortly after delivery. While beef cattle have been selected over time for good mothering traits, which include attention to the calf that enhances calf survival, dairy cattle have been selected with virtually no concern for these traits. Many dairy cattle show very poor instinct for mothering, and in such cases it is difficult to perceive much concern on the part of the dam when the calf is removed.

Under modern dairy management conditions where cows do not calve in an extensive pasture setting and newborn calves are delivered in relatively congested or trafficked maternity pens, there are compelling animal health reasons to separate calves from dams. In the section above concerning infectious disease, the need to reconsider hygiene as a means to minimize spread of infectious agents was emphasized. One of the major areas of concern is the spread of pathogens to newborn calves. As highlighted earlier, baby calf infection rates and subsequent death losses are considerable. Spread of infection to newborn calves is most likely during the hours and days immediately following birth. There are several studies that verify what common sense suggests: the longer the calf is exposed to contaminated environments and adult cows that shed pathogens, the greater the likelihood of calf disease. Current recommendations from various animal health professionals to dairy producers who manage cows in large herds are to separate the calf from the cow immediately after birth, or as soon as possible thereafter, both for the health of the individual calf and to minimize the endemic spread of diseases throughout the herd.

With all of the preceding discussion of why it makes sense to separate newborn calves from dams right after delivery, it remains a liability of modern dairy management methods that this process must induce at least some degree of animal distress. There are reasons to believe that this distress is not as great as it might be for animals with well-established maternal/neonatal bonding, or for animals that are bred and selected for strong maternal characteristics. Nevertheless, it would be foolish to suggest that this is not a viable animal welfare concern. It seems more realistic to say that there are reasons for the practice that have to be balanced against the potential of animal suffering. On smaller dairies, some producers do find ways to allow much more extensive contact between dams and offspring than are afforded in large-scale, more confined dairy settings. Producer advocates of more "natural" calf housing and rearing practices can also boast very good animal health when some of the other predisposing causes of infectious disease are well managed. Specifically, this requires that producers assure that the dam mothers the calf, that the calf suckles adequately from the dam to get the benefit of colostrum ingestion, that the calf is born in a clean and relatively open environment, and that cows in the herd have low rates of infectious disease occurrence. These types of prerequisites are extremely difficult to achieve except on small dairies with considerable investment of personnel effort.

Newborn Calf Care

Even if one accepts that early separation of calves and orphan rearing are reasonable practices, there is another side of the calf-rearing issue that is routinely overlooked and that seems to be a much bigger animal welfare problem than the orphaning process *per se*. The implicit assumption in current calf rearing systems is that humans assume the role of the dam and properly care for the newborn. In my mind, this is a much bigger question than that discussed above. It seems fair to say that modern calf raisers very commonly fail to meet the standards of any reasonable natural cow mother. The ideal is for newborn calves to receive good mothering, which at a minimum includes drying the haircoat after delivery to ensure a thermal protective barrier, stimulating the calf to rise and move, encouraging suckling and colostrum consumption, and seeking or providing for a sheltered environment. These simple aspects of calf care are routinely ignored in many dairy settings. Many calves are retrieved from the calving pen and placed into other holding or housing facilities to be looked at or fed at a later time. In fact, many people leave the calves with the cows to avoid having to do these chores, assuming the cow will show good maternal instincts. Dairy cows are not selected for maternal traits, and this default mode is inappropriate, because leaving the calf to be cared for by a dam that may or may not provide good mothering is effectively a plan for inadequate care. The responsibility for calf care clearly falls to the producer and dairy management personnel, either by assuring that cows provide such care and intervening if they don't, or simply adopting a routine policy of having the care provided by humans as surrogate mothers. Having shouldered the responsibility of rearing baby calves, it is imperative that the task be done properly. To optimize calf survival, especially in cold or inclement weather, this means automatically providing a heat lamp and deep bedding so that calves are sheltered from the elements. Calves should be dried off, stimulated to move, provided warm fluids in the form of first milking colostrum as quickly as possible, and provided a shelter of adequate design and cleanliness.

A critical feature of newborn calf care is colostrum feeding within hours after birth. This first milk of the dam provides fluid, extremely high-quality nutrition with many micronutrient elements, and components that support the calf's naïve immune system to enhance infectious disease resistance. A large dairy survey that focused on dairy calves (NAHMS, 1994; Wells, Dargatz, and Ott, 1996) provided solid evidence that calves left with cows to nurse their colostrum frequently failed to achieve adequate supply and experienced higher death rates than calves fed colostrum by humans. This could be explained by a failure of dams to adequately mother the newborn calf, by large udders with teats that are difficult for calves to find and suckle, or by the production of voluminous colostrum with inadequate immunoglobulin concentration that makes it difficult for calves to consume sufficient immunoglobulin mass. All of these circumstances occur in modern dairy cows selected for high milk production. The study findings reinforce the notion that modern dairy cows do not always serve as good mothers and that dairy personnel should take the responsibility of providing appropriate calf care to enhance neonatal survival. Producer education efforts over the last decade have focused on the positive impact of colostral management on calf health and survival. A subsequent survey suggests that colostrum provision is more carefully managed than it was half a decade earlier, mainly due to these educational efforts (NAHMS 2002). This is encouraging because it suggests that educating producers about the benefits of management practices that increase calf health and well-being will improve calf care.

During episodes of cold or inclement weather, calf care practices become even more important because these young animals are more susceptible to environmental challenges than their more mature counterparts. Strategies to provide protection from the elements should be especially targeted toward smaller calves, calves that experience dystocia (birthing difficulty), calves that aren't doing well, or any calf in extremely cold weather.

Whether a calf can maintain body heat depends on a combination of factors, including sufficient feed energy to withstand the cold, sufficient thermal insulation, dry hair, wind speed, humidity, good nutrition, and physiological soundness. Extremely important is appropriate housing; the hutch structures must be windproof, watertight, well ventilated, and properly positioned so the elements are coming from the back or sides. It is very important that calves be well bedded. This kind of environment retains the heat more, retains the dryness, and blocks the wind so the calf can maintain itself in the cold. In some circumstances, calf jackets or blankets may be warranted. Simply placing a calf in a hutch without concern for these other details may not be enough to protect it from extremes of weather conditions.

Calves exposed to prolonged cold need additional energy to maintain body heat production. Some dairy calf feeding programs fail to meet these needs during bouts of cold weather. In these circumstances, calves utilize their meager body fat reserves quickly for heat production, and then may die from starvation rather than the cold itself. This "starving calf" problem is common and happens when young calves, typically between two and four weeks of age, are not yet eating much solid feed. Such calves are still reliant upon fluid feeding for energy. If they are only provided a fixed amount of milk replacer, instead of an amount proportional to body weight, they are in danger of undernourishment. The likelihood of this problem increases in situations where the producer elects to feed low-quality replacer to save cost. A producer might feed a lower quality/lower-fat-content replacer to a 70-lb calf sufficient for survival, but when that same amount is continually fed to a 100-lb calf, in cold weather, the calf can suddenly die at the critical two-to-four weeks of age. This scenario is particularly tragic because the reasons for curtailing milk feeding in such cases are economically based. The lower-fat replacers are more economically priced, and it is also more costly to feed three or more times a day to increase the volume fed.

Calf Feeding and Nutrition

As discussed above, calves can be, and typically are, weaned from fluid feed by four to eight weeks of age, but it should occur only if they are consuming sufficient solid feed for their survival and growth. The most compelling reason to wean calves to solid feed is that fluid diets are quite costly, both due to the cost of the feed ingredients (milk or milk replacer) and due to the labor cost. Conversely, solid-feed diets are fairly economical. Therefore, the primary reason to convert calves to a solid diet is an economical one, although it is also apparent that calves grow faster and have fewer health problems once they have been weaned to solid diets. This last statement and the feeding practices used to wean calves early warrant closer scrutiny.

Calves at birth are unable to digest solid feeds and require milk for nutrition like other mammals. The development of the rumen from a nonfunctional stomach compartment in the neonate into the preeminent digestive organ of adult cattle requires consumption of small amounts of solid feed that deposit in the undeveloped rumen and initiate the process of microbial fermentation in this stomach compartment. As the rumen grows in size and its bacterial fermentation processes become more robust, the calf can consume increasing amounts of feed and derive increasing nutritional support from the feed. The industry standard for calf age at weaning is currently about eight weeks of age because most calves are consuming sufficient solid feed for their maintenance and growth by that time. It is appealing to think that current calf nutrition programs are providing an optimal fluid diet for the first eight weeks, while calves gradually increase solid feed consumption during that time. Unfortunately, this is not what actually occurs, and it is fair to say that baby calves on milk diets are substantially underfed.

For several reasons, the diet calves receive prior to weaning is very restricted. Feeding calves milk or milk replacer by bucket or nipple feeder has been common practice on most dairies for over 50 years. Such feeding is time and labor intensive and the fluid diet is relatively expensive. Under natural conditions, a baby calf left with its dam would typically nurse six to eight times per day and consume 16 percent to 24 percent of body weight in fluid milk. To bucket feed dairy calves similarly would be a very time-consuming and costly process. Thus, most calves are fed only two times a day. The maximum amount most calves are provided at a feeding approximates 4 percent to 5 percent of body weight because higher volumes can be associated with digestive disturbances. This means that most calves receive a maximum of 8 percent to 10 percent of body weight as fluid feed per day. Given the normal nutrient density of fluid milk, this provides only enough energy for body maintenance plus a small amount of growth. Calves fed in this manner may be expected to gain approximately 200 g/day, compared with approximately 1 kg/day for calves fed ad libitum. The problem of poor growth is particularly true for calves fed milk replacer compared to their milk-fed counterparts because the energy density in most milk replacers is less than that in whole milk. In other words, the most common calf-feeding practices do not provide optimal nutrition. In fact, they are so close to being true starvation that in some circumstances calves may indeed die from lack of energy in colder weather, as discussed above. There is a method to this madness, however. Part of it is playing the game of rearing calves for the least cost, but another aspect is that maintaining calves in a fairly hungry state induces them to begin solid feed consumption more quickly. This in turn means the calves can be weaned at the earliest time.

The observation that calves grow better after weaning is probably less a tribute to the benefits of solid feed than the fact that before weaning the calves are relatively starved. This method of calf rearing has evolved over such a prolonged time that most producers actually believe that 8 percent to 10 percent body weight feeding of milk is optimal for the calf, despite the evidence that the calves remain very lean and are at high risk of disease. In fact, this system did not evolve with the best interests of the calf in mind; rather it evolved as the least cost, lowest labor input solution. Recent research, directed at the question of how to feed calves for optimum growth and health, has begun to demonstrate to producers that the extra cost of a higher plane of nutrition for baby calves may be well worthwhile as a wise investment in the health, growth, and future productivity of calves. Furthermore, there are feeding strategies that have been demonstrated to meaningfully benefit the calf and still allow weaning at a desirable early age, such as feeding the calf more energy during the first weeks of life and then decreasing fluid feeding to encourage solid feed intake later. It is hoped that in the near future the methods of calf feeding will be directed toward the best interest of the animal, rather than the lowest cost for time and feed investment (Davis and Drackley, 1998).

Bull Calf Management

The last topic I'd like to address under the heading of calf management practices is the management of newborn bull calves. Calf management has tended to receive less attention by dairy producers than some other management concerns. This is probably due to the fact that calf problems are further removed from revenue generation than some other issues, such as cow health and milk quality. Bull calves and their management are often yet lower on the priority list. Since the development and widespread use of artificial insemination as a means of breeding milk cows, plus the adoption of selective breeding strategies to improve genetics for milk production, most bulls are not destined to be used as breeding animals. Yet approximately 50 percent of calves are males, and therefore producers have a large number of animals born each year that will not play a role in milk production. Some producers raise bull calves to be sold or slaughtered, but the majority of dairy producers prefer to sell bull calves early in life to decrease the feed, housing, and management costs that rearing these animals would require. Bull calf economic value has tended to be very low. In some times, the market for these calves has been poor enough that it costs more to sell the calf at auction than the selling price received. It is difficult to marshal appropriate management attention to bull calves that will not become production animals on the dairy, and frequently bull calves receive very poor attention. Unfortunately, this can lead to significant morbidity and mortality that can go unnoticed except to the buyer (veal operations and dairy beef rearing units). Clearly it is appropriate to treat bull calves like heifers in attending to their needs as newborn animals, that is, provide them with colostrum, warmth, and nursing care, as described above. Unfortunately, many producers are guilty of overlooking these needs because the effects of poor bull calf management are not a major economic liability, and subsequent poor bull calf health and survival are likely to be someone else's problem. It is important for dairy producers to realize that it is an ethical obligation to care for newborn bull calves with the same attention afforded to heifer calves, even when the economic reward is limited or nonexistent.

BIRTHING AND CALF DELIVERY PROBLEMS

Probably because newborn calves are not the major direct source of revenue for dairy producers, it appears that calf delivery and newborn calf management are undervalued as areas of concern. The problem of dystocia (calving difficulty) has been almost ignored. Very few dairy producers incorporate breeding strategies to decrease dystocia occurrence or have delivery management and newborn-calf management protocols that specifically address the problem. Dystocia is defined as delayed or difficult parturition, and its effects are highly variable depending on the severity of the problem. In affected calves, dystocia produces trauma and asphyxia that decrease calf vitality, predispose to disease, and may result in stillbirth or neonatal mortality. Affected dams may develop reproductive tract problems that impair reproductive function, and in severe cases, trauma and paralysis can result in euthanasia or culling.

Perhaps as a result of the inattention the dairy industry has paid to calving difficulty, the rate of dystocia in dairy animals is substantially higher than in beef cattle. National surveys show that approximately 3 percent of beef cows and 17 percent of primiparous beef heifers, with a total of 4 percent of cattle across all age groups, need calving assistance. In sharp contrast, the average for all dairy cattle is 18.4 percent assisted deliveries and dairy first-calf heifers require assistance for almost 32 percent of calvings (NAHMS 1994; NAHMS 1997a). As described above, infectious disease is typically considered the main cause of dairy calf morbidity and mortality, and national surveys estimate that on average 35 to 50 percent of all dairy calves will be treated for illness and 10 to 13 percent will die prior to eight weeks at time of weaning. However, most producers do not monitor calf death losses that occur before calves are identified in official records. Stillbirth incidence is typically not included in evaluation of dairy calf mortality, and calves that die prior to 24 hours of age are grouped with stillbirths. Since most calf loss estimates exclude still-birth losses, they underestimate the magnitude of newborn dairy calf health problems. Estimates from some studies, including unpublished work we have conducted at CSU, suggest that loss of calves less than one day of age, attributable to calving difficulty, approximately equals the death loss of calves beyond a day of age. This equates to approximately 50 percent of all calf deaths, very similar to estimates of the distribution of beef calf losses. Such an estimate also reflects the trend seen in neonates of other species. This means that the current estimates of dairy calf losses, although very high, only represent half of the story, since this other proportion of losses is typically not tallied.

Calving area management, delivery management, and newborn calf management should be extremely important areas of dairy management focus. Events that occur here can affect calf morbidity and mortality, treatment costs, transmission of herd disease agents (including zoonotic pathogens), dam health and reproductive performance, and ultimately the cost/benefit of replacement heifer rearing. The combined effects of all of these on dairy health and productivity should be profound. Furthermore, dairy replacement heifer raising is the second leading expense for dairy operations, behind feed costs for the lactating herd (Webb 1992). Yet attention to this area of management has been lax. It appears that the short- and long-term benefits of newborn calf health or the costs of calving management problems have not been clearly identified and conveyed to producers. Thus, dairy producers have failed to see economically compelling reasons to direct valuable time and management to changes in these areas. Because calving occurs year-round in dairy operations, it is easy to overlook insidious, ongoing losses unless they are measured and monitored. Looking at this situation from an animal welfare perspective presents a sobering picture. Here is a welfare concern that seems to be all but ignored, and yet, if addressed in a meaningful way that decreased animal losses, could derive substantial benefit to the animals plus improve economic returns for the producer.

In the cow-calf segment of the beef cattle industry, where calf production is the primary source of revenue, dystocia has been surveyed, monitored, and found to be the single most important factor predisposing to disease and death in calves. Although the more severe dystocia deliveries account for the greatest losses, even mild dystocia has been shown to impact calf health and survival. Producer management includes considerable focus on calving management and strategies to decrease dystocia occurrence and impact. Simple methods for increasing calf viability include straightforward nursing care techniques applied promptly to all calves suffering dystocia birth, such as warming, drying, provision of extra colostrum, shelter, stimulation, oxygen delivery, and extra mothering attention. In contrast, dairy animals are not rigorously selected for calving ease or calf vigor, and management is not directed at reducing dystocia risk or effects on baby calves. Despite the fact that dairy AI sires are evaluated for calving ease, most producers preferentially select bulls based on transmission of increased production traits. Except for the dairies involved in AI bull evaluations, most dairies do not even report dystocia occurrence as part of their record keeping. Few dairies have adequate protocols in place for employees to manage the delivery of calves properly, and these dairies often provide little or no supplemental care to calves born with difficulty. This set of management steps could be used to reduce the incidence of dystocia and to decrease the impact of dystocia on newborn dairy calves when it does occur. An increased focus on calf welfare as the reason to institute improved animal management strategies could greatly improve dairy animal well-being.

CULLING AND DEATH LOSS

Evaluation of the reasons that cows leave a herd, the condition of the cows that leave, and the causes of cow death loss provides insight into animal welfare. In an idealized setting, cows might only leave a herd because they die or cease production from old age. In reality, this is unusual and there are many other potential reasons for cows to be sold out of a herd. In situations where a maximum number of animals have been achieved on an operation, some animals may be sold to another operation for milk production. As described at the beginning of the chapter, the number of dairy operations in the United States is decreasing, while the remaining farms are typically increasing in size. In this scenario, many herds are selling some or all of their animals, while other operations are acquiring animals and trying to decrease the number of animals that leave the farm. In a production setting, cows could be electively culled and sold for slaughter if their level of milk production is low, in order to make room for more productive cattle. Injury and disease are major reasons for removal of animals from a herd, even when the herd is expanding and when it is undesirable to lose herd members.

The recent national survey of dairies in the United States (NAHMS, 2002) showed that approximately 25.5 percent of dairy cows left herds permanently during 2001, and that approximately 6 percent of these cows were sold to other dairies, while 94 percent were culled (i.e., sold and not returned to milk production, sent for slaughter). The reasons cows were culled included mastitis and udder problems (27 percent of culled cows), lameness or injury (16 percent), other disease (6 percent), reproductive failure (27 percent), and poor milk production not related to these other problems (19 percent), while other miscellaneous reasons accounted for about 5 percent of culling. Therefore, on average, the overwhelming majority of dairy cows leaving farms are not fit for sale as dairy production animals, and approximately 50 percent of these cows are leaving because of disease or injury problems, rather than being selectively removed because of low fertility or milk productivity.

A partial view of the welfare of culled dairy cows can be obtained from recent audits of cows at slaughter (National Cattlemen's Beef Association, 1994, 2000). These audits showed high rates of significant problems in dairy cull cows that affected their health ante mortem, and decreased their value as slaughter animals. Visible abscesses were identified in 13 percent of culled dairy cows, while 80 percent had bruised tissues identified at slaughter. Approximately 12 percent of dairy cattle went to slaughter with intact horns, which has been shown to increase the risk of injury to nonhorned cattle. Approximately 1 percent of cows were considered disabled, which may have occurred during transit to the slaughterhouse or because of health- and/or dystocia-related reasons. Almost 5 percent of dairy cows had very poor body condition at the time of slaughter (extreme lack of weight/flesh). All of these findings were identified in the study as relevant concerns about the slaughter value of the cows.

More important, however, they represent potentially avoidable problems that speak clearly to the issue of animal welfare. Most of these problems must occur in any population at some level, and it would be unrealistic to think that injuries and other health problems could be completely avoided. Furthermore, the population of animals studied was that group selected for removal from the herd precisely because they had problems that made their retention in the herd undesirable. However, the frequency of occurrence of these problems suggests that there are substantial improvements to be made in animal health monitoring, handling and transportation of dairy cattle, and prompt removal from the herd before the animals are severely emaciated. Improved injection methods, improved handling facilities, improved recognition and assessment of disease, uniform dehorning practices, removal of animal injury risks, and improved decision processes that provide for humane euthanasia to prevent animal suffering from incurable disease problems are all achievable goals. Such improvements would not only enhance the quality of slaughter animals, but also substantially decrease animal welfare problems. The fact that the majority of cows that leave a herd do so because of problems, rather than because of undesirable production, and further, that a high percentage of these cows have significant slaughter defects speaks poorly for the welfare of dairy animals. Most of these problems can be improved with attention to a variety of management changes.

Besides being culled for slaughter or sold for dairy production on another farm, the other major reason a cow drops out of the production population is on-farm death. The NAHMS 2002 survey shows that approximately 5 percent of cows die on the farm each year. This is a very high death rate compared with that of beef cows or feedlot animals, where death rates are estimated between 1 percent and 1.5 percent. Unknown reasons accounted for the largest percentage (20 percent) of dairy cow deaths, followed by calving difficulty problems (17 percent), mastitis (17 percent), and lameness or injury (14 percent). Information was not collected in the survey to suggest what percentage of these deaths were sudden occurrences, without warning, versus what percentage represented animals with more prolonged illness. However, it seems clear that there is room for improvement in detection and diagnosis of disease and need for prompt and appropriate treatment decisions to avoid suffering in animals. Furthermore, this high death rate suggests that there are significant risks for life-threatening illness on dairy farms. The reasons for these risks and the methods for identifying and treating or humanely euthanizing affected animals should be closely scrutinized. There is a high likelihood that these statistics demonstrate some substantial problems in overall animal health monitoring and maintenance. The need for improved methods to avoid dystocia and for training in methods to alleviate dystocia have been discussed above. There are many other health management and training procedures that would be very beneficial in avoiding animal mortalities.

BOVINE GROWTH HORMONE

Bovine growth hormone, or bST (recombinant bovine somatotropin), can substantially increase milk production when administered to dairy cows. Advances in biotechnological methods allowed the large-scale production of bST. Its ability to induce higher production in dairy cattle was the focus of considerable research throughout the 1980s. During the process of drug approval for use of bST in commercial milk-producing animals, there was considerable controversy surrounding questions about its potential to produce ill effects in the treated animals and in humans that consumed their milk. Furthermore, there was debate about the ultimate benefit the product would derive, since national milk supply has been adequate or above for many years, and milk prices to producers are negatively affected by increased supply. Despite these controversies, the corporation seeking to market the drug won approval, and bST is currently administered to approximately 22 percent of U.S. milk cows (NAHMS, 2002).

During the approval process, numerous concerns were voiced about the possibility that cows receiving bST would suffer from increased occurrence of metabolic problems associated with the extra demand for energy for increased milk production. There were also concerns about increased occurrence of mastitis. Indeed, such problems were reported to occur, both in clinical trials conducted before approval and in some herds after the drug was approved and marketed. The corporation successfully argued against the importance of these concerns to win approval of the product, and subsequently employed numerous dairy consultants to help implement use of the drug on farms and to combat the occurrence of these problems. Since that time, no trials have shown definitive evidence of animal health problems associated with bST use. It was argued that metabolic problems occurring in treated animals were the result of poor nutritional management, and that these problems could be circumvented. The corporate-sponsored consultants have helped implement management improvements on farms utilizing the drug, and these changes may be responsible for minimizing expected problems and, perhaps, for improving production more than the drug effects *per se*.

At present there is little reason to believe that the use of bST, when administered to cows under the appropriate management, provides a significant animal welfare concern. One still might question whether it is in the long-term best interests of the dairy industry in the United States to use bST to provide increased milk production. Some producers have certainly benefited financially from its use in the short term. However, this is a product without a problem to solve, because milk production nationally has been at or above demand levels, which depresses the price of milk at the producer level. If milk price remains at, near, or below the cost of production, the economic forces described above will continue to drive changes in the dairy industry that can have some negative effects on dairy animal welfare. Whether there are any negative human health impacts will be difficult to discern, and no long-term studies were conducted to answer this question because the corporation was successful in arguing that there shouldn't be any. If public concern about the use of production-enhancing drugs in dairy cattle intensifies, the dairy industry will be the long-term loser. The only long-term beneficiary of the use of bST appears to be the corporation that produces and markets it, because there are no apparent benefits to the cows, the dairy industry, or the consuming public. In my opinion, morally relevant concerns exist about the use of bST, but they are not based on overt animal welfare issues.

DEHORNING AND TAIL DOCKING

Dehorning and tail docking are two specific management practices that attract attention from an animal welfare perspective. These practices are similar in that they represent procedures that alter the anatomy of dairy animals, but they are very different in the type of challenge they pose to animals and the dairy industry.

Horned animals pose a threat to animal and human health because of the relatively close contact dairy cattle have with their herdmates and their human handlers. Although dairy animals are neither extremely aggressive nor extremely territorial, they normally express both types of behavior in many routinely encountered situations. It is well documented that injuries from horned animals can be avoided by dehorning, and the practice is widely accepted and seems well justified. Therefore, the relevant welfare issue that relates to dehorning is not so much whether it is practiced, but how it is performed, and how pain and subsequent morbidity are avoided. Simply stated, any surgical dehorning procedure (where the skin is cut and the horn bud removed) is clearly an invasive and painful procedure. Furthermore, the open wound that remains after surgical dehorning not only is prone to infection, but also is a source of residual pain for days after the procedure. For these reasons, performing a surgical dehorning without appropriate anesthesia is a major problem for the baby calf. The longer the dehorning is delayed and the older the calf at the time of surgical dehorning, the more profound the associated problems become. If the procedure is performed after calves are more than three months old, a bony projection has begun to grow into the base of the horn and typically the frontal sinus is opened during the dehorning, which dramatically increases the risk of infection and calf morbidity and suffering.

There are straightforward and widely accepted means to minimize dehorning problems. These include dehorning with a bloodless procedure (chemical or cauterizing) to avoid subsequent wound infection, dehorning at a very early age (within several weeks after birth) to avoid substantial horn development and innervation, and using appropriate anesthesia and analgesia to avoid and minimize pain. It is worth noting that the bloodless methods of dehorning avoid or minimize pain and discomfort. Even hot-iron dehorning (commonly performed with an electric hot-iron device), which clearly produces pain at the time of application, appears to leave little or no residual pain, perhaps because the nerves are destroyed. Shortly after electric/hot-iron dehorning, calves will again seek out human attention, while calves clearly avoid humans after surgical dehorning. Thus, while local anesthesia is still clearly desirable for hot-iron dehorning, the pain seems to be more transient and subsequent use of analgesia seems less important. The use of bloodless methods, applied early in life, decreases calf morbidity associated with the procedure, and these methods have become increasingly well accepted within the industry. A recent dairy survey (NAHMS, 1996) estimates that approximately 50 percent of producers now use the bloodless procedures. This leaves the more problematic procedures still in wide use, but it is my impression that welfare issues associated with dehorning are becoming less important as producers are made aware of the value of the more desirable methods and adopt them. This shift should be enhanced by education and encouraged by veterinarians and other consultants because it is clearly in the best interest of the animals and the operation to use the best and least harmful procedures.

Tail docking of dairy cattle has been fairly widely used in New Zealand and Australia, but has only been adopted by some U.S. dairies over the last decade or so. The procedure removes the lower third to two-thirds of the cow's tail. This can be accomplished by applying a strangulating elastic band, by applying a cauterizing cutting implement (hot-knife), or by surgical means. Tail docking can be performed during calfhood or later in life. Several studies have evaluated different tail-docking methods and demonstrated minimal discomfort when the procedure is properly performed, but the most innocuous method appears to be banding. Tail docking is practiced to improve cow cleanliness and worker comfort by eliminating the possibility of a cow swinging a manure covered and urine soaked tail. Some proponents have maintained that the procedure improves udder health and milk quality by improving cow cleanliness. Some milking parlor arrangements put the milkers directly behind the cow as they work with the udder and the milking equipment, and it is easy to see that tail docking does eliminate tail contact in that situation. Numerous concerns about tail docking have made the procedure controversial. Even if the procedure itself does not produce overt animal suffering, it does deprive the animal of a normal anatomical component that is useful for fly avoidance, temperature regulation, and visual communication with other cows. Furthermore, there are alternative practices that can accomplish the same goals this procedure is designed to achieve, specifically, housing management to avoid manure accumulation on tails, tail switch trimming to shorten the tail without amputation, and milking parlor design that helps keep the tails out of contact with workers.

Recent reviews of published studies (Berry, 2001; Quaife, 2002; Stull et al., 2002) report no significant benefit to cows or workers that can be attributed to the procedure. That is, there is currently no evidence that supports the claims made by proponents of the procedure. This presents an interesting problem for the dairy industry, or at least for those in the industry who practice or endorse tail docking. Although there appears to be no gross animal suffering associated with the practice, there is also no clear justification for it. As one recent article title states, "Tail docking makes little sense" (Quaife, 2002). In this situation, dairy producers seem to have little to gain and much to lose in terms of public appraisal of their care for their animals. The current research does not identify clear problems with the procedure, but public opinion can be greatly influenced by perception. It's difficult to envision that the perception of the benefits of tail amputation can be favorable, particularly without compelling evidence of a benefit for the affected animals.

DAIRY VETERINARIANS AND ANIMAL WELFARE

Animal health issues figure prominently in any discussion of dairy animal welfare because health and welfare are intimately associated. This being true, it seems obvious that dairy veterinarians are well positioned to positively impact dairy cattle welfare via their role as health care providers and consultants. Veterinarians have opportunities to monitor health events, to help evaluate the impact of nutrition and housing management on animal well-being, to establish treatment and culling protocols, to train workers in animal handling and treatment procedures, and to provide producers and managers with objective assessments of current welfare status plus goals and methods for improvement. Unfortunately, it appears that only a small minority of dairy veterinarians actively pursue animal welfare improvement as an objective of their work. Many more seem content to fill the role of service providers rather than welfare consultants and advocates. It is my strong impression that many veterinarians find it very convenient to assume the attitude that economic efficiency and maximum milk production are the overriding goals of the dairy industry. In turn, this makes it easy to further assume that certain levels of animal disease and discomfort that can follow from particular attitudes and management practices are acceptable trade-offs. In particular, some practitioners may fear that voicing strong concern for animal welfare may alienate or antagonize their clients. It is rewarding to see that certain issues, such as facility design that enhances cow comfort, are being recognized as key links between animal well-being and herd productivity. It is hoped that veterinarians will increasingly see the opportunities available to promote dairy animal welfare as strong components of the service they provide.

DAIRY PRODUCERS AND WORKER TRAINING

One of the common attributes of dairy producers emphasized in the first part of this chapter is their well-established ethic of caring for their animals. I can honestly say that virtually every dairy producer I know sincerely cares about the well-being of his or her animals and works to assure that the animals are well cared for. Unfortunately, this does not mean that dairy animals always fare well or that they really receive optimal care. The numerous concerns presented in the preceding discussion highlight areas where dairy animal welfare is frequently compromised. Some of the reasons are lack of knowledge or tools to deal with the problems, lack of recognition that a problem exists, and possible conflicts between economic constraints and ideal management practices. However, I believe that an equally or more important challenge to improving animal welfare in modern dairy operations relates to the problem of dealing with individual animal welfare on operations of increasing size. In many cases, it is not the owner who identifies and manages individual animal problems. Increasingly dairy animals are handled and managed by employees, and in turn these employees frequently do not have the same background, training, or perceptions of the owner. In such circumstances, it is easy for producers to believe that observations are made and actions are taken as they would personally do them, while in reality it is not the case. Few dairies have active worker training programs that meaningfully educate workers about key principles of livestock care and that then follow up with evaluations of performance at periodic intervals. In many cases, the owner and the worker may not communicate well because of language and cultural barriers. I believe that one of the most important means of improving dairy animal welfare is the development and implementation of effective worker training programs. Many of the issues discussed above highlight this need in the areas of calf care and management, calf delivery management, disease recognition, and treatment procedures.

SUMMARY

The dairy industry has undergone steady and remarkable change over the last several decades. Numerous factors have stimulated and shaped these changes, but an overwhelmingly important feature has been the demand for increased economic and business efficiency. This tends to force dairy producers to prioritize economic considerations above animal welfare concerns as they make management decisions. Currently, dairy operations in the United States vary widely in size, geographic location, facility design, and management, with a trend toward larger size and migration to the western arid states, although there are still many dairies in traditional dairy regions that follow more traditional management practices. With these changes have come new challenges to animal well-being in addition to some of the older ones. The dairy industry has not had to face some of the extreme criticism that has been focused on other, more industrialized animal production systems. Nevertheless, there are areas of concern that should be addressed, and most of these can be improved via education, research, and appropriate management changes. Dairy producers would benefit the welfare of their animals by increasingly making animal welfare a top priority, on par with the priority awarded to economic efficiency in the production system. There are numerous examples of management improvements that would positively impact animal well-being and also improve dairy productivity. Dairy veterinarians can play an important role in helping to educate and advise their clients, monitor for animal welfare problems, and guide implementation of improved management strategies. There is a very real need for improved training of dairy farm workers because it is more commonly the workers than the owner/operators who directly implement animal care and welfare procedures.

REFERENCES

Bailey, KW. *Marketing and pricing of milk and dairy products in the United States.* Iowa State University Press, Ames, 1997.

Berry, SL. Milking the golden cow—her comfort. J Am Vet Med Assoc 219(10):1382–1387, 2001.

Blayney, DP. The changing landscape of U.S. milk production. Statistical Bulletin No. 978. Economic Research Service, U.S. Department of Agriculture. June 2002. URL: http://www.ers.usda .gov/publications/sb978/sb978.pdf.

Chase, LE. Cold stress in dairy cattle. In: *Encyclopedia of dairy sciences*, Roginski, H, Fuquay, JW and Fox, PF, eds. Academic Press, Boston, 2003, 2582–2592.

Davis, CL and Drackley, JK. Liquid feeding programs. In: *The development, nutrition, and management of the young calf.* Iowa State University Press, Ames, 1998, 259–282.

Greenough, PR and Weaver, AD. *Lameness in cattle*, 3rd ed. W.B. Saunders Co., Philadelphia, 1997.

Kahler SC, and Zielinski H. Raising contented cattle makes welfare, production sense. J Am Vet Med Assoc 218(2):182–186, 2001.

NAHMS. Beef '97, parts I and II: Reference of 1997 beef cow/calf health and management practices. Report from USDA:APHIS:VS, National Animal Health Monitoring System, Fort Collins, CO, #N233.697, #N238.797, 1997a.

——. Dairy 2002, part I: Reference of dairy health and management in the United States, 2002. Report from USDA:APHIS:VS, CEAH, National Animal Health Monitoring System, Fort Collins, CO, #N377.1202, 2002.

——. Dairy heifer morbidity, mortality, and health management focusing on preweaned heifers, part D, Report from USDA:APHIS:VS, National Animal Health Monitoring System, Fort Collins, CO, #N129.0294, 1994.

——. Digital dermatitis on U.S. dairy operations, Dairy '96 Study, Report from USDA:APHIS:VS, CEAH, National Animal Health Monitoring System, Fort Collins, CO, #N231.597, 1997b.

——. Management practices on U.S. dairy operations, parts I–III, Dairy '96 study, Report from USDA:APHIS:VS, CEAH, National Animal Health Monitoring System, Fort Collins, CO, #N200.696, #N210.996, #N212.1196, 1996.

National Cattlemen's Beef Association, Colorado State University. Final Report of the National Non-Fed Beef Quality Audit. 1994.

——. Final Report of the National Market Cow and Bull Beef Quality Audit. 2000.

Northeast Regional Agricultural Engineering Service. Animal behavior and the design of livestock and poultry systems. Ithaca, NY, 1995.

Organization for Economic Cooperation and Development. *Agricultural policies in OECD countries, monitoring and evaluation 2002.* OECD Publications Service, Paris, France, 2002.

Quaife, T. Tail docking makes little sense. Dairy Herd Management 10:70–72, 2002.

Smith, BP. *Large animal internal medicine*, 3rd ed. Mosby, Inc., St. Louis, 2002.

Staples, CR and Thatcher, WW. Heat stress in dairy cattle. In: *Encyclopedia of dairy sciences*, Roginski, H, Fuquay, JW, and Fox, PF, eds. Academic Press, Boston, 2003, 2592–2604.

Stull, CL, Payne, MA, Berry, SL and Hullinger, PJ. Evaluation of the scientific justification for tail docking in dairy cattle. J Am Vet Med Assoc 220(9):1298–1303, 2002.

Webb, DW. Replacement economics. In: *Large dairy herd management*, Van Horn, HH and Wicox, CJ, eds. Am Dairy Sci Assoc, Savoy, IL, 1992, 434–440.

Wells, SJ, Dargatz, DA and Ott, SL. Factors associated with mortality to 21 days of life in dairy heifers in the United States. Prev Vet Med 29:9–19, 1996.

12

Production Practices and Well-Being: Swine

Timothy E. Blackwell

BACKGROUND

Fifty years ago sows and pigs were housed outside in dirt lots with simple shelters to protect them from the weather. These outdoor systems worked well on sandy soils with adequate drainage. On heavier soils, the rooting behavior of the pigs combined with normal rainfall and snowmelt turned these pasture systems into impassable mud lots. To correct this, gestating sows and growing pigs were moved to concrete lots with open-sided or fully enclosed shelters. The work of manure handling, bedding, and feeding was done by hand. This labor-intensive form of livestock rearing ensured that sow and pig inventories remained low. The advent of fully enclosed barns, partially slatted floors, liquid manure systems, and automated feeding allowed for a significant increase in the average size of swine farms.

The moderate environment inside the newer barns encouraged producers to farrow year-round and to wean pigs at less than six weeks of age. This increased output from these more-expensive facilities. Sows were housed in small groups with three to four sows per pen. These small groups of sows fought among themselves at mixing and feeding times occasionally resulting in serious injuries. To put an end to these injuries, producers housed gestating sows individually to ensure adequate feed, water, and freedom from fighting.

In these modern production systems, grower pigs were housed in groups of 10 to 20. The pen floors were composed of a slatted area for dunging and a solid area for resting and feeding. Producers became frustrated with the dunging habits of grower pigs in these pens as pigs commonly dunged on the solid floored areas. New pens were constructed with fully slatted floors to ensure that pigs remained clean regardless of their dunging habits. Each improvement in facility design increased the fixed costs of production, and greater productivity was needed to pay the bills. Earlier weaning of pigs provided an opportunity to increase sow productivity but required more sophisticated nurseries and nursery diets for the younger pigs. This cycle of improved production systems requiring increases in productivity to be profitable continues.

Modern swine facilities are sometimes associated with a decreased standard of welfare for sows and pigs. Welfare concerns in these systems fall into two categories. One category is welfare issues associated with the "unnatural" environment in which domestic pigs are raised. This is exemplified by hogs that live their entire lives on steel, concrete, and plastic floors in overcrowded and unstimulating environments. The second category of concerns relates to the pain and suffering associated with certain husbandry practices.

These practices range from castration and tail docking of piglets to the killing of unproductive animals. Such procedures can cause unnecessary distress to swine if stockpeople are not adequately trained and provided with the necessary resources to prevent or relieve pain. This chapter will review both categories of welfare concerns and suggest alternatives to some controversial practices. The chapter is divided into sections according to the age of the pig or the production area in the barn.

GESTATING SOWS

Housing Systems

Many of the changes in sow and pig housing have improved swine welfare but they have also produced new problems. One area of swine production receiving an increase in public scrutiny is the system of individually housing pregnant sows in two foot by seven foot gestation stalls.

Individually housing sows during gestation ensures that each sow receives an appropriate amount of feed, liberal access to water, and protection from aggressive herdmates. However, gestation crates restrict the movement of sows and make lying in a prone position difficult for larger, older parity sows.[1] Sows were originally placed in these restrictive but secure environments to improve their welfare and productivity. To that extent, gestation crates have succeeded. However, the restrictions on freedom of movement in these stalls created new problems including:

- Difficulty in identifying lame or diseased individuals due to the restricted range of movement and behaviors that can be observed within the confines of a gestation stall
- Vocalization and anxiousness at feeding time when large numbers of sows are individually hand-fed
- Decreased bone density due to a lack of movement[2,3].
- Boredom due to the barren environment and the restricted amount of nutritionally balanced, highly concentrated diet fed daily
- Excessive noise caused by the banging of the metal crates as sows move around inside them
- Difficulty in achieving normal resting positions for larger sows[1]

Gestation stalls resolved the problems associated with housing small numbers of sows in groups. Uneven feed distribution, fighting, and injuries were no longer of concern to producers. Instead, new problems with boredom and lack of exercise existed. Stockpeople, animal scientists, and engineers have addressed the concerns associated with crated gestation housing. Two different approaches to solving the problems have been developed.

One approach utilizes sophisticated computerized feeding technology to reduce aggression at feeding time (fig. 12.1). In computerized feeding systems, the sows are housed in groups and each sow is equipped with a transponder that identifies the individual to a central computer. The computer is programmed to determine how much feed an individual sow should be fed during each 24-hour period. The sows access their feed by walking

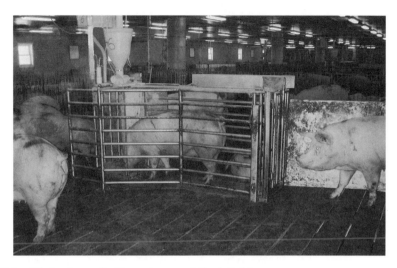

Figure 12.1.   Electronic sow feeding system on a fully slatted floor.

into a gated, computerized feeding station. The gates of the feeding station are electroni-cally controlled so that only one sow can enter the station at a time. When a sow walks up to the entrance to the feeding area, a scanner identifies the sow's transponder. If that sow has not already consumed her allotted portion of feed for that 24-hour period, the gate swings open and the amount of feed to which she is still entitled slowly trickles into the trough. As soon as she leaves the feeding station, the slow flow of feed ceases so that the next sow cannot eat the previous sow's ration. A sow can enter the feeding station as often as she wants until she has consumed her allotted ration for that day. After that, entry is de-nied or if entry is allowed, access to feed is prevented. Sows exit the station through a gate at the opposite side of the station from where the other sows are waiting to enter.

The number of sows in a group is based on the recommendations of the manufacturer regarding the capacity of the feeding station. Depending on the model, one feeder may be adequate to feed between 40 and 60 sows. The lounging area for the sows may be a straw-bedded pen (solid manure system) or a partially or fully slatted pen (liquid manure system).

Another system to feed sows in group housing is based on floor feeding. Stockpeople and scientists working to find a solution to the problems of gestation crates made an important dis-covery. When 3, 4, or 5 sows are housed together, they fight whenever they are fed. However, larger groups of sows do not fight at feeding time. In a small group, 1 or 2 dominant sows pre-vent 1 or more subordinate sows from consuming feed. However, in larger groups of 10 to 30 or more sows, it is impossible for 1 or 2 dominant sows to guard all of the feed that is spread over the floor for the entire group (figs. 12.2 and 12.3). In these larger groups, all sows real-ize that the most efficient approach is to concentrate on eating. In these systems, time spent establishing dominance over another sow at feeding time translates into feed lost. Sows learn not to fight when fed and to concentrate on getting their share of the available ration.

In all loose housing systems, some aggression between sows occurs when groups are initially assembled or reassembled in the pens. This dominance aggression lasts for one to four days after mixing and operators report that it is decreased when

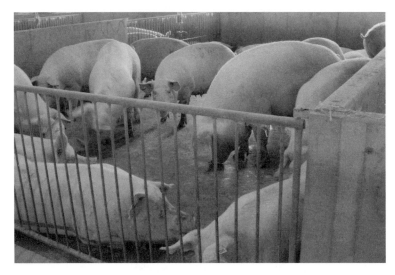

Figure 12.2.   Floor feeding system on a partially slatted floor.

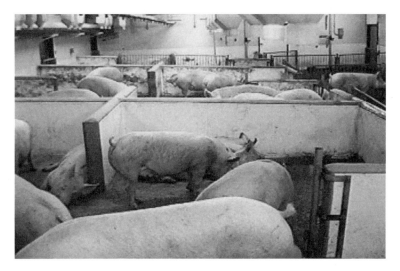

Figure 12.3.   Floor feeding system with partially slatted floor and partial walls in the feeding area.

- sows are grouped according to size;
- a boar is included in the group;
- sows are given extra feed (full fed) directly after mixing;
- sows are mixed late in the day and lights are turned off immediately afterward;
- straw, hay, or toys are provided as a distraction;
- combinations of the above are used.

Fighting between sows primarily involves slashing with the incisors over the shoulder areas causing superficial lesions that normally heal without treatment in 7 to 14 days (fig.

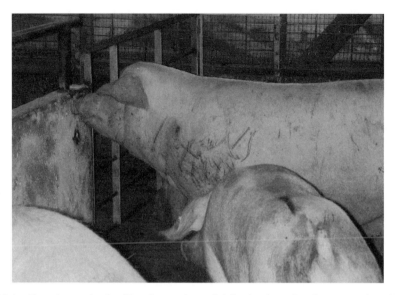

Figure 12.4.   Scratches on the shoulder of a sow due to fighting in a loose-housing system three days after grouping sows together.

12.4). Almost half of all sows may show evidence of having been involved in fighting 1 to 2 days after mixing. These shoulder scratches heal within 10 to 14 days and are barely visible two weeks after mixing.[4]

Loose housing systems for sows vary considerably. Pen designs, management, flooring type, and feeding systems all influence the amount of space each sow should be allotted. Guidelines for space requirements for sows and gilts are given in table 12.1.[5]

An example of a floor plan for a loose housing system utilizing liquid manure is shown in figure 12.5. The plan is based on allowing 25 sq. ft. per sow and is cheaper to build than standard gestation housing using gestation stalls. Small amounts of hay or straw may be fed on the floor or from hay racks mounted to the wall to provide some environmental enrichment. Sows may be fed in this system once or twice daily.

Table 12.1.   Recommended Pen Floor Space Allowances for Replacement Gilts and Sows

Body weight		Partial slats (0.054 * BW$^{.667}$)		Solid bedded (0.059 * BW$^{.667}$)	
Kg	Lb	M^2	Sq. ft.	M^2	Sq. ft.
100–150	220–330	1.5	16	1.7	18
150–200	330–440	1.8	19	2.0	22
200–250	440–550	2.1	23	2.3	25
>250	>550	2.3	25	2.6	28

Note: For calculations, body weight is in kilograms and the resulting answer is in square meters.

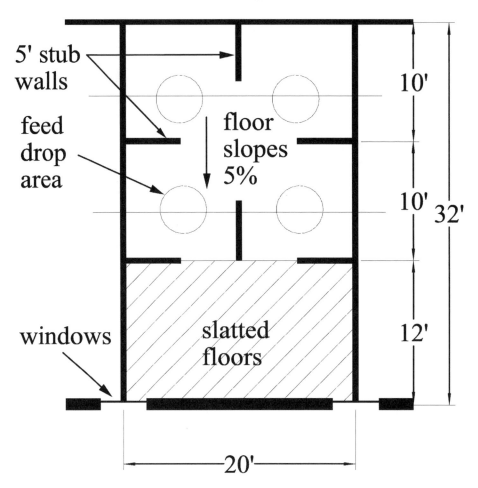

Figure 12.5.   Group pen design for 25 sows using a liquid manure system developed at the Arkell Research Station in Guelph, Ontario. Two feed augers are used to drop feed across two lines on the solid floor. Waterers are mounted or hung over the slatted dunging area.

Nonambulatory or Downer Sows

Nonambulatory or downer sows occur in all types of housing systems. Sows most often have trouble rising and walking during the period from one day to two weeks after weaning possibly due to the extreme metabolic demands of lactation.[2,3] However, sows may "go down" during the breeding, gestation, or lactation periods. The reasons for downer sows are many and often times the exact cause is not determined. A metabolic disease may weaken a sow to the point where she no longer has the strength to stand. Other times, traumatic or infectious arthritides are to blame. Unfortunately, in the majority of cases, the reason that a sow cannot rise is undetermined.

Acute and chronic arthritis is one cause of lameness in sows and gilts. Acute arthritis may respond to treatment with antibiotics and anti-inflammatory drugs. If chronic arthritis progresses to the point where a sow can no longer stand on her own, there is seldom a response to treatment. In such cases, the sow should be euthanized immediately or taken to slaughter as soon as possible. Affected individuals must be kept comfortable prior to slaughter. Unfortunately, only a limited number of the analgesic drugs available to veterinarians will alleviate pain without creating drug residues at slaughter.

The attitude of stockpeople toward sick and injured animals on the farm is crucial.[6,7] It is important that nonambulatory sows and other high-maintenance individuals not be considered an inconvenience in an already busy workday. Animals in distress should not be attended to at the end of the day "if there is time." Animals requiring treatment must be given priority during the workday to ensure unnecessary suffering does not occur. If such attention is deemed financially or physically impossible, affected animals should be euthanized immediately.

FARROWING AND NURSING SOWS

Sows are held in farrowing crates from a few days prior to parturition until the litter is weaned. Pigs are usually weaned between 16 and 28 days of age on most North American swine farms. Although confinement in farrowing crates is as restrictive as gestation crates, the sows appear to tolerate confinement in farrowing crates better. Confinement during gestation occurs when a sow would normally be moving around and foraging, and therefore may be more stressful than the restriction of movement that occurs during the lactation period. Loose-housed lactating sows do not move far from their litter during the first one to two weeks after farrowing.[7,8] Since feed is readily available in the farrowing crate, a major stimulus for the sow to leave her litter after the first week is also eliminated.

A major problem with farrowing crates is that the restrictive environment and the lack of bedding material eliminates any possibility for the sow to express her natural nest-building behavior prior to farrowing. Allowing a sow freedom of movement during or after parturition increases the risk that newborn pigs will be laid on by the sow. "Laid ons" are especially problematic in older, heavier sows with large litters, when very small pigs are part of the litter. Farrowing crate designs that increase freedom for the sow while protecting newborn pigs from crushing have been developed. However, in most of these systems, the problem of denying a sow the opportunity to express her innate nest-building behavior remains. Providing nest-building material and room to build a nest requires a solid floor and, therefore, a solid manure-handling system. Such systems are labor intensive and difficult to keep clean compared to systems using conventional farrowing crates that have fully slatted floors and no nest-building substrate. Cost-effective nest-building substrate that can be incorporated into a liquid manure system is needed if we are to allow sows to express their natural behavior while maintaining the advantages of liquid manure systems. One producer has designed his own turn-around farrowing crate, placing small amounts of shredded newspaper in the crate prior to farrowing. No problems with the liquid manure system have resulted from the use of the shredded paper (fig. 12.6).

Other causes of compromised welfare in sows include heat stress, dystocia, lameness, and infectious disease. The majority of diagnoses and treatments on modern swine farms in North America are done by the stockpeople who take care of the animals. Veterinary

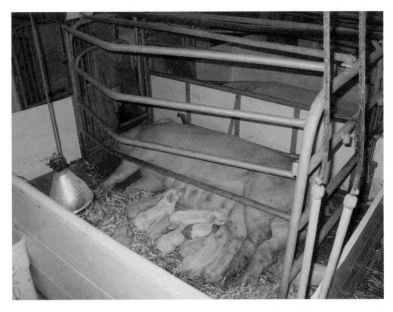

Figure 12.6.   A producer-designed farrowing crate allowing the sow the ability to turn around within the crate. Shredded newspaper is added prior to farrowing to help decrease chilling in piglets and possibly serve as a substrate for nest-building (Photo courtesy of Erik Van Grootheest, designer and builder, Fergus, Ontario).

input on many operations is limited. It is therefore critical that owners and employees of swine farms be sensitive to animal pain and distress and have the appropriate skills and tools to relieve animal suffering when it occurs.

Heat Stress

Heat stress in late gestation or early lactation can be reduced by increasing evaporative cooling of sows. In warmer climates, automatic drippers or misters are commonly installed in the farrowing house so that sows can be kept damp to facilitate cooling. Some farms utilize large evaporative cooling units on the air intakes to lower the temperature inside the farrowing house, breeding and gestation areas. In climates where heat stress is less common, stockpeople spray the sows with a garden hose two to four times per day during hot weather to cool the sows. These preventive measures pay for themselves as sow mortality can increase sharply during summer heat spells and a sow and her litter are generally valued at over $500 U.S.

Prolapsed Uteri and Dystocias

Prolapsed uteri in sows cannot be avoided but should be treated by amputation of the uterus or euthanasia of the sow shortly after discovery. Severe dystocias in sows requiring Caesarean section are rare since litter-bearing species do not often have problems giving birth. Occasionally, a pig does become lodged in the birth canal causing distress to the mother and often the death of that pig and those pigs that were immediately next in the birth order. Although sows often give birth to the retained pig eventually, the increase in time spent farrowing tires the sow and may lead to complications such as metritis. Attending as many farrowings as possible is the best method to avoid this problem. A clean vaginal exam, assistance with delivery of easily reached pigs, and treatment with oxytocin when indicated will decrease farrowing times and associated complications.

Inducing sows to farrow with prostaglandins and oxytocin is done to bring sows into labor during normal working hours so that assistance is more readily available if required. There may be increased piglet mortality due to inducing sows more than two days prior to their natural due date,[9] and in any induction system, some sows will not farrow during the workday as intended. The advantages and disadvantages of induced farrowing must be evaluated on a farm-by-farm basis to decide whether natural or induced farrowings minimize neonatal deaths and sow discomfort.

Infectious Disease and Anorectic Sows

Infectious diseases are rare in mature sows, although outbreaks of viral infections in naïve populations do occur. Bacterial infections are sporadic and most commonly affect the reproductive tract or joints. If a lactating sow is suffering from a disease, milk production often declines and nursing pigs may be malnourished. Feeding artificial milk replacer formulated for pigs supplements the sow's milk production and prevents starvation in piglets.

Occasionally, sows become anorectic during lactation and are reluctant to rise. Remarkably, these sows continue to feed their litter despite minimal feed and water intake. There is reluctance among some producers to treat anorectic sows since they are often shipped to slaughter as soon as their litters are weaned. There is no clear economic advantage to a producer to treat these individuals when they are feeding their litters adequately. The risk of drug residues at slaughter also discourages treatment. Stockpeople should work with their veterinarians to establish treatment protocols that take into account the need to provide necessary medical therapy to such sows while avoiding residues at slaughter. Veterinarians must establish appropriate treatment protocols for disease situations where short withdrawal times are necessary.

Sow Lameness

Lameness, if untreated in sows, causes serious welfare problems. Degenerative joint disease, traumatic injuries, and infectious arthritis are three common causes of lameness. Lame sows often do not respond to treatment, particularly when kept in either gestation stalls or competitive group-housing systems. Affected sows recover more rapidly when housed in pens with good traction and negligible risk of fighting or other behaviors that inhibit healing. Unfortunately, hospital pens are becoming less common on modern swine farms and, as a result, sows may remain in their gestation stalls or loose-housing pens when lame. There is a strong economic incentive to keep a lame, pregnant sow until she farrows, and this can lead to welfare problems.

It is imperative that a lame sow be treated appropriately to minimize pain. Unfortunately, there are few licensed analgesics with which to treat lame sows. Most analgesics must be used in an extra-label manner requiring a veterinary prescription and accompanying extended withdrawal time. Often operators want to ship lame sows to slaughter soon after their litter is born, thus making long withdrawal times problematic. Therefore, pregnant sows due to be culled because of lameness are seldom treated with analgesics. If lameness in a pregnant sow is treated with analgesics, it may be acceptable to house the sow until the litter is born and/or weaned. However, if the lameness does not respond to treatment, the sow should be euthanized. If a treated sow has weaned her litter but stopping treatment for the length of the withdrawal period will cause the sow to be uncomfortable during transportation, euthanasia instead of transportation is indicated. Every swine farm should have a policy regarding lameness in sows and other maladies that have the potential to cause significant welfare problems.

Sow Mortality

Mortality in sows varies greatly from farm to farm. Sow mortality can be as low as 2 percent and as high as 15 to 20 percent.[10] Sow mortality occurs most frequently around the time of farrowing and is often highest during hot weather.[11] Causes of mortality vary and include heart failure, shock, heat stress, septicemias, and ulcers.[12] Consistently high sow mortality (greater than 6 percent) is a cause of concern from both an economic and an animal welfare perspective.

Investigations to date have often been unsuccessful at determining the cause or causes of high mortality on sow farms. Mortality may be higher in crated gestation units where it is more difficult to identify sick or injured individuals due to the limited range of behavior they are able to display. Provided a sick or injured sow consumes her allotted ration within 24 hours, there may be little indication to the stockperson that anything is wrong. Even sows off feed may be treated with one or two days of "wait and see" in hopes that they will recover without treatment. This approach has proved successful often enough to become a standard procedure on many farms. Unfortunately, this procrastination delays the treatment of individuals affected with serious illnesses and may contribute to suffering and above-average sow mortality rates.

NEWBORN AND SUCKLING PIGS

Newborn and suckling pigs present unique welfare challenges. From parturition to weaning, young pigs are very vulnerable to environmental insults, injuries, and infectious diseases.

Early Weaning (Less Than 15 Days)

Decreasing the weaning age of piglets can create welfare problems. In pasture farrowing systems, pigs were weaned at six to ten weeks of age. When pig production moved into fully enclosed buildings, weaning age began to decrease. Piglets were weaned four to five weeks after birth to increase reproductive efficiency of the sow and to decrease the chance of disease transmission from the sow to her litter. Weaning age has been advocated as low as 12 to 14 days of age but in most modern intensive systems today, it varies between 15 and 20 days postfarrowing.

The amount of distress suffered by piglets at weaning is associated with the quality of the nursery facilities, diet, and management. Under good management conditions, minor fighting and reduced appetites occur in piglets during the first two days after weaning and mixing. Following this adjustment period, distress in early weaned pigs is not often observed.

Mortality

Common causes of death in newborn piglets are chilling, enteritis, starvation, and crushing.[13] These four syndromes may occur together in a single piglet. A chilled pig that cannot compete adequately for its mother's milk will begin to starve, then scour, and become so weak that it is unable to move out of the way when the sow lies down. The smallest pigs in the litter are most susceptible to chilling, starvation, enteritis, and crushing. Bacterial septicemia is the next most common disease in suckling piglets.

Good management practices can reduce neonatal piglet mortality from all causes to less than 10 percent of pigs born alive. However, it is important, regardless of the mortality rate, to ensure that the suffering of sick or weak pigs is minimized. Moribund pigs should not be left to a natural or, more accurately, an agonal death. Appropriate treatments where needed and timely euthanasia when indicated are necessary to reduce suffering in sick and weak piglets. The use of carbon dioxide chambers or blunt trauma to the head are recommended methods of euthanasia in nursing piglets.[14] However, it should be noted that blunt trauma to the head is an inexact method and therefore the chances are greater that an instantaneous and painless death may not be achieved. In addition, the use of blunt trauma as a method of euthanasia although readily available, inexpensive, and of little or no risk to the operator, can be distasteful to perform or to observe. The use of carbon dioxide chambers is a safe and effective method of euthanasia more likely to be widely accepted by professional stockpeople.

Welfare problems are created on some larger farms when bonuses are paid for the total number of pigs weaned. This can encourage some well-meaning farrowing room attendants to prolong the life of some pigs that are unlikely to survive the next stages of the production cycle. If a separate growing area is not available to address the needs of these high-maintenance, weaker individuals, they should be humanely destroyed.

Routine Procedures Performed on Suckling Pigs

It is common practice on many modern swine farms to inject iron, dock the tails, and clip the needle teeth of baby pigs within 48 hours of birth. Most male pigs are castrated within 10 days of birth. Inguinal hernias are often surgically corrected at the time of castration. On some farms, injections of antibiotics and vaccines may also be given before pigs are three weeks of age. These procedures are performed by the barn staff and it is rare for any analgesia or anesthesia to be used.

Despite these invasive procedures, suckling pigs demonstrate minimal signs of distress immediately following any of the techniques listed above. Often a pig that has been castrated and injected with iron will return to nursing the sow directly following these procedures. Some observers believe that the greatest discomfort occurs several hours after castration or tail amputation and is associated with the inflammatory response that results from these insults. Although traditionally procedures such as tail docking or castration have been performed without analgesia, it is unlikely that in the years to come the swine industry will be able to justify this practice to consumers. Stockpeople may argue that piglets show few signs of pain immediately following tail docking or castration, however most will admit to noticing evidence of pain or discomfort several hours after the procedures were performed. Analgesia should be administered before or, at the very least, at the time of surgery to reduce pain and inflammation caused by these procedures. At present, a cost-effective and practical system of providing analgesia to neonatal pigs for such procedures does not exist. This may be a lucrative area of research for pharmaceutical companies to pursue.

A few farms have experimented with eliminating some of the procedures mentioned above. Although clipping needle teeth is important to decrease injuries due to fighting in suckling pigs, damage to littermates is normally small provided that cross-fostering is not performed after pigs are one day of age. Recent work has demonstrated that the benefits of cross-fostering older pigs may not outweigh the negative effects resulting from the need to reestablish a dominance hierarchy within the litter every time an individual is added or removed from the group.[15] If the benefits of later cross-fostering are minimal at best, clipping needle teeth may be a procedure that can be eliminated on many farms.

It is unclear how effective tail docking is in preventing tail biting in pigs. Although many farms have demonstrated moderate success in leaving tails intact, the occasional outbreak of tail biting on these farms has convinced most producers to routinely dock tails.

In many European countries as well as in Australia, pigs are not castrated and only intact boars are sold. There is reluctance in the North American market to accept intact boars at slaughter because the risk of boar taint is greater in the heavier market weights that are preferred. Work continues in identifying nonsurgical approaches to eliminating boar taint in intact males at heavier slaughter weights.

NURSERY PIGS

Piglets are commonly weaned from the sow at between 15 and 20 days of age on North American swine farms. Improvements in housing facilities and diets for young pigs have decreased many of the stresses endured by pigs at weaning. On well-managed modern swine farms, pigs grow as well after weaning at 20 days as they would grow if weaned at a later date. Welfare concerns nevertheless exist.

Fighting

Dominance aggression occurs whenever pigs are put into new social groups. Some swine farms keep litters together at weaning and build nursery pens to hold single litters of pigs. More commonly, litters are mixed at weaning into larger groups of 15 or more pigs per group. Occasionally, groups of pigs at weaning are sorted by age, weight, or sex, but most often they are grouped without regard to any of these factors with the exception that occasionally the smallest pigs in a weaning group are housed together.

Regardless of the penning arrangement, newly weaned pigs fight for one to three days to establish a hierarchy within the pen. Injuries resulting from this fighting are normally minor and superficial and seldom require treatment.

Failure to Thrive Syndrome

A small percentage of pigs weaned at almost any age may fail to gain weight normally after weaning. Although the reason for this is occasionally a recognizable pathology, often no reason for the failure to thrive syndrome is found on postmortem examination. A diagnosis of starvation is often made, although the pig came from a pen with ad lib access to feed and water and thriving pen-mates. Occasionally, if such pigs are removed from the pen and are placed in another environment, they begin to eat and gain weight. The reason for this failure to thrive syndrome is unknown but may represent an inability of some pigs to adapt to a new environment postweaning. On some farms, early identification of such pigs and movement to a nurse pen or hospital pen that may contain a different diet and a different social structure has been shown to reverse the syndrome.

Boredom and Vices

Common vices in nursery pigs include navel sucking, urine drinking, and ear and tail biting. Causes of these vices are unknown. Many hypotheses have been proposed to explain why these behaviors occur. These include mineral and protein deficiencies in the diets, lack of water, boredom, crowding, temperature fluctuation, genetic predisposition, stress, and others. One major problem in studying vices in recently weaned pigs is an inability to consistently reproduce these behaviors under experimental conditions. As a result, the majority of information on these vices comes from observations and reports from the field. It is nearly impossible to draw conclusions from these sporadic and varying field outbreaks. Pigs weaned into comfortable environments with adequate access to water and appropriate diets are less likely to demonstrate abnormal behaviors. Toys or substrate in which to root have been used to enrich the environment of newly weaned pigs without consistent results. Should practical methods to enrich the environment of newly weaned pigs be found, the health and productivity of recently weaned pigs will likely improve.

Diseases

Diseases in weaned pigs are relatively common. The change in diet and environment at weaning combined with the natural decline in passive antibody titers acquired through colostrum place young pigs at risk of infectious disease.

The most common disease affecting pigs during the first week after weaning is diarrhea.[16] A number of different bacteria and viruses are capable of causing diarrhea in weaned pigs. Some of these pathogens are highly virulent and contagious and cause severe enteritis under even the best management conditions. However, most infectious enteric diseases in recently weaned pigs can be controlled by careful attention to diet formulation and presentation. The tendency of young pigs to eat very little during the first 12 to 24 hours after weaning and then to compensate by overeating provides an ideal environment for enteric disease to occur. Proper diet formulation, liberal access to water, and delivery of small amounts of feed at carefully spaced intervals (three to six times a day for the first three to five days after weaning) can dramatically reduce the incidence of postweaning diarrhea in pigs.

Besides enteric diseases, recently weaned pigs may be affected by rhinitis, pneumonia, dermatitis, arthritis, meningitis, septicemia, viremia, and other illnesses. For each disease, the infectious agent and predisposing factors causing the illness must be identified and a cost-effective strategy of treatment and prevention applied. A close working relationship with the herd's veterinarian is essential to devise an appropriate strategy for disease control.

Prompt attention to the treatment and prevention of disease is routine practice on nearly all swine farms because of the significant economic costs associated with disease. However, animal welfare concerns may arise following an outbreak of disease when a small number of survivors fail to thrive. These individuals recover from the disease but are so severely affected that they cannot compete with the healthier pigs in the pen. Whether suffering from compromised lungs, severe chronic arthritis, stomach ulceration, or other problems, these pigs deteriorate over a period of days, weeks, or months. Having worked hard to treat and nurse sick pigs back to health, the stockperson may be hesitant to give up on any individual that "recovered."

To avoid this situation, in addition to protocols for dealing with disease outbreaks, every swine farm should have a protocol for dealing with "poor doers" or wasting pigs. These individuals should be humanely destroyed, placed in separate hospital pen facilities, or sold to special markets where individuals specialize in raising weak and recovering pigs. Although occasionally such pigs respond to nursing care and a special environment, oftentimes they do not respond sufficiently to be profitable and humane destruction is indicated.

Space Allotments and Crowding

Facilities are a significant component in the overall costs of raising pigs. It is an economic necessity in pig farming as in most other businesses to maximize the use of all capital investments. Therefore, space allowances for pigs are often determined by measuring the highest return on investment at various stocking densities. It might be assumed that maximizing individual growth rates would correlate closely with maximum economic returns. However, most economic models show that overall farm profits increase when pens of pigs are crowded to a point where maximum average daily gains are slightly decreased.[17] Pens of pigs crowded to a point where individual pig performance is slightly reduced produce more total kilograms of gain per pen, thus increasing total profit per pen.

The welfare of pigs is more complicated than simple measurements of average daily gains and feed efficiencies. It is important to note that tight profit margins will always force producers to maximize returns by running all facilities at their maximum income-generating potential. Only legislation dictating space allowances for pigs will change current pig-stocking densities.

Pen Design, Behavior, and Sleeping Times

Pen design and group size are as important as total space allotment when evaluating pig welfare. A 5 ft. by 6 ft. square weaning pen with 10 pigs per pen or a 6 ft. by 12 ft. pen with 24 pigs per pen each allows 3 sq. ft. per pig. However, square or nearly square pens make it difficult for pigs to establish separate sleeping, eating, dunging, and activity areas. It is also difficult for pigs in such pens to escape dominance aggression.

Weaning pens should allow all the pigs to eat together at the same time for the first three to five days after weaning and should have "quiet areas" where pigs can rest without constant disturbances or interruptions. Pens that are two or two and half times as long as they are wide with feeding and drinking stations placed together at the same end of the pen allow pigs to rest in one area without disturbances from pen-mates that are eating or drinking. Nursing piglets eat and rest approximately 24 times a day.[18] Ad lib feeding in square weaning pens eliminates any possibility of maintaining eating and sleeping patterns similar to those that existed prior to weaning. The inability to rest undisturbed can be a serious stress on newly weaned pigs. Slowly changing feeding patterns from group feeding to ad lib feeding while creating an environment with separate sleeping and activity areas is important for pig health, productivity, and welfare.

Pen Environment: Barren Versus Complex

Pens for pigs are made up of four walls, a floor, a feeder, and a drinker. This simple design is economical to build and easy to clean. However, there is little to occupy the pig's attention. Toys added to pens with weaned pigs are often used for one to two weeks after introduction and then ignored. There is no clear evidence at this time that positive affects on pig health or productivity result from the addition of toys or other objects, such as straw, to the finishing pen environment. Although it appears obvious that pigs enjoy investigating novel objects, after a period of time, the novelty disappears and the objects are ignored. Fresh straw provided as either bedding or for recreational purposes provides material for rooting, chewing, and playing. The cost of the straw and the increased labor required to remove the soiled straw makes this practice uneconomical in most systems.[19] The added costs associated with using straw in pig production are not of concern in countries where the use of bedding is mandated by law. In these countries, the costs are the same for all farms. In countries where the use of bedding is not required, improvements in swine welfare may more practically be achieved by designing pens that maximize pig comfort and provide opportunity for exploratory activity. Rectangular pens with easily delineated areas for feeding, drinking, dunging, and socializing and separate areas for sleeping should be the basis of any pen design. Designs that allow the use of recreational straw or toys while maintaining the advantages of a liquid manure system may be the ideal. Properly designed toys for pigs may be able to affect behavior within a pen by better defining sleeping, dunging, and activity areas.

Temperature

Maintaining the correct temperature for a pen or room of pigs can be difficult as both size of pig and metabolic rate vary from one pig to another or from one pen of pigs to another. It is difficult to establish one temperature that is suitable for all the pigs in an air space. Therefore, it is advisable to group pigs in the pens by size and weight and provide some form of supplemental heat (heat lamp or heat pad) for smaller pigs that require higher temperatures. Sick pigs need higher room temperatures compared to their healthy counterparts. The two most common mistakes made when setting the temperature for weaned pigs are (1) establishing one temperature for a room of pigs that vary significantly in health, size, or weight, and (2) setting the room temperature based on a predetermined target rather than on signs of pig comfort or discomfort. Animal caretakers sometimes pay closer attention to the number on a thermostat than they do to signs of heat or cold stress in the pigs themselves. The ideal temperature for any pen of pigs is that temperature at which pigs rest comfortably without evidence of temperature stress. Chilled pigs pile on top of each other, while heat-stressed pigs have increased respiratory rates and lie on their sides without touching other pigs. Comfortable pigs lie on their sides or stomachs in contact with their pen-mates or a pen divider.

Anesthesia, Analgesia, and Anti-Inflammatories

Nursery pigs seldom require anesthesia. The majority of surgical procedures such as tail docking, castration, or hernia repair are performed while piglets are nursing the sow. Occasionally, a hernia repair is performed after weaning or a "missed" testicle is found in a weaned pig requiring late castration. These surgeries are often performed without anesthesia and, perhaps more significantly, without analgesia. The lack of user-friendly and cost-effective products to provide anesthesia or analgesia in such situations is the reason these procedures are performed without chemical pain control. The limited demand for anesthetics in swine means that there is little economic incentive for a pharmaceutical company to create, test, and market such products. Veterinarians are reluctant to prescribe extra-label analgesics unless they have sufficient information to recommend withholding times prior to slaughter. However, veterinarians should identify effective extra-label analgesics for swine and determine appropriate withdrawal times. Veterinarians should make producers aware that these products are available to provide pain relief for swine and that relieving pain improves recovery rates. Providing analgesia is both good business and good husbandry.

Euthanasia, Downer Pigs, and Casualty Pigs

The majority of discussions on animal welfare in swine production are complex issues where many factors must be considered before reaching a decision. With regard to compromised hogs, there is little room for discussion. Sick or injured hogs must be rapidly identified. Every sick or injured pig should have a presumptive diagnosis made, and an established farm protocol should be in place to deal with each category of injury or disease. Some problems in pigs may require a single injection without need for any further treatment or nursing care. In other cases, prompt movement to slaughter is indicated. Other diseases or injuries may require that a pig be removed to a treatment area where it no longer needs to compete for feed or water and where it will not be disturbed by healthy pen-mates. Some injuries or diseases require euthanasia of the affected pig. Each farm must have a treatment protocol, complete with stopping rules when treatments have proven ineffective, and euthanasia or slaughter protocols for pigs that cannot return to productivity. Under no circumstances should pigs be allowed to suffer and die without treatment or euthanasia.

FINISHING OR FATTENING PIGS

Pigs are commonly moved from the nurseries to the finishing or fattening barns when they reach 45 to 60 lb (20 to 27 kg) of body weight (approximately 8 to 10 weeks of age). In wean-to-finish barns, young pigs are moved to a pen at 9 to 14 lb (4.1 to 6.4 kg) of weight (18 to 21 days of age) and are held there for 20 to 26 weeks until they reach slaughter weight at around 240 to 280 lb (109 to 127 kg). Many of the same problems and welfare concerns that affect nursery pigs affect finishing pigs, although some problems are more common in older pigs.

Mixing and Fighting

Fighting among pigs when they are grouped in the finishing barn is related in part to whether pens of pigs in the nursery are kept together in finishing pens or whether they are resorted. The establishment of a dominance hierarchy in a finishing pen normally takes from one to two days and serious injuries are rare. Occasionally in finishing barns, several pigs will begin fighting one pig in a pen. The reason for this is not clear, but serious injury or death can occur within an hour if the "picked on" pig is not removed.

More commonly, finishing pigs will fight when the social hierarchy within the pen is disturbed. Maximum returns to the producer exist within a narrow range of slaughter weights. Because pigs in a pen do not all fall within this market-weight range at the same time, pigs are sorted out of a pen for market over a two- to six-week period. Each removal of market-weight hogs can stimulate the creation of a new dominance hierarchy in that pen of pigs. To maximize barn utilization during the shipping process, several partially full pens are combined to allow other pens to be emptied out for cleaning and restocking. This also stimulates fighting.

Producers employ different techniques to minimize aggression associated with unstable social groups. In areas where different markets are available for different weights of market hogs, producers can wait until a significant proportion of hogs falls within the highest weight range desired by one packer. At that point, the producer can begin shipping the heaviest hogs to that buyer while shipping lighter pigs to packers that prefer lighter-weight carcasses. In this way a larger percentage of pigs can be removed from the barn at one time, and pigs do not need to be shipped for another two to three weeks until a significant number again falls within the highest weight category. For such a system to work, producers must be in an area with access to a number of packers with a range of requirements for weights of slaughter pigs.

Another approach to reduce aggression resulting from disturbances in pen social structure is to mix pigs immediately before the lights are shut off and give them extra feed, different feed, or some form of toy, such as an old tire or bowling ball, to distract them from aggressive behavior. When all-in, all-out barns are stocked at less than 25 percent capacity, pigs are sometimes moved to a less-expensive barn that may contain one or more simple, large, straw-bedded pen(s). The move to a novel environment and to larger pen size is reported to decrease aggression when mixing late-stage finishing pigs. Unfortunately, there are few trials documenting the effectiveness of any of these techniques.

Vices

Vices are distinct from aggressive behavior in pigs. Although tail biting causes injury, it is not aggressive behavior.[20] Tail biting has been associated with deficiencies in diet, boredom, crowding, poor ventilation, and other factors. One theory suggests that when a pig's environment is deficient or uncomfortable, the pig begins exploratory behavior to seek relief from the stress or stresses in the environment. In modern hog housing systems, this exploratory behavior has few outlets for expression. There is no opportunity to find something else to eat, a warmer place to lie down, or a less-crowded environment. As a result, a pig seeking an outlet for its exploratory drive in a pen of pigs may focus on the other pigs. Tails, even docked tails, are a favorite outlet for pigs seeking to satisfy their exploratory drive.

Many treatments for tail biting have been tried. One of the more successful is to change the ration or to flavor the ration fed to the pigs. A common and inexpensive method to affect ration flavor is to increase the salt content of the feed. Oftentimes the salt content is doubled provided that this does not raise the total salt content of the ration above 1 percent. Free-choice water must be available at all times in such situations. Changing the ration or flavor of the ration often stops tail biting for up to two weeks. After this time, if the cause of the tail biting has not been identified and corrected, the tail biting usually resumes. Additional changes to the ration can buy additional time, but ultimately the cause must be corrected or tail biting will continue.

In some "outbreaks" of tail biting, only one animal may be at fault. Ten or more pigs in one pen may all have their tails bitten by one pen-mate. Other pigs in the pen may sniff or even chew an already damaged and bleeding tail but removal of the single offender can stop the problem.

Another vice of growing pigs is ear biting. Ear biting is likely an aggressive act when it occurs immediately after pigs are mixed in a pen. Biting an ear is an effective method to move a pig away from a limited resource such as feed or water. There should be at least one water nipple for 10 to 15 pigs and flow rates should be not less than 500 ml or one pint per minute.[21] The amount of feeder space is very dependent on feeder and pen design, but commonly one feeder space per 8 to 12 pigs is recommended.

Other vices in pigs are rare. They seldom cause significant welfare concerns.

Diseases

Respiratory and enteric diseases are the most common diseases of fattening pigs. Diseases can be a significant welfare concern if appropriate treatment and prevention practices are not implemented. There are many causes of respiratory and enteric disease in pigs caused by viruses and bacteria. Some infectious agents are sufficiently virulent to make pigs sick single-handedly, while others require additional factors to produce disease. For example, swine influenza virus alone can cause serious respiratory disease and high fever for several days in mature pigs. On the other hand, many bacterial pathogens require viruses, mycoplasmas, or other stressors before they can initiate a disease process.

The occurrence of some diseases in growing pigs is difficult to avoid. Therefore, barn workers must be trained to recognize common swine illnesses. Stockpeople must know how to provide prompt treatment for infected pigs and effective prophylaxis for pigs at risk of disease. Occasionally, recovered pigs do not return to a productive state of health and grow very slowly, if at all. These pigs can become a welfare concern if their compromised state of health or size causes them problems in a group of larger, stronger, and healthier pen-mates. If such pigs are not growing at a comparable rate, they may respond to removal to an appropriate hospital pen that is designed to increase the pig's chances for recovery. If an appropriate hospital pen does not exist on the farm or no reasonable hope for return to productivity or profitability exists, severely affected pigs should be shipped to a salvage market or euthanized.

Space Allotments and Environment

The space allotted to finishing pigs is a compromise between maximizing individual animal productivity and maximizing whole-farm profitability. Although these two parameters are correlated, they are not the same. The code of practice for the care and handling of pigs in Canada recommends 8.7 sq. ft. (0.81 m^2) for a 240-lb (110 kg) pig on a fully slatted floor, 9.7 sq. ft. (0.90 m^2) on a partially slatted floor, and 11.1 sq. ft. (1.03 m^2) on a solid floor with bedding (table 12.2).[5] The requirement for increasing space associated with increasing the proportion of the pen with solid flooring is established to allow for certain areas of the pen to be used as dunging areas and therefore unavailable for other activities. In addition, solid-floored pens require more room in the summer months to allow for heat dissipation.

Finishing pens are normally simple designs with few objects to attract the interest of the pig. The simplicity of the pen design minimizes cost and improves the ease of cleaning after the pigs leave the pen. The lack of objects for pigs to investigate in these pens is considered by some to be a form of environmental deprivation. However, when novel objects

Table 12.2.   Recommended Pen Floor Space Allowances for Growing Pigs
Based on Body Weights[667]

Body weight		Fully slatted		Partial slats (0.039 * BW.667)		Solid bedded (0.045 * BW.667)	
Kg	Lb	M²	Sq. ft.	M²	Sq. ft.	M²	Sq. ft.
10	22	0.16	1.7	0.18	1.9	0.21	2.2
20	44	0.26	2.8	0.29	3.1	0.33	3.5
50	110	0.48	5.2	0.53	5.7	0.61	6.6
75	165	0.62	6.7	0.70	7.5	0.80	8.6
90	198	0.70	7.5	0.78	8.4	0.91	9.7
100	220	0.76	8.2	0.85	9.1	0.97	10.4
110	242	0.81	8.7	0.90	9.7	1.03	11.1

Note: For calculations, body weight is in kilograms and the resulting answer is in square meters.

are placed in pens of pigs, interest in these toys wanes after one to two weeks or even sooner if the objects become soiled. No production benefits are associated with the addition of such objects to finishing pens, although some producers believe the addition of some type of material to chew may discourage tail biting. On most farms, the time and effort involved in adding, cleaning, and replacing these toys are seldom considered of value.

Pen Design and Behavior

Finishing pens should be approximately two to two and half times as long as they are wide to allow pigs the opportunity to organize them into separate activity areas. One section of the pen should contain both the feed and the water supply and will be an area of constant activity during the day. One or more corners of the pen will usually be used as dunging areas. Spindle gating between pens allows pigs to see and socialize with pigs in adjoining pens, and activity and dunging are more common in these areas. It is important that an area separate from the dunging, socializing, and activity areas is available for sleeping. Young growing pigs need and want rest. If a pen is designed so that there is constant traffic from one end to the other, as occurs when ad lib feeders are placed at opposite ends of the pen from the drinkers, there are few places where pigs can rest undisturbed during the day. This is a source of stress and aggravation for pigs and may contribute to vices such as tail biting.

Although pigs appear to enjoy and benefit from straw-bedded pens, the reduction in labor and improved cleanliness of the pigs in partial or totally slatted finishing floors makes it unlikely that the industry will return to solid manure systems. At present, pen designs that allow pigs to eat, drink, sleep, explore, and socialize freely are a reasonable target for the immediate future. A small amount of recreational straw that would not interfere with a liquid manure handling system is likely the practical ideal.

In finishing pens without bedding, temperature and pig comfort must be closely monitored. The absence of bedding means that pigs can avoid chilling only by lying in close proximity to other pigs. Occasionally, the social hierarchy in a pen causes the weakest pigs, who may be most in need of supplementary heat, to lie away from the main group, thus further exacerbating the smaller pigs' problems with thermoregulation. Strict attention should be paid to pigs in modern finishing barns to ensure that the environmental conditions are suitable to all individuals in the pen. If individual pigs do not thrive in their pen environments for whatever reason, they must be removed to a hospital or isolation pen where their specific needs can be addressed.

Anesthesia, Analgesia, and Anti-Inflammatories

It is uncommon for market hogs to require anesthesia, although there may be rare circumstances involving prolapsed rectums, hernias, or injuries where surgery is indicated. Most commonly, such pigs are sent for salvage slaughter, as cost-effective, safe, and efficacious anesthetics with approved withdrawal times for pigs are not readily available.

Analgesics or anti-inflammatories are used in swine medicine to treat injuries, arthritis, or other painful conditions. In most countries, the choice of products is limited and veterinarians are required to prescribe medications extra-label. This requires veterinarians to establish accurate withdrawal times for animals that may be within days or weeks of slaughter. In many countries, the swine practitioner's only possibility to control pain is a limited selection of steroidal and nonsteroidal anti-inflammatory drugs. Nevertheless, it is the veterinarian's responsibility to ensure that safe and effective analgesic protocols exist on all farms.

Moving Swine

Modern swine production occurs in distinct production areas. Almost all farms have separate farrowing rooms, nursery rooms, finishing rooms, and breeding/gestation rooms. This compartmentalized system of production provides superior disease control while minimizing cost and maximizing space utilization. The grouping of animals by stage of production combined with increasing farm size has made it necessary to move pigs weekly or semiweekly. These animals range in weight from 13-lb (6 kg) nursery pigs to 550-lb (250 kg) sows. Although some work has been done on methods to move slaughter pigs onto and off of trucks, there is little practical information available on moving sows into and out of gestation and farrowing crates and moving pigs from one area of production to another. Injuries to stockpeople and to the livestock occur when pigs are moved, and it is often a stressful event for both the pigs and the handler. Not enough is known about pig behavior in swine facilities to recommend standard methods for a stockperson to use to move pigs. Unfortunately, animals that are reluctant to move toward their intended destination are often driven in the desired direction with a combination of force and negative stimuli. The result is most often exhaustion and frustration for both the handler and the pigs.

A combination of appropriate facility design and stockperson training can minimize the stress and exertion of pig movement. Proper lighting, alley width, flooring type, and other factors are critical if pigs are to move easily from one location to another.[22]

One form of on-the-job training in animal movement is the following: When pigs fail to move the way the stockperson intends, the stockperson should ask, "What am I doing wrong?" Often stockpeople wonder instead, "What is wrong with these pigs?" The answer to the second question is that nothing is wrong with the pigs. They are responding naturally to the stimuli that the stockperson is providing. Answering the first question is the key to improving stock handling on a farm.[23]

An example of the above occurs when a stockperson wants to empty a pen of pigs. A commonsense approach is to open the gate and get behind the pigs and drive them out of the pen using the pigs' natural flight zone to move them forward. However, the nature of pigs makes them reluctant to explore new territories when being pressured from behind. Pigs feeling pressure are likely to keep whatever is pressuring them in sight, thus causing them to circle past the open gate and around to the back of the pen behind the handler. The more pressure the pigs feel, the more they seek the safety of the back of the pen. The pigs are responding naturally to their flight zone but do not immediately realize that the open gate offers relief from the pressure. A different approach to emptying the pen is based on the natural curiosity and "follow the leader" instincts of pigs. A handler that quietly opens the pen gate and stands just to the side of the open gate will draw the attention of the most curious pigs in the pen. Curiosity brings these pigs toward the handler and the open gate. After exploring the stockperson for a few seconds these lead pigs see the open gate and usually proceed through it to the alleyway. As the first pigs exit, the next most curious pigs follow and soon the group instinct draws even the most reluctant pigs through the gate to join their pen-mates. The result in the first case, where one attempts to drive the pigs, is often a frustrated stockperson and frightened pigs. In the second case, the stockperson watches the natural curiosity of some pigs and the herd instinct of other pigs empty the pen without any strenuous effort on his or her part.[23]

If the use of electric prods, yelling, or pushing pigs to facilitate movement is viewed as a failure on the part of the stockperson, continued improvement in swine handling can be expected. If the use of such techniques is seen as a standard practice in pig handling, then the routine movement of swine on a hog farm will continue to be a source of stress to both the pigs and the stockpeople.

Feed and Water Restrictions Prior to Slaughter

Limiting access to feed and water prior to slaughter is a standard practice on many farms. The feed given to hogs the day of slaughter is considered wasted as it often ends up in the offal bins. Pigs fed immediately prior to loading on a truck will sometimes regurgitate feed during transportation. It is also less likely that accidental punctures of the intestines will occur during evisceration if the intestinal tract is not filled with ingesta at the time of slaughter. There is no justification for withholding water prior to slaughter. Most jurisdictions allow market hogs to go between 24 and 36 hours without feed or water but insist on resting, watering, and feeding hogs if time between loading and slaughtering exceeds this. An increase in the prevalence of gastric ulcers in hogs held off feed for as little as 12 hours has been documented in some studies[24] but refuted in others.[25] As slaughtering facilities become larger and more efficient, access to smaller, local slaughtering facilities will decline and longer shipping distances will become the rule. Humane transportation codes that ensure adequate space for all pigs to lie down during transport, restrictions on total transport times, and protection from heat and cold stress have been established in most hog-producing countries. Nevertheless, transportation and handling at slaughter facilities remain areas where welfare problems arise. Monitoring of large numbers of pigs as they are unloaded and during lairage will be easier as hog slaughter becomes increasingly centralized in fewer, larger plants. With a heightened emphasis on pork quality, the well-established relationship between pig welfare prior to slaughter and meat characteristics should ensure that packers, producers, and transporters share a common interest in delivering well-rested and nonstressed hogs to the abattoir.[22]

Miscellaneous Topics

Owner-Operator Attitudes and Desensitization

One of the most potentially damaging coping mechanisms a stockperson can develop is one of desensitization. Desensitization is the failure to respond compassionately to the suffering of an animal or animals. Desensitization of stockpeople occurs on both large and small swine farms but for different reasons.

Small family farms can be profitable but relentless occupations. These farms often have unique and creative methods to deal with the daily tasks in swine husbandry. As a result, it is difficult to teach another person to operate these farms. For this reason, the entire family seldom gets away from the farm for a full day let alone an extended holiday. Tired and overworked stockpeople can begin to ignore minor cases of lameness or tail biting and then even more serious welfare problems as enthusiasm for a job demanding 7 days a week, 52 weeks a year wanes. The never-ending work that comes from caring for livestock can cause deterioration in the standard of welfare over time. This happens if the overworked stockperson reduces part of the workload by becoming desensitized to the needs of the animals.

The inability of the owner-operators of a family swine farm to leave the farm is a major factor in the move to larger swine operations. Large farms with multiple employees can schedule work hours so that all employees have days off each week as well as some form of extended holiday.

Unfortunately, desensitization of employees on large farms also occurs but for different reasons. Desensitization in any size of farm is a coping mechanism for stress and on large farms the greater numbers of animals on site mean sick and dying animals are always present. To cope with the daily sicknesses and deaths on these farms, employees become desensitized to the suffering around them. On both large and small farms, when labor is stretched to its maximum, it is difficult to justify spending time to treat or care for individual suffering pigs.

Employees quickly grasp the priorities of the barn manager. The willingness of an owner or manager to allow animals to suffer on a farm tells employees that pain and suffering is not of the same importance as ensuring that feed is properly mixed or that pigs are sorted correctly. As a result, sick and injured pigs must cope with their afflictions, while employees are forced to cope with the sight of compromised animals. Employees who are unable to deal with this workplace environment terminate their employment, while other workers desensitize themselves to the needs of the pigs. This desensitization process leads to a lowering of swine husbandry standards, a decrease in stockmanship, and ultimately lost productivity and profitability.

Good stockpeople react to the suffering of animals and good stockpeople are key to profitability on a swine farm. When a manager establishes a work environment where animal suffering is tolerated, stockmanship skills and production efficiencies decline. Therefore, all farms must have standard operating procedures for treating sick animals, including the use of analgesics and anti-inflammatories where indicated. Part of these standard operating procedures should be guidelines for stopping treatments that are not proving efficacious. For example, a standard procedure for treating pneumonia in a pig could be daily injections with a certain antibiotic. If no improvement is noted after two to three treatments, the protocol might dictate a change to a second specific antibiotic or to call the herd veterinarian. A complete treatment protocol also contains information on when to stop treating a pig and when euthanasia is indicated. Such protocols can help prevent employees from becoming desensitized to the needs of sick or injured pigs.

Ear Hematomas

Hematomas of the ears of pigs occur as a result of trauma. Head shaking due to mange mites, biting by other pigs, or injuries from poorly designed equipment or penning can all lead to rupture of blood vessels and bleeding under the skin of the ear. Affected pigs have grossly distorted ears and may have a difficult time obtaining feed from conventional feeders because of the pain associated with pushing the affected ear against the feeder. Lancing the ear to remove the clotted blood and bandaging the ear against the head is the most effective and humane treatment for this condition. Amputating the ear by use of elastrator bands placed around the base of the ear has also been advocated. Elastrator bands have been associated with increased levels of stress and discomfort when used for castration or tail docking of lambs.[26] It is likely that a similar situation exists in regards to the ears of pigs and this approach to correcting hematomas should be discouraged. Ideally, the cause of the hematomas should be identified and corrected so treatment of the condition is no longer indicated.

Casualty Pigs, Euthanasia Techniques, and Reluctance to Euthanize

One of the most serious welfare concerns in modern swine production is the casualty pig. Barren environments, high stocking densities, temperature fluctuations, infectious disease, and other stressors may be debated in terms of the seriousness of their welfare implications. However, the suffering of an individual animal that is left in a pen of herd-mates but is unable to compete for feed, water, or a resting place is indisputable. It is imperative that all farms have hospital pens to house such individuals until the animal is cured, slaughtered, or euthanized. Hospital pens should be purposefully constructed to facilitate the treatment and recovery of pigs housed therein. If a suitable hospital pen is not available, immediate euthanasia may be indicated for severely affected individual pigs. Strict rules and timelines must be established when treating sick individuals so that pigs are not allowed to languish in a debilitated state at risk of suffering an agonizing death.

Euthanasia is an important component of swine welfare but a task avoided by most caring stockpeople. The decision to euthanize an animal is usually made because the animal's pain or suffering cannot be controlled or because treatment or additional treatment is not likely to be cost-effective. The decision to euthanize can be difficult when the stockperson has tried unsuccessfully to treat the illness in the pig and as a result has developed a closer attachment to that pig than to the rest of the herd. The stockperson may view euthanasia as a personal failure to adequately care for a pig. The decision to perform the unpleasant task of euthanasia is therefore postponed with the hope that "a little more time" will make a difference. For these reasons, pigs may suffer unnecessarily because clear rules about when to euthanize a pig are not established.

All farms must have a policy on the euthanasia of sick or unprofitable pigs. Those involved in raising pigs should be allowed input into the policy on humane destruction. It is often best if one person on the farm has the task of euthanizing pigs. This person should volunteer for this job because they both understand the importance of the work and feel able to deal with the stress of the job. The task of euthanasia should never be assigned to someone against his or her will.

Carbon dioxide is effective to euthanize small pigs and captive bolt guns work well to euthanize larger pigs. Information on the humane destruction of swine is available.[14] A clear euthanasia policy is key to humane animal rearing.

Welfare Audits

Various methods of assessing the welfare of swine on farms have been proposed.[27] Proponents of welfare audits range from animal rights activists to niche marketers. Many factors influence pig welfare, and a number of different production systems could potentially provide adequate welfare for swine. An audit system that is both fair and objective across all management systems and barn designs has been difficult to devise. Welfare audits need to be able to factor in both the number of animals in distress as well as the severity of the distress. It is relatively easy to measure factors such as space allowances, morbidity, mortality, temperature, vices, lameness, cleanliness, and the availability of food and water. Problems arise in interpreting scores assigned to these criteria and in determining the cutpoint between acceptable and unacceptable welfare standards. Most of these systems are based on subjective assessments of objective measures. For example, is it worse to have 5 percent of pigs slightly lame or 1 percent of pigs severely lame?

Welfare audit systems may not be the best method to improve the welfare of swine in modern production systems. Audits can be designed to be either accepting or critical of standard practices in hog production. The industry prefers an audit system that favorably scores the majority of farms. Animal rights groups prefer the opposite. A more pragmatic approach to improving swine welfare and satisfying consumers is to designate specific husbandry practices as prerequisites to sell pigs within a marketing system. The European Union requires group housing of gestating sows because this is consistent with the ethics of the European consumer. Regulations such as these create large improvements in animal welfare provided that alternate systems are available to replace systems deemed unacceptable.

Reporting Animal Welfare Problems

Many people are reluctant to address animal welfare problems on farms. There are understandable reasons for this reluctance. A person who observes substandard swine welfare may believe the owner or manager of the farms is experiencing problems of either a financial or personal nature causing a short-term downturn in the normal husbandry standards on the farm. Or the observer may be reluctant to report animal distress for fear the owner will suspect the source of the complaint. Often only the local humane society is designated to respond in such situations, and it may not have people on staff familiar with swine production practices. At other times people do not report welfare problems because they just do not want to get involved.

The swine industry in each state, province, or region should set up an animal welfare committee to address animal welfare issues on farms. This committee should work to establish and enforce minimum husbandry standards. The committee should be an advisory board for both pork producers and humane societies. It should send out its own investigators if a complaint is received. This system provides swine producers the opportunity to monitor welfare complaints and become part of the solution to swine welfare issues. Delegating this task to a voluntary organization such as the local humane society may not be in the best interests of swine producers.

Surgical Procedures Performed by Lay Personnel

Traditionally, owners of livestock or those employed by the owners have performed certain surgical procedures on farm animals. Swine farm owners or employees routinely castrate, clip needle teeth, notch ears, and dock tails on nursing piglets. Occasionally on smaller swine farms and commonly on large farms, the need arises for more invasive surgical procedures. Inguinal hernias and retained testicles occur more frequently on large production units because of the greater number of animals on site. On smaller farms, veterinarians perform these surgeries because the need for these operations is so rare that producers do not acquire the necessary expertise or confidence to do the surgeries themselves. On large-scale hog farms, the relatively common occurrence of these problems has prompted lay staff to attempt the surgeries themselves. Although many barn workers become adept at these procedures, they seldom administer preoperative, intraoperative, or postoperative analgesia.

Although it is legal for such invasive procedures to be performed by barn staff, it should be the herd veterinarian's responsibility to ensure that appropriate analgesia is used, that surgical techniques are adequate, and that the success ratio is comparable to that of the veterinarian. These same criteria should be applied to any procedure on the farm that can cause unacceptable suffering in pigs. Examples of procedures that require regular veterinary audits include detusking of mature boars, castration of pigs over two weeks of age, delivering pigs from a sow with dystocia, cryptorchid surgeries, inguinal hernias, and euthanasia.

Issues such as dry sow housing tend to dominate discussions on the welfare of swine in modern pig production. However, a poorly performed hernia repair or the ineffective killing of a cull pig causes immense suffering in individual animals and can lead to very negative images of the swine industry in the public eye. It is important to review all potentially painful procedures performed on pigs on a farm. The attending veterinarian and stockpeople involved should be confident that all practices meet an acceptable standard of animal care.

SUMMARY AND CONCLUSIONS

Swine production is evolving toward larger and more intensive forms of production for both economic and social reasons. The need to constantly improve the efficiency of pork production together with the desire of modern swine farm owners and employees to have time off has fueled the development of larger swine farms. The size of a farm does not correlate with the well-being of the pigs housed therein. Swine welfare problems occur on smaller holdings due to financial restrictions or due to overworked family members that become desensitized to animal suffering. Large farms can have problems related to an unstable workforce or a management system that emphasizes profits over individual animal welfare.

Solving welfare problems on swine farms involves identifying welfare concerns, searching out the root causes, and finding practical methods by which to alleviate animal distress. Farm owners as well as all those employed on the farm should understand that improving swine welfare improves worker morale, farm profits, and the overall image of the industry. Animal agriculture must stop reacting defensively to concerns regarding the welfare of domestic livestock. Livestock industries, instead, must encourage open dialogue concerning animal welfare issues. To form a basis for such dialogue, livestock commodity groups should establish local industry-based reporting systems to address welfare concerns raised by the public.

Animal agriculture must give up the concept that "educating the public" regarding modern livestock farming practices is the answer to alleviating consumer concerns over the welfare of swine on today's pig farms. This approach will not bring an end to the public's natural aversion toward practices such as the housing of sows in gestation crates or performing invasive surgeries without analgesia. Educating the public in most situations is little more than a desperate effort to maintain the status quo. It translates to: "Trust us. We know what we are doing and you don't." This insults consumers and portrays the industry as arrogant and uninterested in what consumers care about. In a free market system, when customers want something from the producers of goods, it is bad business to respond by trying to convince the customers that they don't want or can't afford what they are asking for. This is a sign of an industry in decline. If consumers in large numbers want a product that an industry is capable of producing, then the industry must deliver or die.

The swine industry can address the welfare concerns of consumers. Consumers are not stupid nor do they need to be educated because they no longer come from farms. Consumers know what they want and will respond positively to industries that take their requests to heart. It is time to get on with the business of producing the pork our customers want. We have always been successful in this regard. There is no reason not to continue with our success.

REFERENCES

1. Anil, L., Anil, S.S., and Deen, J. 2002. Evaluation of the relationship between injuries and size of gestation stalls relative to size of sows. JAVMA 221: 834–836.
2. Spencer, G.R. 1979. Animal model of human disease: pregnancy and lactational osteoporosis; Animal model: Porcine lactational osteoporosis. Am J Pathol 95:277–280.
3. Marchent, J.N., and Broom, D.M. 1996. Effects of dry sow housing conditions on muscle weight and bone strength. J An Sci 62:105–113.
4. Zurbrigg, K., Animal Health Surveillance Technician, Ontario Ministry of Agriculture and Food. Personal Communication. November, 2002.
5. Connor, M.L. 1993. Recommended code of practice for the care and handling of farm animals. Pigs. Agriculture and Agri-food Canada publication 1898/E; 13.
6. Gonyou, H.W. 2001. Pig welfare and large systems. Proceedings Western Canadian Association of Swine Practitioners Conference; 82–89.
7. Ebner, J. 1993. Group-housing of lactating sows. Studies on health, behaviour and nest temperature. Thesis. Swedish Univ. Agr. Sci. Dept. of Anim. Hyg. Report 31.
8. Halverson, M. 1997. Swedish deep-bedded group nursing systems for feeder pig production. Department of Sustainable Agriculture. Swine System Options for Iowa. Iowa State University, Ames; 6.
9. Britt, J.H., Almond, G.W., and Flowers, W.L. 1999 Diseases of the reproductive system. In Diseases of swine, 8th ed., eds. Straw, B.E., et al. Iowa State University Press, Ames; 893.
10. D'Allaire, S., and Drolet, R. 1999 Culling and mortality in breeding animals. In Diseases of swine, 8th ed. Iowa State University Press, Ames; 1008.
11. D'Allaire, S., Drolet, R., and Brodeur, D. 1996 Sow mortality associated with high ambient temperatures. Can Vet J 37:237–239.
12. D'Allaire, S., Drolet, R., and Chagnon, M. 1991.The causes of sow mortality: a retrospective study. Can Vet J 32: 241–243.
13. Spicer, E.M., Driesen, S.J., and Fahy, V.A. 1986. Causes of preweaning mortality on a large intensive piggery. Aust Vet J 63: 71–75.
14. Anon. 1997. On farm euthanasia of swine. Am Assoc Swine Pract. and National Pork Producers Council. Bulletin # 04249–4/97.
15. Straw, B.E. 1997. Veterinary practice: art, science, and politics. In: Proc Am Assoc Swine Pract. Quebec; 1–31.
16. Svenmark, B., Nielsen, K., Willeberg, P., and Jorsal, S.E. 1989. Epidemiological studies of piglet diarrhoea in intensively managed Danish sow herds. Acta Vet Scand 30:55–62.

17. Edwards, S.A., and Armsby, A.W., Spechter, H.H. 1988. Effects of floor area allowance on performance of growing pigs kept on fully slatted floors. Anim Prod 46:453–459.

18. Klopfenstein, C., Farmer, C., and Martineau, G.P. 1999. Diseases of the mammary glands and lactation problems. In: Diseases of swine, 8th ed., eds. Straw, B.E., et al., Iowa State University Press, Ames; 841.

19. Koomans, P. 1981. Open front piggeries with and without straw. In: The welfare of pigs; Current topics in veterinary medicine and animal science, ed. Sybesma, W. Martin Nijhoff Publishers; 11:171–177.

20. Van Putten, G. 1969. An investigation of tail-biting among fattening pigs. Br Vet J 125:511–517.

21. Anon. 1998. Tri-state swine nutrition guide. Bulletin 869–98. The Ohio State University.

22. Grandin, T. 1996. Factors that impede animal movement at slaughter plants. J Am Vet Med Assoc 209:757–759.

23. Lidster, N. DNL Farms Consulting. White Fox, Saskatchewan, Canada. Personal Communication. June, 2002.

24. Lawrence, B.V., et al. 1998. Changes in pars esophageal tissue appearance of the porcine stomach in response to transportation, feed deprivation, and diet composition. J Anim Sci 76:788–795.

25. Eisemann, J.H., et al. 2002. Effect of feed withdrawal prior to slaughter on prevalence of gastric ulcers in pigs. J Am Vet Med Assoc 220:503–506.

26. Kent, J.E., Malony, V., and Graham, M.J. 2001. The effect of different bloodless castrators and different tail docking methods on the responses of lambs to the combined burdizzo rubber ring method of castration. The Veterinary Journal 162:250–254.

27. English, P.R., and Edwards, S.A. 1999. Animal welfare. In: Diseases of swine, 8th ed., eds. Straw, B.E., et al., Iowa State University Press, Ames; 1008, 1067–1076.

13

Maximizing Well-Being and Minimizing Pain and Suffering: Sheep

Cleon V. Kimberling and Gerilyn A. Parsons

The tacit compact mutually binding betwixt man and the animals he domesti-
cates implies a duty connected with an interest to both parties. Man fur-
nishes to them food and protection, and enables them to pass a few years of
comfortable existence; they repay him with their lives or their services.
—John Bradbury, *Travels in the Interior of America*

The shepherd traveled along with the sheep across the western United States. During this time, the shepherd provided protection from predators, and searched for better grazing and water sources for the flock's overall health and well-being (fig. 13.1). During this time, there was often conflict between sheep owners and cattle owners over grazing rights. This increased the stress level of the sheep even over the natural environmental stresses (e.g., predators, drought).

Sheep have played a vital role in the settlement of America from the pilgrims to the settlement of the western United States. As noted in *American Sheep Trails* by E. N. Wentworth,

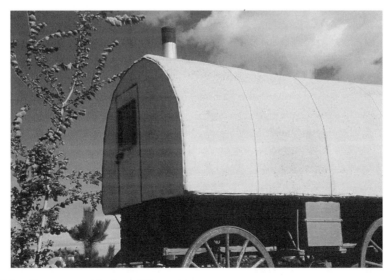

Figure 13.1.   Sheep camp at the turn of the century.

271

> Trails of the shepherd, searching fresh grasses for his flock, led to every corner of the most remote canyon and precipice. No hunter, explorer, or scientist has penetrated the obscure parts of our western mountains and forests with the frequency, thoroughness, or methodical regularity that has characterized the sheepherder. Flock master and flocks alike have participated in, or created, the long series of situations that have welded us into the nation of today.

The domestication of sheep has played the most vital role in the advancement of the human race of any animal, providing humans with fleece and hide for protection from the elements, and milk, cheese, and meat for daily nourishment.

Wentworth continues:

> The trail of sheep leads out of the centuries. Its primitive traces emerge dimly from the rocks and dusts of ancient Asia. During the Old Stone Age the western tribes of that continent were following bands of wild sheep, back and forth with the seasons, adapting their own convenience to the whims and necessities of the grazing flocks. What unsung individual first demonstrated the greater ease of guiding and herding the wild sheep of that country, as compared to the long pursuits of hunter, will never be known, but his contribution to human history parallels that of man who first controlled fire. The tending of flocks forced mankind to plan for the future, and initiated property values.
>
> When Neolithic man drove back the Cro-Magnons in Western Europe, about 10,000 B.C., he brought with him domestic livestock—sheep, goats, cattle and dogs. The most ancient relics suggest that the first food animals to arrive were the flocks of sheep, and apparently they were thoroughly tamed by that date. As centuries passed, ovine hooves traveled or intersected the courses of Jason and Ulysses, Alexander and Hannibal, Leif the Lucky and Columbus. The trail of sheep marked the world's trade ways, and the course of empires followed routes first stirred by the patter of the flock.

Ancient to modern-day, history is documented with the close association of sheep and humans, and the shepherd's close attention to the health and well-being of the flock and the individual animal. Over the centuries, sheep and humans have joined in commensalisms benefiting both parties. Ancient findings in Switzerland show that sheep lived in the same quarters with the humans. In many parts of the world, the commensalisms between sheep and humans still exist with both relying on the other for a sustainable existence. During the latter half of the twentieth century, the raising of sheep in the United States has become extremely diversified. Modern-day people have capitalized on the ability of sheep to utilize roughages and terrain that other animals cannot, then shift to a completely different diet and environment for finishing.

SELECTION

If we are to expect a lifetime of healthy productivity for our flock, we must first determine what we expect from the individuals within the flock. We may have a vision in mind, but the first and utmost duty is to do a complete assessment of the resources available to carry out the vision. After assessing the nature of the environment, feed, and water resources, we must answer the question of how we best coordinate these things to optimize the health and well-being of the flock and individuals. It is best if we document our goals and parameters in writing and use them for guidelines. It is even better if we review this document on a systematic basis. There will be times when we review these goals that they may need to be revised. The environment, water and feed resources, and physical facilities will have a great influence on selection of the breed and type of animals we pick. Individual animals vary greatly within a breed, but there are breed characteristics that are very dominant. For example, the Dorset is known for its ability to breed out of season; the Rambouillet is noted for its gregariousness and hardiness; the Poly-pay for its out-of-season breeding and multiple offspring; the Warhill for its hardiness, twinning, and mothering instincts. The list goes on.

HEALTH CONSIDERATIONS

Before the productive cycle begins, we must assure that the females and males are free of diseases that will compromise health, well-being, and production.

Ovine Progressive Pneumonia

The basic flock must be free of *ovine progressive pneumonia (OPP)*. This disease is a slow, insidious disease that eventually (1) destroys the lungs (a nonfebrile pneumonia); (2) compromises the mammary gland (a condition known as hard-bag), which in turn leads to starvation of the lambs; (3) develops into a periarticular arthritis, which causes lameness and carcass condemnation; (4) may be presented as a nervous form causing incoordination. The nervous form is infrequently seen in the United States.

The disease is caused by a lentivirus. The word *lenti* means slow. It takes months to years for the disease to develop. It sometimes takes months for the immune system to seroconvert or become positive. The young lamb may become infected from the mother's colostrum, and the serum may not test positive until the animal is 8–12 months of age. Once the disease starts developing in the system, it is progressive. There is no treatment, no vaccination, or no improvement once infection has commenced. In some management systems, there is not a dramatic loss of individual production as other conditions are responsible for the ewe being eliminated prior to the signs of OPP production loss. It takes dedication and diligence to eradicate the disease once it is in the flock. When purchasing animals, *only purchase animals from an OPP-clean flock.*

If your flock has OPP, the only way of eradicating the disease is by testing and removal of the test-positive animals. This could take a number of repeated tests to remove the test-positive animals, and an annual test to assure that all carriers have been identified. If the flock is infected, the first test should be done prior to the breeding season. Remove all of the positive animals and retest prior to lambing to remove any that have seroconverted during gestation. This should be done until there are no seropositive animals. An annual test should be conducted prior to lambing to assure the flock remains OPP free.

The disease is transmitted from the mother to her offspring primarily via the colostrum and milk. *Never keep replacements from a test-positive ewe.* Often there are new testing procedures that become available. Check with your local veterinarian or your extension veterinarian to determine the most appropriate test in your situation.

Caseous Lymphadenitis

Caseous lymphadenitis (CLA) is another slow-developing disease that compromises production and is responsible for condemnation of the entire carcass or parts of the carcass. The disease is caused by the bacterium *Corynebacterium pseudotuberculosis.* The organisms establish infection in the lymph nodes developing into abscesses. The rupture and drainage of the superficial abscesses contaminate the environment and are the source of further infections. The organisms enter the body through scratches, abrasions, cuts, and punctures. There is some indication that the organism can enter through the digestive and respiratory tract. The lymph nodes at the point of the mandible just under the ear are probably infected from the organisms gaining entry through abrasions in the mouth caused by rough feeds. There are often superficial abscesses at the point of the shoulder or the stifle joint. These infections probably arise from scratches or cuts in the area of the infected lymph node. Contaminated shearing combs are often the source of transmitting the infection during the shearing operation. Internal abscesses are often seen in the mediastinal lymph nodes between the lungs and in the mesenteric lymph nodes in the abdomen. They can also be found in the kidney, liver, lungs, and mammary gland (figs. 13.2, 13.3).

Once the environment is contaminated, it is difficult to control the transmission. Thorough cleaning and disinfection is the key to control of transmission. Any ewe with obvi-

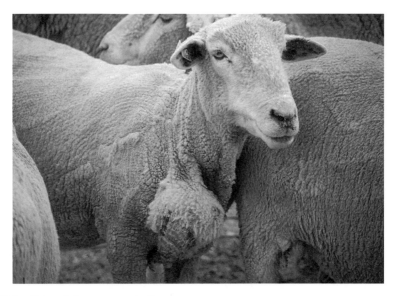

Figure 13.2.   External abscess on neck of ewe.

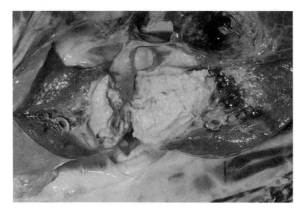

Figure 13.3.   Internal CLA abscess found in the liver of a ewe.

ous external abscesses should be removed from the flock. There is no effective treatment. The disease is not an immediate threat to the life of the animal but causes weight loss and a reduction in productivity with eventual death or condemnation of the carcass.

If the disease is diagnosed in the flock, it is best to start a vaccination program. Vaccinate all animals that are to remain as permanent breeding animals. These should be revaccinated in a month then given an annual booster vaccination. The new replacements should receive two vaccinations initially, then annual boosters thereafter. The vaccination *will not cure* an existing disease but will aid in prevention of new cases.

Contagious Ovine Footrot

Contagious ovine footrot is a devastating disease causing lameness and severe loss in production. The disease starts with a moist lesion between the claws, which eventually undermines the sole and wall of the hoof. In advanced cases, the sole and wall of the hoof may separate leaving the underlying distal part of the toe exposed. There is a very distinct, foul odor. Two organisms work in conjunction to produce the disease. *Dichelobacter nodosus* is the limiting organism. *Fusobacterium necrophorum* is in the environment of all areas where livestock are kept, and during wet conditions, sets up a favorable environment between the toes for the *D. nodosus* to invade. Without this organism, the disease will not take place.

D. nodosus lives in the necrotic tissues under the sole and wall of the hoof and contaminates the moist soil anywhere the sheep walk. This is usually around watering tanks, feed bunks, ponds, or streams where the sheep tend to congregate. Other sheep pick up the infection by walking through the contaminated ground. The ground that becomes contaminated by an infected sheep will remain infective for about 10 days to 2 weeks, after which time the organism will die. This fact is important to keep in mind when trying to eradicate the disease. Prevention is the key. Do not purchase animals from an unknown source. Purchase only animals from a reputable breeder that does not have contagious ovine footrot in his or her flock. Isolate all sheep that are brought onto the property for a minimum of one month, and observe closely for any signs of lameness or other abnormalities. There is an approved vaccine for contagious ovine footrot. There are two major drawbacks to this product. The efficacy is low, and it leaves a granuloma (or knot) at the site of injection. Treatment is time-consuming and requires extreme dedication to detail. Contact your veterinarian immediately for assistance if you suspect contagious ovine footrot in your flock (fig. 13.4).

Foot Abscesses

Foot abscesses are often confused with contagious ovine footrot (fig. 13.5). They are caused by trauma to the soft tissue around the hoof or puncture to the sole of the foot. The

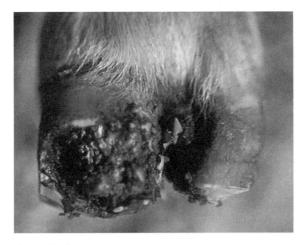

Figure 13.4.   Contagious ovine footrot.

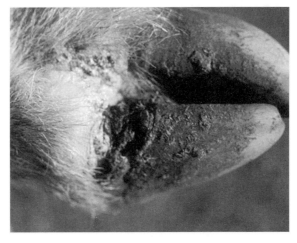

Figure 13.5.   Foot abscess.

organism is the same one that established the proper environment for the *D. nodosus* that causes contagious ovine footrot. In cases of foot abscess, there is swelling and redness of the joint just above the coronary band. This may abscess just above the coronary band and drain pus that has no odor. If left untreated, the infection will invade the joint and cause permanent lameness. The joint will become enlarged, thus the term "bumble foot." This condition can often be avoided by not grazing stubble or other rough materials that may cause damage to the soft tissues of the foot. Early treatment with tetracyclines is usually effective. The condition is not contagious and does not spread from one sheep to another. This is more a condition of the environment and management.

Mastitis

Mastitis can be a leading cause of starvation in the newborn lambs. Mastitis is an inflammation of the udder caused by bacteria. The most common organisms causing mastitis are pasteurella, streptococcus, staphylococcus, and *E. coli*. These organisms can build up in the environment during lambing and cause infection. The source of new infections is often a ewe that had mastitis the previous season and that breaks with mastitis at lambing time. The udder is inflamed (hot, red, swollen, and painful) and the milk is loaded with the causative organisms. The lamb tries to nurse, gets a mouth full of the infective milk, and is rejected by its mother because of the pain. The lamb becomes hungry and robs milk from another ewe, transferring the organisms to another susceptible mother.

Early detection, treatment, and isolation are essential to prevent transmission to other ewes. One of the early signs is lameness in the rear leg. It is common for only one-half of the gland to be affected. The ewe will appear to be lame on that side as she tries to avoid touching the affected gland with her leg when she walks. Once a ewe has been infected, there is formation of scar tissue in the gland. This replaces normal productive mammary tissue and is the source of infective microorganisms during future lactations. It is therefore best to identify ewes that have been treated for mastitis and eliminate them from the flock at the end of the season. Mastitis is best controlled by strict adherence to sanitation and removal of all previously infected ewes. Prior to the breeding season, the udder of each ewe should be thoroughly examined by palpation for any abnormalities. The ones with an abnormality should be removed from the flock.

PARASITE CONTROL

Internal Parasites

Internal parasites cause more loss of production than any other condition. These little monsters eat away at the productivity of the animal. There are three major groups of internal parasites. The most important group is the roundworms or gastrointestinal nematodes. This group affects grazing sheep in all parts of the world causing severe economic loss. The flatworms include liver flukes and tapeworms. The liver fluke has a limited distribution as it depends on a specific snail to complete its life cycle. Tapeworms have a wide distribution, some of which pose significant human health concerns. The group of coccidia causes severe diarrhea, production loss, and death in lambs. The ewes develop immunity to coccidia, but they usually remain a carrier contaminating the environment transferring the infection to the lamb. It is far beyond the scope of this chapter to go into specific details of the internal parasites.

Unless the parasite burden is extremely high, there may be no apparent signs of production inefficiency. Moderate to high levels of parasite infestation are noted by lack of performance, such as weight gain and milk production. A slight to moderate diarrhea may be one of the early indications of a parasite burden. As the burden increases, the diarrhea may intensify. In the case of *Haemonchus* infestation, commonly referred to as the "barber pole" worm because of the blood in the worm's intestinal tract, there is an anemia in the animal. This is often mistaken for pneumonia as there is a rapid respiration due to the lack of the blood's capacity to carry oxygen. In these cases, the mucous membranes will be extremely pale. There are a number of internal parasites that cause damage to the stomach and intestine of sheep (fig. 13.6).

If you own sheep, it is a given that you must have a parasite-control program. To control these parasites and assure the health and well-being of your flock, you must design a control program specifically for your flock and its environment. You must become familiar with the life cycle of the particular parasites in the flock and build a control program for those parasites. A control program is designed to reduce the buildup of parasites on the pasture during the grazing season. Older animals that have been exposed to parasites build a certain amount of immunity. If the parasite buildup on a pasture becomes extremely high, this can overwhelm the immune system causing extreme production loss and, in some cases, death of the animal.

In the case of *coccidiosis,* it is wise to reduce the level of oocyst production in the ewe with one of the coccidiostats (Amprolium or Decoquinate). Coccidia are extremely hardy in the environment making thorough cleaning of the lambing quarters necessary prior to the lambing season. Prevention of fluke infestation requires avoiding areas where the spe-

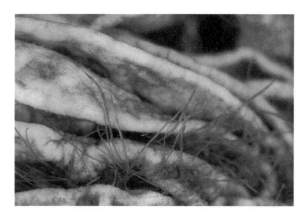

Figure 13.6.   *Haemonchus* infestation in the abomasum.

cific snail resides. This may require fencing of certain lowland areas that are inhabited by the snail. There is no treatment available for the immature form of the snail. The adult causes liver damage resulting in Blacks Disease (*Clostridium novyi*), causing death or liver condemnation at slaughter. The adult form can be treated with Albendazole or Ivermectin F. Always follow label instructions. Certain tapeworms are insignificant to the production efficiency of the ewe while others pose health and production problems. *Taenia multiceps* and *Echinococcus granulosus* are two tapeworms of sheep that are zoonotic to humans. In these cases, it is extremely important to control the parasite in the dogs and not allow dogs or wild carnivores to feed on any sheep carcass.

There is a great deal of good information on parasite control programs. *Treatment is only a part of the answer* to an effective control program, so seek the help of a professional to assist you in designing a program for your flock. Timing and rotation of pastures, even rotation with seasonal forages are an important part of the control strategy.

External Parasites

External parasites are ubiquitous. They are everywhere in multitudes causing irritation and discomfort resulting in production inefficiency. During the summer grazing season, we often see sheep huddled with their heads together and their muzzles close to the ground. The reason: they are being tormented by flying insects. This one is usually the fly that causes nose bots (*Oestrus ovis*). These flies deposit the larva onto the nasal secretions. The larva then migrates up the nasal passage to the nasal turbinates where it matures into a large bot. These bots overwinter in the nasal passage, feeding on the host and causing extreme irritation. They drop onto the ground in the warm season and mature into adult flies to complete the life cycle. Nose bots are extremely irritating. There will be a lot of clear to blood-tinged nasal secretion. If you observe an infected group of sheep, there will be a lot of sneezing due to the irritation of the bots. Diagnosis of the condition is by close observation of the sheep for excessive nasal discharge and sneezing. A normal sheep does not sneeze. Ivermectin is a very effective treatment. Ivermectin drench is approved for sheep and is the treatment of choice. Follow the label instructions.

There are a number of species of mosquitoes that torment sheep, some of which transmit disease. At one time, our knowledge was that West Nile virus (WNV) only affected horses. The WNV has the ability to mutate and change its characteristics. The strain of WNV that we have in the United States has been shown to infect ruminants causing clinical signs. Our knowledge of WNV in sheep, at this point in time, is very limited. A midge, *Culicoides veripennis*, is the insect that transmits the blue tongue virus (BTV) to sheep (figs. 13.7, 13.8). In North America, the *Culicoides* midge is the only known vector in the transmission of the blue tongue virus. The seasonal variance of blue tongue (BT) relates to availability of the vector. In America and other parts of the temperate zone, the disease occurs during late summer and early fall. During summers of high rainfall, the disease appears early in the season. *Culicoides* breed in many habitats, particularly damp, muddy areas, running streams, and fecal matter. Because of nocturnal feeding habits, the *Culicoides* attack the host sheep on night pastures or open pens. The female *Culicoides* feeds

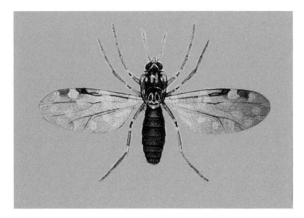

Figure 13.7. *Culicoides veripennis.*

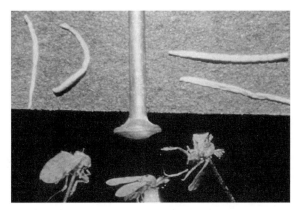

Figure 13.8. *Culicoides veripennis* actual size (directly below pin) compared to a straight pin and grass blades.

on a sheep or cow that has the blue tongue virus in its blood. The virus replicates in the *Culicoides,* and in 7–10 days is in the salivary gland of the *Culicoides* available to infect the next animal on which the *Culicoides* feeds. These midge females take a blood meal every 3 to 4 days during their life, which can be up to 70 days. The disease is character- ized by a high fever and damage to the capillaries, small blood vessels, in the mouth and coronary band area. The damage causes blood to spill into the tissues resulting in a bluish coloration, thus the term *blue tongue.* The coronary band above the hoof will become in- flamed causing lameness. As the disease progresses, the lesions in the mouth become raw, open sores making eating extremely difficult (fig. 13.9).

In some cases, the lips, muzzle, and ears will become edematous from the leakage of serum from the damaged blood vessels. The disease can be economically devastating due to interruption of breeding, periods of infertility, lack of conception, and fetal death or ab-

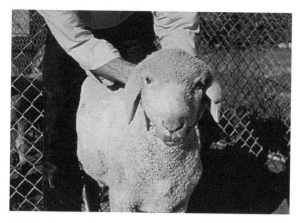

Figure 13.9.   Ewe with blue tongue; note swollen ears and muzzle.

normalities. Prevention is difficult, as the only licensed vaccine is for strain 10. There are at least five strains of BTV in the United States. Each strain is antigenically separate meaning that the vaccine will only protect for one, strain 10. The *Culicoides* is a night feeder and prefers open areas. It is therefore beneficial to house sheep at night to prevent the *Culicoides* from feeding and transmitting the BT virus. Treatment is directed toward supportive therapy and tender loving care.

Fly strike is another complicating factor of a heavy burden of internal parasites. The diarrhea produced by the internal parasites causes soiling of the wool in the perianal area. This is a perfect environment for the fly to lay eggs. Injuries that break the hide resulting in bleeding or serum exudates are also excellent places for fly strike. The eggs hatch in a matter of hours and the larvae feed on the tissue under the wool. If untreated, the maggots spread quickly causing severe irritation and damage to the skin, eventually leading to death of the animal. Prevention is by keeping the perianal area free from fluid fecal material, and treating all injuries with a fly repellent. In treating cases, the wool must be removed to expose the infested area before treating with an approved insecticide.

The *sheep ked (Melophagus ovinus)* is a wingless fly that spends its entire life cycle on the sheep (fig. 13.10). It feeds on the surface of the skin, unlike a tick that engorges on blood, producing severe irritation. Sheep will rub on fences or any object to relieve this irritation. This results in wool damage from broken fibers and loss of wool. The feeding also produces a lesion on the skin causing serum exudates. This mats the wool with serum. The condition is known as cockle. The damage to the hide and wool reduces and oftentimes causes complete loss of value. A heavy ewe may roll onto her back to scratch and relieve the irritation. If the ewe is unable to right herself, she will die in a few hours. If you find a ewe on her back, a reason may be irritation from sheep keds.

If the infestation is light, there may be no indication of the problem. Shearing time is the optimal time to examine all animals for the presence of keds. This is also the optimal time for control. If keds are found on only one individual, all of the flock *must* be treated

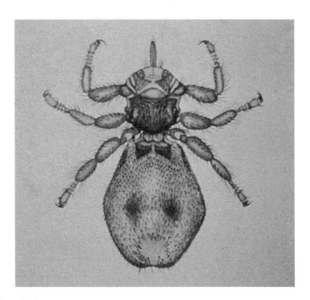

Figure 13.10.   Sheep ked.

including the lambs. Ectrin and X-par are two synthetic pyrethrums that are approved for this use. These are available in pour-on form and are most effective when applied at shearing. Ectrin is mixed with water and applied topically down the back of the animal. It is sometimes difficult to determine if an animal has been missed. Producers often mix common food coloring in the solution making is easier to see which animals have been treated. Follow label instructions for mixing, dosage, and application. Sheep keds are not known to play a role in the transmission of disease.

Ticks are obligate ectoparasites of most types of mammals and birds, wherever these animals are found (fig. 13.11). There are over 850 species of ticks. They have a life cycle that may involve a number of stages on different host animals. Each stage feeds on a particular host, drops off, and molts, maturing to the next stage where it will feed on another host. The mature tick feeds, drops to the ground, and lays its eggs to start the cycle again. There are some one-host ticks that feed only on one specific host to complete their life cycle, while others have as many as three hosts. They are exclusively bloodsucking in all feeding stages. Ticks transmit a great variety of infectious agents plus cause allergic reactions, and they can cause paralysis from the toxins in the saliva.

The tick species and various habitats make tick control extremely difficult. If ticks are a problem, it will be necessary to identify the tick and seek professional help to develop a control program. The main reasons for tick control are to protect the sheep from irritation and production losses, formation of lesions that can become secondarily infected, damage to hides and udders, toxicosis, paralysis, and infection with disease agents.

Mites in sheep are commonly referred to as mange, which causes severe irritation and therefore loss of production (figs. 13.12, 13.13). There are five types.

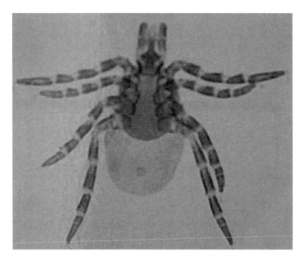

Figure 13.11.   Deer tick.

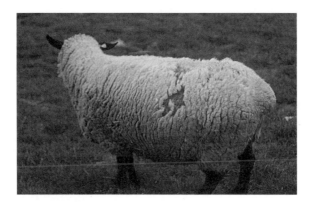

Figure 13.12.   Loss of wool due to mange.

1. *Sarcoptic mange* is rare in sheep and is reportable to the state and federal veterinarian in the United States. It affects the nonwool skin, usually starting on the head and face.

2. *Chorioptic mange* is common in Europe, New Zealand, and Australia during the winter. It has been eradicated in the United States and is reportable to the state and federal veterinarian.

3. *Psoroptic mange (sheep scab)* is reportable to the state and federal veterinarian but no cases have been reported in the United States since 1970. Sheep scab is characterized by large, scaly, crusted lesions, which develop on the wooly parts of the body. It causes intense itching manifested by biting and scratching. Left untreated, sheep often become emaciated and anemic. Ivermectin given twice at seven-day intervals is the treatment of choice.

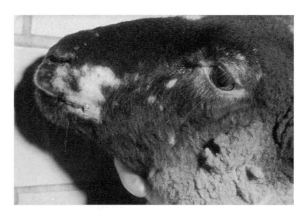

Figure 13.13.   Loss of wool due to mange.

4. *Demodectic mange* has been reported in sheep with lesions similar to those in cattle. It is characterized by follicular papules and nodules. There is no itching but the condition results in hide damage.

5. *Psorergatic mange (itch mite, Australian itch)* is a common skin mite of sheep in many parts of the world. It has been eradicated from the United States. It is a reportable condition. The disease is characterized by intense generalized itching and scaliness, with matting and loss of wool.

Sheep may become infested with the sheep biting louse and three sucking lice: the sheep foot louse, the face and body louse, and the African blue louse.

For the health and well-being of the animal and the future productivity of the flock, make certain that the existing flock and the replacement individuals are free of the above conditions.

NUTRITIONAL MANAGEMENT

Nutritional management is a key factor in the health and well-being of the individual animal and the entire flock. We depend on our power of observation to determine the health and degree of well-being of the individuals within our flock. Sheep are extremely hardy and stoic individuals. It takes a keen observer to note the subtle changes in attitude.

We depend heavily on body condition as the monitor of our nutritional management program. It is impossible to tell the body condition of a sheep with wool without feeling for the covering over the body. This is determined by palpating the dorsal and lateral spinous processes of the lumbar vertebrae and covering over the ribs. Body condition scores run from 1 to 5. We do not want our animals on either end of the spectrum. A moderate condition of 3 is ideal for the animal. If we have animals that are too fat or too thin, we need to adjust our nutritional program accordingly. In the case of the thin animal, we must determine if the cause is nutritionally or physically related or a specific ailment. An excellent reference for nutritional guidelines can be found in the *Sheep Production Hand-*

book published by the American Sheep Industries. This is also an excellent reference manual for all phases of sheep production including health and parasite programs.

Nutrition is composed of five basic elements: energy, protein, vitamins, minerals, and water. Each of these plays an important role in the health and well-being of the animal.

Energy

There are two types of energy requirements. *Energy for maintenance* is necessary for maintaining respiration, circulation, digestion, and other metabolic functions. *Energy for production* is necessary for work, growth, reproduction, and lactation. Energy is derived from carbohydrates, fats, and excess protein. Energy sources for sheep come from forages, grains, and a multitude of plants. Many species of plants are high in protein and fats, both of which can add to the energy source. Sheep are extremely versatile in utilizing a wide variety of plants as an energy source. Sheep are great biological agents for weed control. Most plants in the growth phase make good quality forages. The quality of plants decreases as they mature. The quality of harvested forages depends on the stage of maturity of the plant, the weather conditions during drying, and the storage from harvest to feeding. The health and well-being of the animal depend on the quality of the feed.

Protein

Protein is essential for sustaining a healthy microbial environment in the rumen for the digestion of low-protein feeds. Without adequate protein, digestion becomes reduced and the animal's condition deteriorates. Basically, protein is essential for growth, reproduction, milk production, and a healthy immune system. Adequate protein is essential for optimal wool production.

Vitamins

Vitamins play an important role in the health of any animal. All sheep require dietary vitamins A, D, and E. These vitamins are contained in the normal feed sources.

> *Vitamin A.* Plants do not contain vitamin A as such but contain beta-carotene, which the sheep convert into vitamin A. Any of the green leafy forages are an excellent source of beta-carotenes. Except for yellow corn, all grains and concentrates are a poor source of beta-carotene. As grasses mature and dry, they lose the beta-carotene. If the sheep graze good green forage or are fed good green hay, the liver will store vitamin A for a period of time. The storage time in the liver is dependent upon a number of stress factors. For example, transportation stress and the stress of severe winter storms and feed source will deplete the liver stores of vitamin A rapidly. Vitamin A is essential for the development of healthy tissues in the body. Deficiency of vitamin A may be exhibited in growth retardation, retained placenta, bone malformation, reproductive failure, and night blindness.

The newborn lamb is void of vitamin A. It is therefore necessary that it receive vitamin A via colostrum. Vitamin A is essential for the healthy development of the lining of the respiratory and alimentary tracts of the newborn lamb. It is essential that the ewe have an adequate supply of vitamin A during gestation. The vitamin A is transferred to colostrum during the last stage of gestation.

Vitamin D plays an essential role, along with calcium and phosphorus, in the development and maintenance of a healthy skeletal system. Sun-cured hays are an excellent source of vitamin D, whereas grains and dehydrated hays are poor sources. In most parts of the country, sheep exposed to sunlight generally obtain adequate amounts of vitamin D through ultraviolet irradiation. In confinement operations, vitamin D must be supplemented, especially for fast-growing lambs. The newborn must rely on colostrum for vitamin D.

Vitamin E along with selenium plays an essential role in the maintenance of healthy muscle tissue. A deficiency of vitamin E will be manifested in the lamb as white muscle disease. This condition is characterized by stiffness in the rear legs, tucked-up rear flanks, and an arched back. Severe cases will die of pneumonia, starvation, or heart failure. Necropsy will reveal white streaks in the long muscles of the rear limbs and white striations of the heart muscles. Vitamin E deficiency has been associated with an increase incidence of vaginal prolapse. High-quality legume hay, dehydrated alfalfa, and wheat germ are excellent sources of vitamin E. In some parts of the country, soils are inadequate in selenium. In these areas, both vitamin E and selenium must be supplemented to the ewe and the lamb. A supplement of vitamins A, D, and E is a good management practice.

B vitamins are normally synthesized by the microflora in the rumen. Some high-concentrate rations and those with high sulfur content may destroy thiamine causing a syndrome known as polioencephalomalacia (star gazing). Injection of thiamine is necessary. In conditions where the microflora of the rumen has been compromised from being off feed, injection of B vitamins will often stimulate the appetite.

Minerals

Minerals are an important part of the healthy body. Feed sources contribute most of the minerals required for normal body functions. Some feeds are low in certain minerals and high in others. It is necessary to do feed analysis and meet the needs of the animal by mineral supplementation.

Salt plays an important role in feed intake. A lack of salt reduces feed consumption, ultimately affecting production.

Calcium is the most abundant mineral element in the body, functioning as the structural component of bones and teeth. Calcium is involved in blood clotting, membrane permeability, muscle contraction, transmission of nerve impulses, heart regulation, and secretion of certain hormones, and has a role in certain enzymes. Most roughages are good sources of calcium. Cereal hays and their residues and silage are relatively low in calcium. Legumes are excellent sources of calcium although most grass hay has adequate amounts. Calcium and phosphorus are interrelated in forming and maintaining the skeleton.

Phosphorus is essential for proper bone and teeth development and plays a major role in the optimal performance of the animal, including growth, reproduction, efficiency of feed conversion, appetite, and milk production. Roughages are often low in phosphorus. Many soils are deficient in phosphorus, which is reflected in low levels in plants. Phosphorus levels decline as the plant matures. Most grains are an excellent source of phosphorus. Supplementation of phosphorus can be made with steamed bone meal, mono- and dicalcium phosphate, and defluorinated rock phosphate. High grain rations often lead to a calcium/phosphorus imbalance resulting in urolithiasis in rams and male castrates (wethers). Animals on high-concentrate (grain) rations may require calcium supplementation. Ground limestone is a cheap and excellent supplement. Rations should have a 2:1 calcium/phosphorus ratio.

Magnesium maintains electrical charges across nerve endings. The typical magnesium deficiency is usually seen in the spring when new grass is at its maximum growth and we have the condition known as "grass tetany." This most often occurs in lactating females grazing fast-growing grasses or cereal grains used for pasture in the spring. The condition is characterized by tetany and nervousness, followed by paralysis and death within a few hours. Magnesium is essential in the metabolism of calcium. In certain areas of the country, it may be necessary to supplement with magnesium oxide in the mineral mix. This may only be necessary during the early spring grazing season.

Potassium controls the intracellular fluid and is important in acid-base balance. It is involved in regulation of osmotic pressure, water balance, muscle contractions, nerve impulse transmission, and several enzymatic reactions. It is also essential for energy utilization. Most forages are good sources of potassium, so deficiencies are usually not a problem.

Sulfur functions in the synthesis of amino acids essential in wool growth. Sulfur deficiency results in loss of appetite, reduced weight gain, weight loss, and reduced wool growth. Excessive salivation, lacrimation, and wool shedding may occur. Excess sulfur interferes with copper and molybdenum utilization. It can also reduce selenium retention.

Copper is a critical element in many of the enzyme pathways that regulate the hormones of reproduction, development of the nervous and immune systems, building of healthy skin and hoof growth, and many other functions. Neonatal ataxia, commonly known as "swayback," is a characteristic symptom of copper deficiency in young lambs. Imbalances of copper are often manifested in an acute hemolytic crisis known as "copper toxicity." There is a narrow margin between copper deficiency and toxicity in sheep. Supplements formulated for cattle and swine will often result in toxicity in sheep. This is dependent on the area of the country and the amounts of molybdenum, sulfates, and iron present in the forages and water that interfere with copper metabolism. It is critically important that you know the levels of copper and molybdenum in the forages and feeds in your area.

Iron is the key component in hemoglobin, which maintains oxygen transport throughout the body. Supplementation of iron is rarely necessary, although heavy gastrointestinal parasite infestation (haemonchosis) and loss of blood may result in a secondary iron deficiency anemia.

Iodine is responsible for many metabolic functions. A deficiency manifests itself as goiter in the adult and as woollessness in the lambs. Iodine deficiency in the pregnant ewe may result in stillborn lambs. Many of the inland soils are deficient in iodine requiring the addition of iodine to the salt.

Selenium is an essential component necessary for healthy functioning heart and skeletal muscles. Selenium and vitamin E combine to control nutritional muscular dystrophy (white muscle disease). Many areas of the country are low in selenium requiring supplementation either by injection or through the mineral mixture.

Zinc's primary function appears to be maintenance of normal reproductive activity. Zinc deficiency has been reported to hinder testicular development and cause defective spermatogenesis. In the ewe, zinc deficiency can adversely affect the reproductive process from estrus to parturition and through lactation. It can reduce conception rates and cause high rates of abortions and stillbirths.

Molybdenum is a complex mineral interacting with copper and sulfur in regulating many body functions. The copper-molybdenum ratio is critical in prevention of copper deficiency and toxicity. The normal range is 8:1 to 10:1.

Cobalt functions in the rumen in the synthesis of vitamin B_{12}. Deficiency of cobalt is characterized by a lack of appetite, unthriftiness, emaciation, weakness, anemia, decreased estrous activity, and decreased milk and wool production. The recommended prevention of cobalt deficiency is to supply 1.1 grams of cobalt sulfate or cobalt chloride per 100 pounds of salt. This can be supplied in the trace mineral supplement.

Water

Water is necessary for the regulation of body temperature, for growth, reproduction, lactation, digestion, metabolism, excretion, hydrolysis of nutrients, transportation of nutrients and waste in the body, plus many other functions. Restriction of water intake results in reduced performance and ultimately the health of the animal. It is necessary to provide an ample source of fresh clean water at all times.

Many range operations depend on snow as a source of water. This is a good source that may be the only form of water available. Keep in mind that it takes additional energy to melt the snow, and the moisture content is extremely variable. An ample supply of fresh, clean water and ample feed during lactation will optimize milk production. When possible, water temperature should be between 45 and 55 degrees Fahrenheit for optimal intake.

BREEDING PROGRAM

A well-planned breeding program is essential in saving lives and minimizing stress on the sheep and the shepherd. The gestation period in the ewe ranges from approximately 142 to 148 days. Some may extend a couple of days longer. The start of the breeding period depends on your plans for the future of the offspring. Therefore, plan backwards so the lambs will reach their desired maturity at the optimal time.

Depending on the operation, there are many factors that play a role in when lambing season should start and end. Environmental factors, facilities, availability of labor, and feed supply are a few of the considerations. After you have determined when you want the first newborn to arrive, you back up 150 days to determine when to start the breeding period. Getting things in place for the breeding period will start another 60 days prior to turning in the ram(s). Selection of the ram(s) is extremely important as the male contributes approximately 80 percent of the potential genetic improvement in a flock. In the ram, the 60-day period prior to breeding is very important. It takes approximately 60 days for the completion of sperm development and maturation. Any stress such as transportation, hot and humid weather, infections, and high internal body temperature will compromise semen quality. If the semen quality is compromised for any reason, it will take approximately 60 days to recover. Therefore, avoid stressing your ram(s) during this period and give attention to proper nutrition to maintain a body condition score of 3 (fig. 13.14).

It is advisable to have a breeding soundness examination (including a *Brucella ovis* test) conducted on rams to determine their potential fertility and capacity. Scrotal circumference is extremely important when selecting a breeding ram. Rams with a large scrotal circumference have a greater serving capacity, produce more twins, and influence earlier puberty of the female offspring. A ram with a large scrotal circumference and excellent semen quality can service one hundred or more ewes in a 17-day breeding period. The estrus cycle of the ewe is approximately 17 days. For the sanity of the shepherd and the well-being of the flock, a 34-day breeding program is optimal. Lambing periods that extend beyond 34 days tend to exhaust the personnel resulting in neglect to the ewe and newborn.

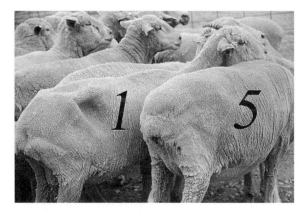

Figure 13.14.   Body condition scores of 1 and 5.

During this same time period, each ewe should be physically examined to determine if she is a qualified candidate to be in the breeding flock. This hands-on physical should include an examination of general condition (freedom from obvious disease), teeth, feet, and udder; and it should determine a body condition score (fig. 13.15).

Any defect should disqualify the ewe as a potential breeder. The ideal body condition score approaching the breeding season should be 2 or 3. About two weeks prior to breeding, the ewes should be placed on an improved ration or better pasture in order to improve the body condition. This is known as flushing. This will result in an increased number of offspring. Vaccinations at this time may include *Campylobacter* and *Chlamydia* for prevention of abortions. Check with your local veterinarian for specific needs of your area.

To shorten the lambing season, one can use the technique of placing a teaser ram with the ewes approximately ten days prior to introducing the fertile ram(s). This tends to group the estrous cycles of the ewes. For this technique to function properly the ram(s) must be out of sight, sound, and smell of the ewes for at least one month.

If the flock size permits, identify each ewe with a unique individual number, place a colored marking harness on the ram(s), and record the date of breeding. At day 18, change the color of the marker and record the dates of any second breedings. This information is extremely valuable at lambing time.

To prevent injuries and deaths, never place ram lambs and older rams in the same breeding groups. It is best to use ram lambs on the older experienced ewes and the older rams with the first-time breeders.

During the gestation period, nutrition should never be compromised. One should follow the nutritional program outlined in the nutrition section of the *Sheep Production Handbook*. It is essential that you check body condition scores on a set periodic basis by palpating a representative sample of the group. Nutrition is critical during the last third of

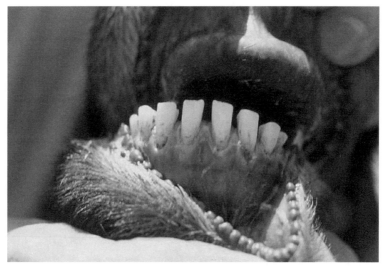

Figure 13.15.   Teeth of a seven-year-old ewe.

gestation, as 70 percent of the fetal growth takes place during this period. This is especially critical for ewes with twins or triplets. This increased nutritional demand continues through lactation. It is a good management practice to examine the ewes using ultrasound to determine the number of fetuses. This is best done between 45 and 70 days of pregnancy. The ewes with twins and triplets should be separated and given a higher concentrate ration to accommodate the increased demands for fetal development. Compromising nutrition may result in absorption of one or both fetuses or lambing paralysis if the lambs are carried to term.

Prior to lambing, a plan should be developed to handle every possible scenario. The lambing area should be prepared well in advance. Equipment, medications, and instruments should all be organized and stocked in a proper place, cabinet, or refrigerator. Approximately four weeks prior to lambing, the ewes should be given a booster of *Clostridium perfringens* types C and D bacterin/toxoid or an eight-way vaccine that contains *C. perfingens* types C and D plus five other strains of clostridia and tetanus. If *E. coli* scours have been a problem, this vaccination should also be administered at this time. This is an excellent time to shear and to control external parasites. The use of a dewormer prior to lambing is also recommended. In many areas, coccidia is a problem. Coccidiostats can be used to lower environmental contamination and potential exposure to the lambs.

MANAGEMENT

Now that we have discussed selection and nutrition of the flock, we will follow a lamb born in the United States today along some of the diverse trails it may take, and note the risks and perils it faces along the way.

Delivery

Coming into this world has its risks of survival during the delivery process. Close attention by the shepherd to the delivery process will save many lives. Closely observing the ewes every 30 minutes is recommended. During the lamb's birth, there are three stages of parturition. If at any time during this process you have a question, don't hesitate to contact your local veterinarian or an experienced shepherd for help. It is very important for the ewe and lamb's health and outcome that everything go well now.

Stage one of the birthing process can last 30 minutes to 2 hours. You will notice the ewe becoming restless, looking for a place to deliver her lamb(s). She will often lie down, then get up and move to another area. Do not let this stage go beyond 2 hours before examining to determine if there is a problem.

In stage two, the ewe will lie down and start abdominal contractions (figs. 13.16, 13.17). If the fetus in not presented and delivered in about 30 minutes, assistance should be given. When giving assistance, restrain the ewe on her left side. It is much more comfortable for her and easier on yourself. You should have a supply of lubricant handy for use if necessary. As with any species of animal, an obstetrical examination must be done very gently to determine why the offspring cannot quite make it to the outside world naturally.

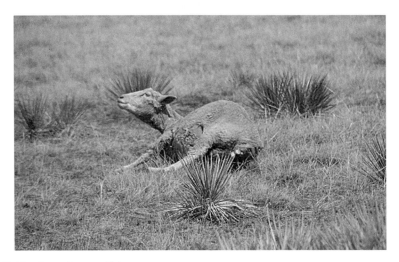

Figure 13.16.   Second stage of labor.

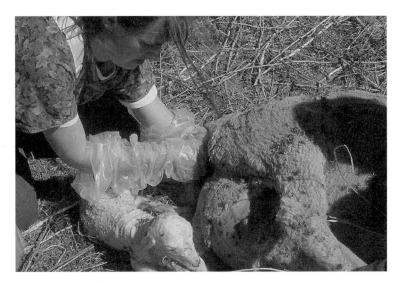

Figure 13.17.   Providing assistance.

Plastic obstetrical sleeves and cleanliness are important for all involved during this time. Many dystocia problems are easily corrected, and delivery is then successful when observed early. Sheep are capable of giving birth to more than one offspring during one gestation period, so there should always be a check for more lambs by balloting or bumping the lower abdominal wall of the ewe to "bump" another lamb.

The third stage of labor consists of the ewe passing the placenta and membranes. This should occur anywhere from ten minutes to five hours after the lambs are born.

After Delivery

What are the chances that the ewe will accept and take care of her offspring? Now that the lamb has made it into the world, its body has a lot of adjusting to do. Arriving from a 102°F environment into a 50°, 60°, or 70°F world, the lamb will shiver and look uncomfortable, wet, and icky. At this point, please don't interfere. Let the ewe take care of cleaning and drying her own offspring. From a distance, observe how the ewe reacts to her offspring. Does she go to it and begin licking and cleaning it? Does the lamb shiver and shake itself from the stimulation by mom? The shivering is normal and shows us the tiny body is working at regulating its own temperature for the first time. Healthy lambs should try shaking their heads, trying to clear their nasal passages. At this point, they should also be able to hold themselves upright while lying down. They will also begin attempts at standing and seeking a spigot at which to fill their stomach with mother's warm colostrum. The mother's attentiveness and care of her newborn during this time is of utmost importance. The ewe licking her lamb will provide stimulation to help the lamb's breathing and circulation. Licking also removes the amniotic sac and membranes, and helps to clean and dry the lamb. Mom and baby need this time and some space for bonding (fig. 13.18).

The first time a young ewe (lamb or yearling) gives birth, she may be uncertain of what has happened and will not know what to do. She possibly will start to wander off to graze, look bewildered at that thing on the ground, and leave. A common mistake among humans is to rush in and swoop up the young to make sure its needs are met. However, most of these ewes will very quickly come back as their natural instincts kick in. With these lambs,

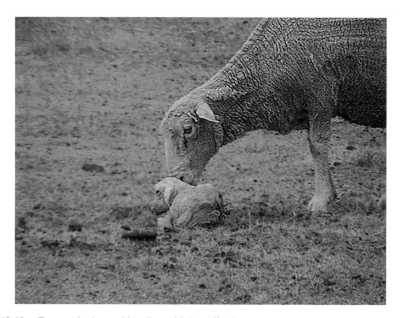

Figure 13.18.   Ewe mothering and bonding with her offspring.

if you are sure the lamb is breathing, shows movement, and tries to get up, keep your distance giving mom a chance to come back. You are one of many stresses to the mother at this time.

If the lamb is a twin, what are the chances that the mother will accept one or both and have the milking capacity to assure survival? It is good management to check the ewe's udder for sufficient milk by stripping out a squirt of colostrum and palpating the udder to determine if any abnormalities exist. If the lamb has not nursed in 30 to 45 minutes, give assistance. To provide this assistance with minimal stress, lay the ewe on her side. Next lay the lamb on its side putting a teat in its mouth and encouraging it to nurse. If this method fails, milk the ewe and feed the lamb via a stomach tube. The lamb must have four to six ounces of colostrum within the first two hours after birth (fig. 13.19).

Throughout the many breeds of sheep, there is a wide range of natural mothering instincts. Some of the breeds have been developed and adapted through time for somewhat specific environments. The Warhill breed, for example, was developed in the state of Wyoming for the sparse range vegetation with low grazing capabilities, for good mothering instincts, and also for the harsh winter weather that often occurs. Some of the breeds are specifically bred for meat production, and because of their body structure, they do not do well out in those same conditions. Depending on your ewe's natural mothering instincts, you will make some of your decisions about where to "lamb out" your herd or flock.

The musts of a proper environment are that it be clean, dry, and well ventilated with adequate space for the number of sheep you have.

If you are using lambing jugs, you need to have ample space so that mom will not step or lie on her young injuring it (fig. 13.20). The environment needs to be kept dry by removing any fetal membranes as quickly as possible after they are expelled. Feed and water the ewes up off the ground. This will prevent the feeds and water from being contaminated with feces and membranes as well as add to the safety of the lambs by preventing unnecessary drowning. If lambs are born in an environment that is cold, damp, drafty, and con-

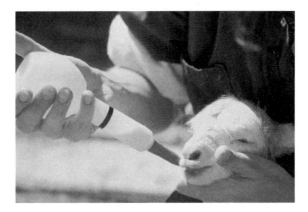

Figure 13.19.   Feeding supplemental colostrum to a newborn.

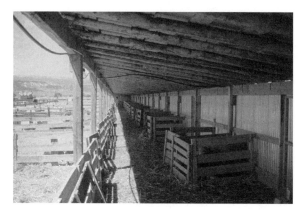

Figure 13.20.   Lambing jugs.

taminated, will they be able to survive the attacks of pneumonia, diarrhea, enterotoxemia, *E. coli,* and viruses? If lambs are born out in the open under a brilliant sky where the sunshine disinfects the birthplace, will the predators eat them alive before their guardian shepherd can protect them (figs. 13.21, 13.22)?

Humans are responsible for minimizing the risks of all these scenarios. Humans are responsible for planning and executing a program and providing an environment to assure the health and safety of the newborn irrespective of the nature of the operation. A written plan for the entire operation will help prevent disasters. Write up a plan for all phases of production, and review this with your veterinarian and sheep extension specialist periodically.

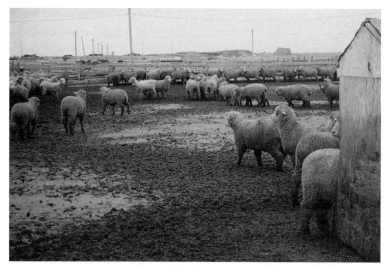

Figure 13.21.   Poor environmental conditions.

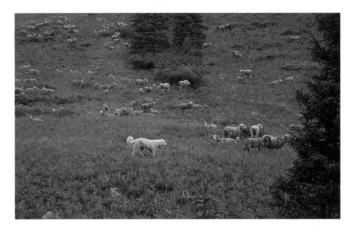

Figure 13.22.   Guard dog at work.

Tail Docking

Now that the lamb has entered this world, has a good mom that feeds it well and looks after it, and a good shepherd that provides it with a good clean environment and protects it from predators, what are its next perils? The next painful encounter will be the amputation of its tail.

Amputation of the tail is done for sanitary reasons and, in some areas of the country, it will help in preventing fly strike and maggots from invading the flesh around a soiled behind. There are many methods for amputation of a lamb's tail. The length at which the tail should be docked has been a controversial subject for many years. The minimum length recommended should be no shorter than at the end of the caudal tail fold (figs. 13.23, 13.24). If docked shorter, it will predispose the lamb to rectal prolapse (fig. 13.25).

Where you live and the season of the year may have a major impact upon the method used. Please research these methods and discuss a best-management practice with your

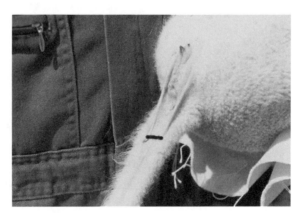

Figure 13.23.   Black line on tail shows minimum length the tail should be docked.

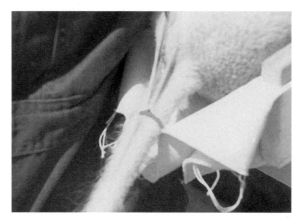

Figure 13.24.   Amputation of tail with elastrator band at 12–24 hours after birth.

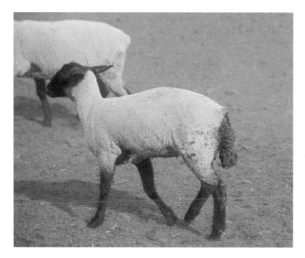

Figure 13.25.   Rectal prolapse.

veterinarian. Regardless of the method, this surgery needs to be done in the first 48 hours of life before the pain receptors awaken. The use of a local anesthetic is not particularly useful this early, as the administration of the anesthetic agent is as stressful to the lamb as the procedure alone. Docking of tails should only be delayed due to inclement weather, illness, environmental sanitation, and nutritional stress. If this surgery is delayed beyond eight weeks of age, the use of a local anesthetic is recommended.

Immunization

Which lambs will become members of the flock that continues the bloodlines of their ancestors and which will be destined for the food chain? In either case, the lambs will need proper immunizations. To keep the handling to a minimum level, carry out as many procedures at one time as possible. The docking of the tail, castration, all immunizations, and marking of each individual healthy lamb are easily done with little stress to the lamb within the first two days of life. When removing a lamb from a jug or small pen, to reduce stress to both mom and baby, a useful tool to use is a modified pitchfork (fig. 13.26).

Using the pitchfork, you scoop and lift the lamb out of the pen. This allows for distance between the ewe and yourself, preventing the ewe and lamb from becoming overly anxious. The number and type of immunizations given are quite variable from producer to producer and region to region. The route of administration for each immunization may also vary (fig. 13.27). Read and follow the labeled directions. Never vaccinate when the animal is wet. Vaccinating wet animals often leads to abscessation. The most commonly used vaccine in sheep is *Clostridium perfringens* types C and D. It is manufactured as a stand alone product or with other Clostridia and/or with Tetanus. To minimize the number of injections, it is preferred to give the combined product. The preferred route of administration

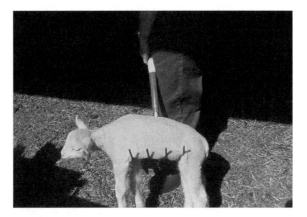

Figure 13.26.   Use of modified pitchfork when handling a newborn lamb.

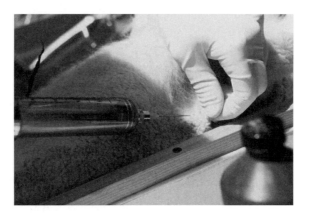

Figure 13.27.   Vaccine being given in the axillary region.

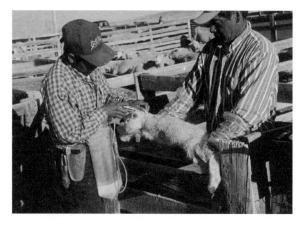

Figure 13.28.   Vaccine being administered SubQ in the neck.

for this vaccine is subcutaneously or SubQ (fig. 13.28). A SubQ injection deposits the product just under the skin. This may be easily done in the axillary region, the loose skin area behind one of the front legs, or in front of the shoulder in the neck region where there is loose skin. Use a clean, short needle with a small bore (20 ga × 1/2 in.) that is sharp. Never put a used needle into the bottle of vaccine or a needle that was used for a different product. When vaccinating several animals at a time, replace the needle often, at least after every 20 animals or as needed when the needle gets bent or burred. Intramuscular or IM injections place the product in the muscle. Never use the leg muscle for IM injections. Administer these in the neck region. For quality assurance, IM injections should be avoided whenever possible, as they cause irritation and ruin the meat in that area.

Another typical route of administration for vaccines is intranasal (fig. 13.29). This is generally used with Nasalgen, a type of vaccine used for the prevention of pneumonia. You simply administer the proper dose through a nasal cannula into one of the nasal passages.

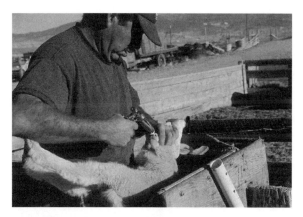

Figure 13.29.   Administration of an intranasal vaccine.

If you have ever encountered a soremouth outbreak on your farm, another immunization you may use is *Ovine ecthyma*. This product contains a modified live virus and should be handled with care. Gloves should be worn whenever using this product, as it can cause a human form of the disease called orf (fig. 13.30). When vaccinating with this product, you quickly scrape an area of skin that is woolless, then brush the vaccine on the scrape. A local reaction will occur on the lamb at or near the vaccination site. Use caution when handling any sheep with contagious ovine ecthyma.

As the Lamb Ages

As the lamb ages, it will continue to need shelter, good nutrition, and protection from predators. Lambs will have the tendency to follow their mothers' grazing habits early and adapt to the forages the mothers have been eating. This is known as imprinting. A large part of the overall health of your flock will be very dependent on your feeds and forages. Special attention to nutrition including vitamins, minerals, and good, fresh water can greatly reduce the incidence of disease. Sheep adapt well to forages that are often unsuited for other livestock. They are very good for use on poisonous plant control, such as with pastures containing larkspur or scrub oak. Sheep can be used to clear pastures of these plants prior to cattle. They serve a mutually advantageous purpose when allowed to graze in the state and national forests. Sheep are excellent for the environment: they clean up and thin the brush and weeds to reduce the spreadability of wildfires, while leaving no damage to the area. However, a "naïve" flock will not do well when subjected to an unfamiliar environment. When sheep move onto unfamiliar forages and feeds, they may search for the greenest, leafiest plant available, which often can be toxic to the naïve flock. Your local extension agent can help you in identifying plants that may be toxic to sheep.

Transportation

The most stressful part of a lamb's existence will probably be transportation. Poor facilities and impatient shepherds that scream, jab, and prod, plus an untrained dog that bites

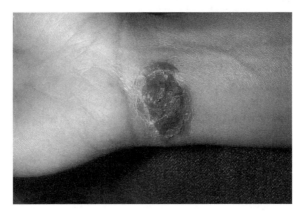

Figure 13.30.   Orf lesion on a human.

and tears the skin add to a lamb's fears of moving on up and into the unknown trailer. Understanding normal sheep behavior can save both time and frustration to the sheep and handlers. Sheep have wide-angle vision, allowing them to see behind without turning their heads. There are some breeds and genetics that reduce this visual zone due to wool blindness. Wool blindness occurs when the sheep has reduced vision due to wool covering the face and eyes. In this case, these sheep need to have this wool carefully trimmed (called facing) (fig. 13.31).

It is very important to select breeding stock with a clean, open face that is free of wool. Sheep have the natural tendency to move toward diffuse light (not bright) and work uphill better than down when moving. Sheep like to see where they are going. Knowing this allows for smoother loading and unloading when shipping large numbers of animals. It is best to use an experienced livestock hauler who has handled and hauled sheep before. To minimize disease, a responsible hauler will clean and disinfect the truck/trailer between each load (fig. 13.32).

When loading sheep into a truck/trailer unit, diffuse lights can be put in the trailer as well as at the trailer entry, at the top of the loading ramp. Likewise, when unloading, the

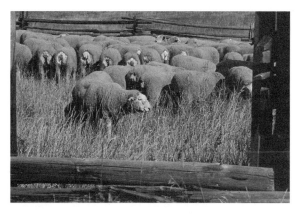

Figure 13.31.   Ewe that has been faced to reduce wool blindness.

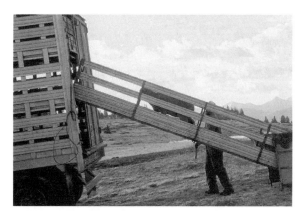

Figure 13.32.   Loading sheep into a truck trailer.

light should be at the lower end of the loading ramp and the catch pen should also be lit. The loading facilities and truck flooring should be solid and nonslippery. The use of bedding or sand can improve this when necessary. Weatherwise, it should be cool, not hot or wet. For these reasons, often sheep will be loaded when it is dark or dusky outside. Sheep should be held off of feed and water for a period of 8 to 12 hours prior to loading and shipping for trips that are going to take 8 to 12 hours. Sheep that will be transported for longer periods should be lightly fed and watered 2 to 3 hours prior to loading. This allows for easier loading and better sanitation (i.e., disease resistance) due to the decrease of urine and feces as well as less wool contamination. Sheep that have been fasted are less likely to lie down, reducing the chance of being stepped on, crushed, and/or suffocated. Avoid overcrowding animals during transportation for these reasons also. When sheep are transported for over 48 hours, the animals should be given a chance to be off-loaded, rested, and given fresh drinking water with electrolytes. This reduces the chance of transport tetany. Transport tetany is a paralytic condition caused by low blood calcium similar to milk fever in the cow.

Regardless of the sex of the lamb, if lucky enough to be in a seed stock flock and selected to carry on the excellent genetics of its ancestors, it will only have its tail amputated and receive immunizations. The lamb will be fed well, kept in a good clean environment free from stress, receive booster shots, and have its toenails trimmed, if needed (fig. 13.33). It will be kept away from strangers who may bring in diseases and be looked after until it is time to join the breeding program.

On the other hand, if destined for the food chain and a male, it will have another painful surgery to remove the testes.

Castration

As with amputation of the tail, it is much less painful and of minimal stress if the shepherd does this operation before two days of age. The lamb will receive a number of shots and dewormers to assure it doesn't get sick during the course of existence. The shepherd will make certain that it is well fed and protected from predators and other harm. The stressful parts of life will be removal from the companionship of mother, being placed in a truck

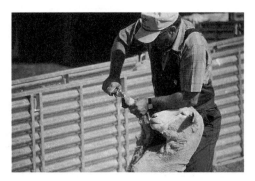

Figure 13.33.   Trimming the hooves.

with 450 other lambs, and transported to a new location for feeding or directly to the processing plant. This is all new to the lambs, and if the person in charge has designed the facilities properly, they will go willingly as directed. A lot of noise and poorly designed alleys with shadows and numerous distractions make it extremely confusing. In some cases, the lambs may stay on the same farm avoiding the stress of being transported to a far away place and presented with food they have never seen before. In all cases, it is nice to have facilities and be handled in a manner that will keep them from being injured.

Show Circuit

If the unfortunate role of entering the show circuit is the card drawn for the lamb, it will have the potential of a life filled with stress. Its tail may be surgically removed to the point that the musculature in the area of the anal sphincter will be disrupted allowing for an increased risk of a rectal prolapse. This lamb may be placed on a diet and training regime and trained as a marathon runner. On show days, it will not have food and water, and it may receive drugs to dehydrate it so that the hide is tight for the judge. It will be trained to brace hard against the shepherd to show off the muscles developed on the treadmill or from being run by the shepherd's dog. It will stand proudly in the winner's circle to the delight of the owner. If a castrated male, it will be auctioned off to some big retail chain as an advertising gesture. If breeding stock, it either will be sold to another or will travel from show to show, being transported in any kind of weather, and eventually might end up back with a small flock used for reproduction purposes. At this point, the lamb will need time to "destress" from all this, prior to the expectations of reproducing, whether male or female. The effects from extreme stress affects the reproductive tract as well, and this can last for some period of time.

RESPONSIBLE OWNERSHIP

Regardless of the operation—whether it be a large range operation, a small farm flock, a hobby fleece producer, a sheep dairy operation, a club lamb producer, or a sheep kept as a pet—the principles and responsibilities of providing a healthy, stress-free environment are the same. The only difference is the magnitude.

Sheep have the unique ability to utilize a variety of forages. This ability gives them a wide range of useful endeavors. Provided with a safe environment, sheep can be utilized for an environmentally safe noxious weed control program, used in forests for control of underbrush reducing the danger of wild fires, or enlisted to clean up the weeds and crop aftermath around the farmstead. Regardless, of the forage and feeds presented, care must be taken to assure a balance providing good clean water plus salt, minerals, and vitamins to maintain a healthy body. Each phase in the life of the sheep has different nutritional requirements. The pregnant ewe has a changing nutritional demand during the various stages of gestation. These demands vary considerably depending on the number of fetuses being carried. Inadequate nutrition in later stages of pregnancy may lead to loss of the fetuses and death of the ewe. Nutritional balance is the most important part of maintaining a healthy body.

Sheep are gregarious in nature. They have a flocking instinct and stay together as a group following a leader. Building on this basic knowledge, handling sheep is very easy. Utilizing a trained lead sheep will make moving sheep unfamiliar with the surroundings much easier. Design the working facility so that it is on a curve and funnels down to a single-file alley (fig. 13.34). A sheep will follow the one ahead of it, if there are no distractions. Make handling facilities with solid sides and eliminate all distractions. The design must be made without sharp corners to avoid bruising. Avoid rough handling. If sheep are not working through the facility, you should stop, take the time to determine the cause of the problem, and make corrections. It is usually the lack of attention to the design that caused the problem.

A good preventive health program will aid in the well-being and minimize the pain and suffering of the animal. Health programs must be designed specifically for each individual flock. Each flock is unique, and management differs with the goals and purpose of the enterprise. The one most overlooked element of a flock health program is that of biosecurity. Introduction of new animals from other sources without an adequate quarantine period (a minimum of 30 days) often introduces new diseases and parasites.

The *Sheep Production Handbook* published by the American Sheep Industries Association has excellent sections on nutrition, handling facilities, health programs, predator control, and many other aspects of maximizing well-being and minimizing pain and suffering of sheep. It is required reading for any responsible sheep owner.

One talent that humans are gifted with is the power of observation. A keen observer can spot the individual that is not well and suffering or the areas that cause stress and pain. It is our responsibility to the animals we own or supervise to provide them with the proper environment, nutrition, and safety so they will lead productive and efficient lives. We are their shepherds.

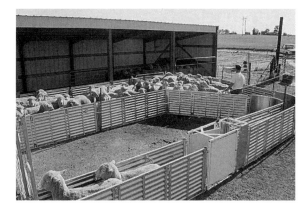

Figure 13.34.   A well-designed working facility.

REFERENCES

1. Kimberling, C: *Raising Healthy Sheep*. 1994. Christian Veterinary Mission. Seattle, WA.
2. SID: *Sheep Production Handbook*. 4:120–248; 12:1001–1015. 1996. American Sheep Industries, Denver, CO.
3. Bradbury, J: *Travels in the Interior of America in the Years 1809, 1810, and 1811*. Repr. of 2d ed. 1986. University of Nebraska Press, Lincoln.
4. Wentworth, E: *American Sheep Trails*. 1948. The Iowa State College Press, Ames.
5. Cheney, J: Colorado State University parasitology lecture series—pictures of internal and external parasites. 1963–2003.
6. Kimberling, C: Colorado State University field trials and investigations. 1965–2003.

14

Welfare Problems of Poultry

Ian J. H. Duncan

INTRODUCTION

Of all livestock species, poultry species are probably kept more intensively, both for meat and for egg production, than any other. In most of the developed world, they are kept in completely controlled environments, under very artificial husbandry conditions, such as in cages or on deep litter, in huge numbers, crowded together in single-sex, single-age groups. This suggests that the conditions under which poultry live and the procedures to which they are subjected may reduce their welfare. This chapter will examine these conditions and procedures and show that this is indeed the case. A chicken's lot (or that of a turkey, or duck, or any other member of a farmed poultry species) is not a happy one.

A consideration of every domestic poultry species is beyond the scope of this chapter. Most of the discussion, therefore, involves the most numerous of the poultry species, the domestic fowl (*Gallus gallus domesticus*) with occasional reference to turkeys (*Meleagris gallopavo*). Welfare problems are considered in the order in which they are encountered by the birds during their lives, that is, from hatchery to slaughterhouse.

In this chapter, "welfare" will be considered as being dependent on what the birds feel. That is, birds that are experiencing negative subjective feelings (in other words, birds that are suffering) will be adjudged to have poor welfare. Birds that are not suffering will be regarded as not having a welfare problem, but this does not preclude the possibility that their welfare might be improved if they could experience positive subjective feelings or pleasure (Duncan, 2002).

CHICK WELFARE

All commercial poultry in the developed world are incubated and hatched artificially. Since all our poultry species are precocial (i.e., they hatch in a well-developed state and are able, to a large extent, to fend for themselves), this means that they are sentient during late embryonic development. The possibility therefore exists for reductions in welfare before hatching. There is no evidence that artificial incubation imposes any particular stress on the prehatch chicks. It is true that under natural incubation, there is some communication between the mother hen and the developing embryos (Vince, 1974), but the absence of this does not seem to lead to problems. In fact, because the processes involved in incubation are so well understood, and because modern incubators and hatchers can control temperature to a tenth of a degree and humidity to a percentage point, it seems likely that the welfare of artificially incubated and hatched chicks is well protected.

After hatching, chicks are heavily "processed." They are handled several times, inspected, sexed, sometimes injected, sometimes sprayed with vaccine, and subjected to a variety of more invasive procedures. To a layperson, the handling of chicks at a hatchery often looks very rough as they are transported along moving belts, picked up, inspected, and tossed into chutes and funnels. However, newly hatched chicks are very resilient. They are extremely light and their down acts both as a shock absorber and parachute. Moreover, they do not show much in the way of fear responses at this stage of their life (Duncan, 1985); they are primed for imprinting, which means they will follow any large and noisy moving object. It is therefore extremely unusual to see any ill effects of handling at the hatchery.

The more invasive procedures, mentioned earlier, are another matter, and there is a distinct possibility that some of these do reduce welfare. For example, most laying hens in North America are beak trimmed or debeaked. Male chicks destined for breeding are "dubbed," that is, they have their combs cut off. Male turkeys are "desnooded" as chicks, that is, they have the fleshy protuberance that hangs over their beaks cut off. Broiler breeder males (the sires of meat chickens or broilers) have a toe cut off each foot as chicks. Many turkeys, male and female, also have a toe cut off as chicks. The reason for all these surgeries is to prevent damage later in life. The appendages causing the damage (the beak or the toes) are cut off or modified so that they cause less damage, and the appendages likely to be damaged (the combs and the snoods) are cut off or modified so that they are less likely to be damaged. It could be argued that all these surgeries are carried out for welfare reasons—in order to prevent pain and injury later in life. However, anesthetics or analgesics are never given, and whenever these surgeries have been carefully investigated, it has been found that there are welfare costs, often involving pain. This is best illustrated using the example of beak trimming or debeaking, although it should be said that this particular surgery is not always carried out while the birds are still chicks.

In fact, neither of these terms—*beak trimming* or *debeaking*—is strictly accurate. When the surgery is carried out on birds in the growing phase, a third of the upper beak is amputated using a sharp heated blade. Alternatively, when the birds are still chicks, the growing tip of the beak can be damaged using a precision machine with a laser beam, a powerful electric spark, or an infrared beam. The end of the beak sloughs off a few days later. The beak of the fowl is well innervated and contains both mechanoreceptors and nociceptors (Breward, 1984). It has been shown that when the beak is partially amputated using a hot-blade debeaker during the growing phase, the severed nerves grow back into the damaged stump and form neuromata (tiny neural tumors), which then send spontaneous pain signals back to the brain (Breward and Gentle, 1985). This appears to be similar to the phenomenon that causes phantom limb pain in human amputees. It has also been found that behavioral changes suggestive of acute pain occur in the two days following surgery, and this is followed by changes indicating chronic pain, which last at least five or six weeks after surgery (Duncan et al., 1989; Gentle et al., 1991). This neural and behavioral evidence suggests that beak trimming reduces welfare through causing both acute and chronic pain. The problem is that beak trimming is carried out for the very good reason of preventing or controlling feather pecking and cannibalism, which can themselves cause great suffering. Faced with this dilemma, what are producers to do? If they do not trim beaks, then feather pecking and cannibalism may cause enormous suffering. If they do trim beaks by conventional methods, the birds will suffer from acute and chronic pain.

The evidence suggests that it is not possible to control feather pecking completely by keeping hens in other, more natural, environments. This can be illustrated by what happened in Sweden. Before joining the European Union, Sweden made a decision to ban battery cages for laying hens. However, the Swedes had previously banned beak trimming. Ironically, they could not get alternative, more extensive husbandry systems to work because of feather pecking and cannibalism problems, and they had to postpone their decision to ban battery cages.

It may be possible to reduce the pain of beak trimming by carrying it out at a very young age, but this does not eliminate pain completely (Gentle et al., 1997).

It is known that feather pecking has hereditary characteristics (Richter, 1954), and that its incidence may have been increased by unintentional genetic selection (Cuthbertson, 1980). It therefore seems likely that the long-term solution to this problem will be a genetic one. Muir and Craig (1998) have shown that it is possible to select against feather pecking using a kin selection method, and they have produced a line of birds that does not require beak trimming. The challenge will be to persuade the primary breeding companies to adopt such a procedure.

There has been little investigation into the welfare costs of the other elective surgeries carried out on poultry. However, Gentle and Hunter (1988) have produced neuronal evidence suggesting that detoeing may be painful at the time of amputation but is less likely to be followed by chronic pain than is beak trimming. There are also reports that toe clipping in turkeys increases mortality and depresses growth (Newberry, 1992; Owings et al., 1972), which strongly suggests that it also decreases welfare.

Chopping off parts of young animals in order to prevent future welfare problems is a very crude solution. These surgeries are all performed without anesthesia or analgesia and, at the very least, will cause some acute pain. In addition, there may well be other welfare costs. Beak-trimmed birds will not be able to explore their environments or preen themselves as thoroughly as intact birds. Dubbing may well cause social problems since it is known that the head region is used in individual recognition (Guhl and Ortman, 1953). Detoeing may interfere with scratching during foraging and cause problems of balance. The poultry industry would do well to question these procedures. Are they all necessary? Are there alternative solutions? Could the procedures be made more humane?

The disposal of unwanted chicks and "hatchery waste" is another potential problem area in the poultry industry. In any hatch of eggs, there will be a small proportion of chicks that are not fit to be sold. They may be malformed or crippled in some way or may not have hatched properly. They may still be alive and should be euthanized by an approved method. Of course, in addition to these unwanted chicks and late-stage embryos, when birds destined for the egg-laying sector are hatched, half of the chicks are male and of no use to the industry. For many years, this was a forgotten or ignored problem; unwanted chicks were dropped into plastic bags and allowed to suffocate. It is now acknowledged that this is completely unacceptable, and improvements are being instituted. To date, the method adopted by most large-scale hatcheries is destruction of the chicks by a macerator designed for the purpose. This seems very violent and is anything but aesthetic. However, it delivers instantaneous death. A much less violent method is gassing. Unfortunately, this is a rather slow procedure since chicks are resistant to high levels of carbon dioxide, which is the gas most often used. There is also some evidence that carbon dioxide is not the ideal gas for this purpose since many animals, including birds, find it aversive (Raj, 1996). Carbon monoxide would actually be much more humane, but it is never used because of the danger to the human operators.

THE WELFARE OF MEAT BIRDS

Birds being raised for meat, both chickens and turkeys, are kept on the floor. Although, traditionally, meat birds have been kept in open-sided and curtain-sided barns in the southern United States, the trend is toward completely controlled environment housing. This allows for better climate control, with respect to both keeping the birds warm when outside temperatures are low, and keeping them cool when it is extremely hot outside.

Without doubt, the biggest welfare problems for meat birds are those associated with fast growth. The environmental conditions may not be ideal, but generally the birds have freedom to move about, they have a substrate in which to forage and dust bathe, fresh food and water are always available, and they are killed at a relatively young age, before aggression becomes a big problem. There is one environmental feature that probably does reduce welfare, and that is day length. Meat birds are typically kept on very long days of about 23 hours with a very short dark period. The idea behind this is to give the birds as much feeding time as possible. In fact, in order to combat problems of fast growth (to be discussed next), some producers are now trying to limit food intake and slow growth by putting the birds on shorter days at first and gradually increasing day length (Classen, Riddell, and Robinson, 1991). However, there is another more important reason for limiting day length and that is to allow the birds to have a proper rest. All young animals need to rest and sleep, and meat poultry may be denied this by keeping them on very long days. In a natural environment, a mother hen and her chicks show periods of great activity alternating with quiet periods when the chicks are brooded by the hen. Malleau, Duncan, and Widowski (1997) have shown that young chicks kept on simulated brooding cycles of alternating 40 minutes light and 40 minutes dark have a far healthier lifestyle than chicks kept on long days. They synchronize their activities, are very active during the light periods, and rest completely during the dark periods.

The incidence of conditions such as skeletal disorders and ascites that accompany fast growth in meat strains of poultry is high (Leeson, Diaz, and Summers, 1995; Julian, 1998). The skeletal problems are diverse, but by far the greatest incidence and severity are seen in the leg bones and include such conditions as tibial dyschondroplasia, chondrodystrophy, and femoral head necrosis (Leeson et al., 1995). Ascites is a condition in which the high demand for oxygenated blood in the soft tissues leads to the heart attempting to pump more blood through the lungs. The right ventricle of the heart becomes distended and unable to function properly, at which point there is back-pressure created in the blood supply system and, because of this, leakage of plasma from the liver into the body cavity causing an edema (Julian, 1998).

It has been estimated that, in broilers, skeletal problems account for 30–40 percent of overall mortality, morbidity, and carcass downgrading and that ascites might be responsible for 5–12 percent mortality (Leeson et al., 1995). But, of course, these conditions are welfare problems as well as production problems because they cause the birds to suffer. For example, there is evidence that skeletal deformities are painful. Broilers with gait abnormalities, when given a choice between two feeds, one of which contained an analgesic, consumed more of the drugged feed than did broilers with no lameness. Moreover, the walking ability of lame birds was improved by this self-administered treatment (Danbury et al., 2000). In another experiment, male turkeys greatly increased their spontaneous movement when administered a drug that reduces pain and inflammation in arthritic joints. These turkeys were later shown to have degenerative lesions of the hip joints (Duncan et al., 1991). These results suggest that the normal behavior of the birds was being inhibited by pain although they were not showing obvious symptoms of pain.

The increasing incidence of fast growth problems such as these in meat strains of poultry indicate that the biological limit of growth is being reached and that it is a mistake to think that we can go on and on selecting for increased growth rate without costs to the bird. It is also a mistake to think that there may be environmental or nutritional solutions to these problems. There may be some short-term, Band-Aid solutions, but the long-term solution will be genetic. McMillan (2000) developed a computer simulation in which the effects of four different genetic selection procedures *for* growth rate and *against* incidence of ascites were compared. None of the procedures resulted in a decrease in the incidence of ascites. All of these procedures resulted in increased growth rate together with an increase in the level of ascites. The primary breeding companies must pay attention to this warning. They need to stop selecting for increased growth and pay attention to the total health of their birds instead.

THE WELFARE OF LAYING HENS

Battery Cages

The battery cage system for laying hens was one of the first intensive husbandry systems to come under attack on animal welfare grounds. Ruth Harrison (1964), in her ground-breaking book *Animal Machines*, was very critical of battery cages, and her opinions were largely supported by the Brambell Report (Command Paper 2836, 1965). Since then, the criticisms have continued and, if anything, have increased (e.g., Singer, 1990; A.J.F. Webster, 1995). In Europe, the movement against traditional cages for laying hens has been so great that, in 1999, the European Union approved a directive (CEC, 1999) to ban cages. Under this directive, traditional battery cages will be prohibited from January 1, 2012, and the only cages allowed from 2012 will be furnished or enriched cages. This directive also sets the standards for all husbandry systems alternative to cages.

In spite of all the criticisms of traditional cages, it should be remembered that they do have certain advantages, and some of these are actually welfare benefits. For example, the original reason why cages were introduced was to separate the birds from their feces, and this confers a substantial hygiene advantage to cages. This has resulted in a much lower incidence of diseases, such as avian TB and various salmonella infections, where the infectious agent is spread via the droppings (Duncan, 2001). Also the small group size in cages is much closer to the group size that hens prefer (Hughes, 1977; Dawkins, 1982; Lindberg and Nicol, 1993, 1996).

In contrast to these advantages, there are many welfare problems associated with cages. Caging prevents the occurrence of several behavior sequences, the most important of which, undoubtedly, is nesting. Nesting or prelaying behavior satisfies the criteria for being a "need" —behavior that if not allowed expression, causes frustration (Hughes and Duncan, 1988; Duncan, 1998). Nesting behavior is controlled by hormonal events that take place at ovulation, about 24 hours earlier (Wood-Gush and Gilbert, 1975). It has been shown that once nesting behavior has been triggered, hens are strongly motivated to seek out a suitable nest site (Duncan and Kite, 1989) and will work very hard to obtain one (Follensbee et al., 1992; Freire, Appleby, and Hughes, 1997). Also, many hens, particularly those of light hybrid strains that are commonly used in North America, show symptoms of severe frustration (Duncan, 1970) in the prelaying period when they are kept in cages (Wood-Gush, 1972; Mills et al., 1985a,b).

Are any other behavior systems inhibited by caging? The ones that have been investigated the most are dust bathing and perching and the evidence regarding them is rather mixed. There has been much debate over whether dust bathing is largely governed by internal factors (e.g., Vestergaard, Hogan, and Kruijt, 1990), and therefore qualifies as a need, or external factors (Duncan et al., 1998), and does not. More recent research has shown that the performance of dust bathing may be motivated by pleasure (Widowski and Duncan, 2000). Therefore, in spite of the conflicting theories on its causation, there would appear to be some welfare benefit in allowing hens to dust bathe, either to reduce their suffering or to increase their pleasure, and they cannot dust bathe in cages. Similarly, hens have been shown to be motivated to roost on perches when they are resting or sleeping, suggesting that their welfare may be compromised when this is prevented, as it is when they are kept in cages (Olsson and Keeling, 2000).

In addition to inhibiting complete behavior systems, the lack of space in battery cages may reduce welfare by preventing hens from adopting certain postures and performing particular elements of behavior. For example, Dawkins (1985) has shown that traditional battery cages are not sufficiently high to allow hens to adopt the standing alert posture that is very common in their repertoire. In addition, the evidence suggests that cages may reduce the incidence of certain behavior patterns such as wing flapping and tail wagging (Nicol, 1987a,b; Dawkins and Hardie, 1989). These findings corroborate earlier preference tests showing that hens prefer more space (Hughes, 1975b; Dawkins, 1981).

There is another way in which the lack of space in battery cages may reduce welfare, and this is by restricting movement and exercise, which contributes to bone weakness in laying hens (Leeson et al., 1995). Caged laying hens sometimes show paralysis around the time of peak production, a condition known as "cage layer fatigue." The condition is caused by fractures of the fourth and fifth thoracic vertebrae that compress the spinal cord (Riddell et al., 1968) and is not seen in noncaged hens that get more exercise. A condition probably related to cage layer fatigue is the bone weakness seen in spent laying hens coming from cages (Rowland et al., 1972; Leeson et al., 1995). At the end of a laying year, hens from battery cages have lower limb bone strength than hens from noncage systems and are at risk of suffering from broken bones (Knowles and Broom, 1990). It has been shown that adding a perch to a cage can increase bone strength (Hughes and Appleby, 1989; Abrahamsson and Tauson, 1993).

In addition to restricting certain behavior, the lack of space in a cage means that hens are crowded together. All the indications are that, at commercial cage densities used in

North America (300–350 cm² per bird in the United States and 450 cm² in Canada), welfare is decreased. In a review of this topic, Hughes (1975a) found that decreased area per bird depresses egg production, reduces food consumption, lowers body weight, and increases mortality. Moreover, there is evidence of an increased stress response with increasing population density (Mashaly et al., 1984). Studies that have examined spacing behavior of hens have shown that, if given the opportunity, they will space themselves farther apart than they can under commercial cage densities (Zayan, Doyen, and Duncan, 1983; Zayan and Doyen, 1985; Keeling and Duncan, 1989). All this evidence suggests that hen welfare is reduced at commercial cage densities.

Forced Molting

After they have been laying eggs for about a year, commercial laying hens start to become photorefractory (i.e., they no longer respond to long days), egg production starts to fall, eggshell quality decreases, and the hen is often overweight. The hen's skeleton has been depleted of calcium through producing many eggshells and is fragile. Of course, if hens were kept under natural daylight conditions, they would gradually go out of reproductive condition and into a molt when day length decreased in the autumn. Commercial hens kept on long days for a year would also gradually go out of lay and molt naturally if they were subjected to short days of, say, eight hours. However, natural molting is a slow process and within a flock of hens there would be a wide range of times for individual hens to complete the molt. Currently, the poultry industry is not prepared to accept this extended loss of production. Therefore, at about 74 weeks of age, hens are sent to slaughter as "spent laying hens" (this happens commonly in Canada and in Europe) or are "force molted," in order to speed up the molting process and get the hens back into reproductive condition for a second and sometimes a third laying year (this is the common practice in the United States).

Forced molting programs usually involve reducing day length to six to eight hours and, at the same time, withholding feed for 10 to 14 days (North and Bell, 1990; Leeson and Summers, 1991). Forced molting shortens the nonproductive period to about eight weeks but results in a huge increase in stress and suffering. Mortality figures give a rough measure of welfare (Hughes, 1975a), and during forced molting, mortality increases dramatically. Dr. Don Bell summarized molting results from 353 U.S. flocks during 1997 and 1998 and found that mortality typically doubled during the first week of molt, then doubled again during the second week (cited by Duncan and Mench, 2000).

However, even apart from mortality, the evidence suggests that hens suffer enormously during forced molting. Chickens have evolved to forage and consume food throughout the day (Savory, Wood-Gush, and Duncan, 1978), so that even a moderate period of deprivation is stressful. Consequently, food deprivation of 10 to 14 days acts as a drastic stressor. It results in a classical physiological stress response (Mench, 1992). Frustration of feeding leads to signs of distress such as increased aggression (Duncan and Wood-Gush, 1971) and the formation of stereotyped pacing (Duncan and Wood-Gush, 1972). Extremely hungry birds also develop stereotypic pecking at objects such as feeders (Kostal, Savory, and Hughes, 1992; Savory and Maros, 1993; Hocking, Maxwell, and Mitchell, 1996). In an experiment in which hens were deprived of food for three days, A. B. Webster (1995) found that cage pecking increased by a factor of three and feather pecking increased by a factor of eight. In a later study, designed to simulate forced molting, A. B. Webster (2000) deprived hens of feed for 21 days. At first these hens showed increased aggression and nonnutritive pecking suggestive of severe frustration and extreme hunger, and later they showed inactivity suggestive of debilitation (Duncan and Wood-Gush, 1971, 1972).

If any other sentient species were subjected to this degree of food deprivation, it would amount to an offense under most states' cruelty to animals laws. The fact that the practice is still accepted in most American states is a grave indictment of the poultry industry.

THE WELFARE OF BREEDERS

Food Restriction of Broiler Breeders

The genetic selection of broilers for fast growth rate has resulted in birds with increased appetites (Siegel and Wisman, 1966). Broiler breeders, that is, the parent birds that produce broilers, have the same huge appetites as their progeny. However, if they were allowed to satisfy these appetites, they would quickly become obese and suffer from all the problems of obesity including low fertility and reduced life expectation (Leeson and Summers, 2000; Renema and Robinson, 2000). They are therefore kept on very severe food restriction from a very early age. Food restriction is carried out for a very good reason: to keep the birds in good reproductive condition and prevent them from becoming obese, a condition that would itself reduce welfare. However, there is a large welfare cost to pay. Broiler breeders, kept according to management guidelines, exhibit behavioral symptoms that indicate greatly reduced welfare (Savory, 1989; Mench and Falcone, 2000). Producers are once again faced with a dilemma; if broiler breeders are allowed to feed to appetite, they will become obese and long-term welfare will be reduced; if they are restricted sufficiently to maximize fitness, then they show symptoms of hunger and extreme distress. It may be possible to alleviate hunger in the short term by diluting the diet with nonnutritive substances such as cellulose (Zuidhof et al., 1995; Savory et al., 1996). However, in order to solve this problem in the long term, primary breeding companies will have to breed parent stock with smaller appetites.

Hyperaggressive Behavior in Broiler Breeder Males

During the 1990s, an increasing number of reports described broiler breeder males as being very aggressive toward females (Mench, 1993). Females were being injured and even killed by this behavior, and fertility levels were plummeting. This behavior is very unusual, because male domestic fowl dominate females passively, and seldom show any overt aggression toward them (Wood-Gush, 1956). As well as being a production problem, hyperaggressive behavior is a welfare problem, because females are being harassed, badly injured, and even killed by males. At first, the problem seemed to afflict males of only one strain, but within a year or two most strains were affected (Millman, Duncan, and Widowski, 2000). This hyperaggressiveness toward females cannot be explained in terms of a general increase in aggression, since game fowl males, which have been bred for fighting and which are much more aggressive toward other males than are broiler breeder males (Millman and Duncan, 2000a), show little if any aggression toward females (Millman and Duncan, 2000b). Food restriction of the males does not seem to be a cause of the increased aggression, either during the rearing phase (Millman and Duncan, 2000b) or during the adult phase (Millman et al., 2000). It has also been shown that broiler breeder males are deficient in certain elements of courtship behavior (Millman et al., 2000). The result is that the females do not react appropriately when males approach, but move away and avoid them (Millman and Duncan, 2000c) and this, perhaps, exacerbates the situation.

At the moment, it is not at all clear how this problem of aberrant aggressive behavior in broiler breeder males has arisen. It almost certainly has a genetic basis. It is unclear whether the courtship deficiency and the hyperaggressiveness are separate or linked problems. It may be that these traits are genetically linked to some production trait, such as broad breastedness, which the breeding companies have been selecting for. On the other hand, it may be the result of a misguided attempt to improve fertility, which is poor in broiler breeders, particularly toward the end of the breeding year. This is due to the males being unable to achieve cloacal contact with the females because of the males' conformation (Duncan, Hocking, and Seawright, 1990). This suggests that the broiler industry is destined to follow the example of the turkey industry, where selection for broad breasts has resulted in males that are incapable of fertilizing females naturally. However, it is commonly thought in the broiler breeding industry that the low fertility is due to decreased libido. So the breeding companies may have been selecting males that approach females very quickly in the mistaken belief that they are very sexy, whereas, in fact, these males are very aggressive.

CATCHING AND TRANSPORTATION

Meat Birds

It was stated earlier that meat birds have a reasonable environment in which to live. However, at the end of their short lives, when they are caught and transported to a processing plant, their welfare is severely compromised. Traditionally, they are manually caught by the legs and stuffed into crates, and the crates are stacked onto trucks. During transportation, the birds may be subjected to extremes of temperature, high carbon dioxide levels, exhaust fumes, sudden accelerating and braking forces, vibrations and traffic noises, all the while being crowded together with other birds that they may not know. At the processing plant, they are pulled from the crates, their legs are thrust into shackles, and they are carried upside-down to a stunning bath.

But do these catching and transportation processes actually reduce welfare? The evidence suggests that they do. For example, surveys on broilers have reported that 10 to 30 percent of birds are injured during these processes (Gerrits, DeKoning, and Migchels, 1985). In addition, laboratory simulations reveal that subjecting birds to catching, handling, and vehicular motion is particularly stressful (Duncan, 1989).

In recent years, a great deal of effort has gone into improving the whole catching and transportation process. For example, chicken-catching machines have been developed that pick birds up from the barn floor and place them in transportation crates very gently. This process causes much less stress and damage to the birds than does traditional manual catching (Duncan et al., 1986). Also, transportation vehicles are being developed that monitor and control the environment of the birds to minimize stress (Mitchell and Kettlewell, 1993; Mitchell et al., 2000). Ideally, the whole catching, transportation, and preslaughter system should be integrated with an automated catching machine placing birds in crates, modules of crates being placed on environmentally controlled trucks, and the crates moving straight into a gas stunning unit at the processing plant (Kettlewell et al., 2000). The challenge now is to get the poultry industry to adopt these methods, since, there will be a substantial cost involved.

Spent Laying Hens

Spent laying hens are hens at the end of their productive lives. It is usually arranged (by manipulating body weight and day length) that laying hens start to lay eggs at about 20 weeks of age. They lay eggs for about a year, at which point it is no longer profitable to let them continue, because of decreasing egg numbers and reduced eggshell quality. Therefore, when the hens are about 74 weeks old, they are either force molted (previously discussed) and kept for a second and sometimes a third laying year, or sent for slaughter as spent laying hens. In any case, regardless of the number of years they have been in lay, all laying hens are eventually slaughtered as spent laying hens.

The disposal of spent laying hens is probably the most serious welfare problem confronting the poultry industry today. It is difficult to gauge just how serious it actually is. However, in a British survey, 29 percent of hens from battery cages were found to have freshly broken bones just before they were stunned (more bones get broken during stunning) and most of this damage occurred as the birds were being removed from the cages (Gregory and Wilkins, 1989). It seems reasonable to conclude that with this incidence of broken bones, there must also have been a high rate of soft-tissue injuries. Spent laying hens in North America are handled no differently, so there is no reason to think that American statistics would be any better.

There are three main reasons for these dreadful figures. First, as discussed earlier, hens kept in battery cages, even for one laying year, have very fragile skeletons (McLean, Baxter, and Michie, 1986; Knowles and Broom, 1990; Norgaard-Nielsen, 1990). In modern, high-producing, laying hens there is such a high demand for calcium for eggshells, that cortical bone as well as medullary bone is used as a source of calcium. This results, at the end of a laying year, in bones that are depleted of calcium and easily broken (Leeson et al., 1995). This bone weakness is exacerbated by lack of exercise in cages (Leeson et al., 1995). The second reason is that traditional battery cages are poorly designed for the removal of hens. Catchers usually grab the hens by a leg and pull them through the cage door foot first. Small doors to the cages result in hens getting their wings or free leg caught as they are being removed. Modern European cages are designed so that the whole front opens up, resulting in a much lower risk of damage (Tauson, 1980, 1989). The third reason is that spent laying hens are worth very little, and so no effort is made to handle them carefully (Broom and Knowles, 1989). The combination of these three factors, fragile skeleton, poorly designed cage, and low value, results in an unacceptably high injury level. The problem is made worse by the fact that journeys to slaughter for spent laying hens are often long because only a few processing plants are prepared to accept spent hens. This means that injured hens may be in pain for long periods of time.

When spent hens reach the processing plant, their problems continue. The tetany and muscular spasms that accompany electrical stunning lead to further bone breakage because their skeletons are so fragile (Gregory and Wilkins, 1989). In order to reduce this, there is a tendency on the killing line to reduce the intensity of the electrical stun. This increases the risk that some hens will not be properly stunned before slaughter. If they are not properly stunned, they do not assume the characteristic posture during tetany and so are at risk of missing the automatic machine that cuts the neck vessels. Unless there is a close inspection of all birds at this stage, some hens may enter the scald tank alive and conscious (Duncan, 1997).

Incidentally, the tendency for the bones of spent laying hens to break during handling and stunning means that processors are very reluctant to develop products that use the meat of spent hens because of the risk of contamination with bone fragments. This reduces the value of spent laying hens even further and means that less care is taken of them in their final hours of life.

The disposal of spent laying hens is proving to be a very intractable problem. There have been many solutions suggested, but to date, none has proved effective. Most of them involve killing the birds on the farm. Of course, the carcasses would not then be fit for human consumption and would have to be composted, and this gives the industry a very wasteful image. The most humane method would be to kill the hens while they are still in the cage, say by gassing them. However, there is a practical problem with this method and that is the mechanical one of removing carcasses from the cages after they are stiffened by rigor mortis. Another suggestion has been to remove the hens from the cages manually and drop them into a vacuum tube that quickly transports them to a macerator outside the barn. However, this would expose the birds to considerable trauma as they were sucked through the tube, and it is unclear whether a macerator, which works well on day-old chicks, could be scaled up to deal effectively with laying hens. Another idea has been to develop a portable gas stunning and killing cabinet (Webster, Fletcher, and Savage, 1996) into which hens could be placed on removal from the cages.

Of course, the cost of humanely disposing of spent layer hens should be factored into the costs of production for eggs. For example, it has been realized that the only way to protect the environment from the dumping of worthless used automobile tires is to add a charge for their disposal when they are bought as new tires. Similarly, an amount should be added to the price of eggs to cover the cost of humanely disposing of the spent laying hens.

Water-Bath Stunning

In most civilized countries, the vast majority of all birds slaughtered, including meat chickens, spent laying hens, and turkeys, are stunned by water-bath stunning before being killed by exsanguination. The exceptions are birds killed according to religious slaughter laws. When water-bath stunning was introduced in the 1950s and 1960s, it represented a huge increase in welfare compared with what preceded it. However, when looked at objectively today, it is not very efficient and not very humane (Duncan, 1997). When birds arrive at the processing plant, they are taken out of the crates in which they have been transported and are hung by the legs on a shackle line. This involves handling (sometimes quite rough handling), which birds find very aversive (Duncan et al. 1989). There is also evidence that forcing birds' legs into metal shackles is a painful procedure (Gentle and Tilston, 2000). The shackle line moves into the processing plant and over a water-bath so that the birds' heads go into the water. An electrical potential between the line and the water should render every bird unconscious. However, there are many variables in the system. Differences in the size of the birds, differences in the conductivity of the birds, changes in the conductivity of the water as it becomes dirty, and other variables, all affect how much current travels through the birds' brains, and therefore how well they are stunned (Duncan, 1997). There is much research going on to try to make this process more efficient and more foolproof (e.g., Raj, 1998, 2000; Fletcher, 2000).

There is, however, an alternative method of stunning poultry and that is gas or modified atmosphere stunning. This method renders the birds unconscious by starving their brains of oxygen. The birds are placed in an inert gas such as argon or a mixture of argon and carbon dioxide (Raj, 1993). More recently, nitrogen, which is much cheaper than argon, has been used for stunning. It has been known for some time that nitrogen is very effective and very humane in inducing unconsciousness (Woolley and Gentle, 1988). It was not used originally because it has the same density as air and so is difficult to contain. However, this problem has been overcome by mixing it with a little argon to make it heavier and so more easily contained in the gassing chamber. Gas stunning has many welfare advantages. Birds are stunned in the crates in which they have been transported, thus avoiding the stress of being shackled while conscious. It has been shown that losing consciousness through anoxia is very humane, being quick and painless (Woolley and Gentle, 1988). In practice, the birds are actually killed by anoxia before being shackled and bled, which means that there is no risk of recovery. Switching from water-bath stunning to gas stunning would add a small cost to the final product. However, there are other commercial advantages. For example, the conditions for the people hanging birds on the shackles is much better, since there is less noise, less dust, more light, and they can stand in a more ergonomically correct position. There is also the possibility that the whole process of shackling dead birds could be automated. Gas stunning also gives a better quality product with less damage and bruising and allows for quicker further processing. It also means that there is a very safe environment for the people working in the slaughter plant, since the gas being used is inert (Raj, 1993; Duncan 1997).

REFERENCES

Abrahamsson, P. and Tauson, R., 1993. Effect of perches at different positions in conventional cages for laying hens of two different strains. *Acta Agriculturæ Scandinavica*, Section A, Animal Science, 43: 228–235.

Breward, J., 1984. Cutaneous nociceptors in the chicken beak. *Journal of Physiology*, London, 346: 56.

Breward, J. and Gentle, M. J., 1985. Neuroma formation and abnormal afferent nerve discharges after partial beak amputation (beak trimming) in poultry. *Experientia*, 41: 1132–1134.

Broom, D. M. and Knowles, T. G., 1989. The assessment of welfare during the handling and transport of spent hens. In: *Proceedings of the Third European Symposium on Poultry Welfare* (Eds. Faure, J. M. and Mills, A. D.), pp. 79–91. Tours, France, French Branch of the WPSA.

CEC, 1999. Council directive for laying down minimum standards for the protection of laying hens kept in various systems of rearing. *CEC Directive*, 1999/74/EG.

Classen, H. L., Riddell, C. and Robinson, F. E., 1991. Effect of increasing photoperiod length on performance and health of broiler chickens. *British Poultry Science*, 32: 21–29.

Command Paper 2836, 1965. *Report of the Technical Committee to Enquire into the Welfare of Animals Kept under Intensive Livestock Husbandry Systems*. London, Her Majesty's Stationery Office.

Cuthbertson, G. J., 1980. Genetic variation in feather-pecking behaviour. *British Poultry Science*, 21: 447–450.

Danbury, T. C., Weeks, C. A., Chambers, J. P., Waterman-Pearson, A. E. and Kestin, S. C., 2000. Self-selection of the analgesic drug carprofen by lame broiler chickens. *Veterinary Record*, 146: 307–311.

Dawkins, M. S., 1981. Priorities in the cage size and flooring preferences of domestic hens. *British Poultry Science*, 22: 255–263.

——. 1982. Elusive concept of preferred group size in domestic hens. *Applied Animal Ethology*, 8: 365–375.

——. 1985. Cage height preference and use in battery-kept hens. *Veterinary Record*, 116: 345–347.

Dawkins, M. S. and Hardie, S., 1989. Space needs of laying hens. *British Poultry Science*, 30: 413–416.

Duncan, I. J. H., 1970. Frustration in the fowl. In: *Aspects of Poultry Behaviour* (Eds. Freeman, B. M. and Gordon, R. F.), pp. 15–31. Edinburgh, British Poultry Science.

——. 1985. How do fearful birds respond? In: *Second European Symposium on Poultry Welfare* (Ed. Wegner, R.-M.), pp. 96–106. Celle, Germany, German Branch of the World's Poultry Science Association.

——. 1989. The assessment of welfare during the handling and transport of broilers. In: *Third European Symposium on Poultry Welfare* (Eds. Faure, J. M. and Mills, A. D.), pp. 93–107. Tours, France, French Branch of the World's Poultry Science Association.

——. 1997. *Killing Methods for Poultry: A Report on the Use of Gas in the U.K. to Render Birds Unconscious Prior to Slaughter*. Guelph, Canada, Col. K.L. Campbell Centre for the Study of Animal Welfare,.

——. 1998. Behavior and behavioral needs. *Poultry Science*, 77: 1766–1772.

——. 2001. The pros and cons of cages. *World's Poultry Science Journal*, 57: 381–390.

——. 2002. Poultry welfare: science or subjectivity? *British Poultry Science*, 43: 643–652.

Duncan, I. J. H. and Kite, V. G., 1989. Nest site selection and nest building behaviour in domestic fowl. *Animal Behaviour*, 37: 215–231.

Duncan, I. J. H. and Mench, J. A., 2000. Does hunger hurt? *Poultry Science*, 79:934.

Duncan, I. J. H. and Wood-Gush, D. G. M., 1971. Frustration and aggression in the domestic fowl. *Animal Behaviour*, 19: 500–504.

——. 1972. Thwarting of feeding behaviour in the domestic fowl. *Animal Behaviour*, 20: 444–451.

Duncan, I. J. H., Beatty, E. R., Hocking, P. M. and Duff, S. R. I., 1991. An assessment of pain associated with degenerative hip disorders in adult male turkeys. *Research in Veterinary Science*, 50: 200–203.

Duncan, I. J. H., Hocking, P. M. and Seawright, E., 1990. Sexual behaviour and fertility in broiler breeder domestic fowl. *Applied Animal Behaviour Science*, 26: 201–213.

Duncan, I. J. H., Slee, G. S., Kettlewell, P., Berry, P. and Carlisle, A. J., 1986. Comparison of the stressfulness of harvesting broilers by machine and by hand. *British Poultry Science*, 27: 87–92.

Duncan, I. J. H., Slee, G. S., Seawright, E. and Breward, J., 1989. Behavioural consequences of partial beak amputation (beak trimming) in poultry. *British Poultry Science*, 30: 479–488.

Duncan, I. J. H., Widowski, T. M., Malleau, A. E., Lindberg, A. C. and Petherick, J. C., 1998. External factors and causation of dustbathing in domestic hens. *Behavioural Processes*, 43: 219–228.

Fletcher, D. L., 2000. Stunning of poultry. In: *Proceedings of the 21st World's Poultry Congress*, Montreal, Canada, 20–24 August 2000. Paper S3.13.02.

Follensbee, M. E., Duncan, I. J. H. and Widowski, T. M., 1992. Quantifying nesting motivation of domestic hens. *Journal of Animal Science*, 70, Supplement 1: 50.

Freire, R., Appleby, M. C. and Hughes, B. O., 1997. Assessment of pre-laying motivation in the domestic hen using social interaction. *Animal Behaviour*, 54: 313–319.

Gentle, M. J. and Hunter, L. N., 1988. Neural consequences of partial toe amputation in chickens. *Research in Veterinary Science*, 45: 374–376.

Gentle, M. J. and Tilston, V. L., 2000. Nociceptors in the leg of poultry: implications for potential pain in pre-slaughter shackling. *Animal Welfare*, 9: 227–236.

Gentle, M. J., Hughes, B. O., Fox, A. and Waddington, D., 1997. Behavioural and anatomical consequences of two beak trimming methods in 1- and 10-d-old domestic chicks. *British Poultry Science*, 38: 453–463.

Gentle, M. J., Waddington, D., Hunter, L. N. and Jones, R. B., 1991. Behavioural evidence for persistent pain following partial beak amputation in chickens. *Applied Animal Behaviour Science*, 27: 149–157.

Gerrits, A. R., De Koning, K. and Migchels, A., 1985. Catching broilers. *Misset International Poultry*, 1 (July): 20–23.

Gregory, N. G. and Wilkins, L. J., 1989. Broken bones in domestic fowl: handling and processing damage in end-of-lay battery hens. *British Poultry Science*, 30: 555–562.

Guhl, A. M. and Ortman, L. L., 1953. Visual patterns in the recognition of individuals among chickens. *Condor*, 55: 287–298.

Harrison, R., 1964. *Animal Machines*. London, Vincent Stuart.

Hocking, P. M., Maxwell, M. H. and Mitchell, M. A., 1996. Relationship between the degree of food restriction and welfare indices in broiler breeder females. *British Poultry Science*, 37:263–278.

Hughes, B. O., 1975a. The concept of an optimal stocking density and its selection for egg production. In: *Economic Factors Affecting Egg Production* (Eds. Freeman, B. M. and Boorman, K. N.), pp. 271–298. Edinburgh, British Poultry Science.

——. 1975b. Spacial preference in the domestic hen. *British Veterinary Journal*, 131: 560–564.

——. 1977. Selection of group size by individual laying hens. *British Poultry Science*, 18: 9–18.

Hughes, B. O. and Appleby, M. C., 1989. Increase in bone strength of spent laying hens housed in modified cages with perches. *Veterinary Record*, 124: 483–484.

Hughes, B. O. and Duncan, I. J. H., 1988. The notion of ethological "need", models of motivation and animal welfare. *Animal Behaviour*, 36: 1696–1707.

Julian, R. J., 1998. Rapid growth problems: ascites and skeletal deformities in broilers. *Poultry Science*, 77: 1773–1780.

Keeling, L. J. and Duncan, I. J. H., 1989. Interindividual distances and orientation in laying hens in groups of three in two different sized enclosures. *Applied Animal Behaviour Science*, 24: 325–342.

Kettlewell, P. J., Hampson, C. J., Berry, P. S., Green, N. R. and Mitchell, M. A., 2000. New developments in bird harvesting, live haul and unloading in the United Kingdom. In: *Proceedings of the 21st World's Poultry Congress*, Montreal, Canada, 20–24 August, 2000. Paper S3.13.01.

Knowles, T. G. and Broom, D. M., 1990. Limb bone strength and movement in laying hens from different housing systems. *Veterinary Record*, 126: 354–356.

Kostal, L., Savory, C. J. and Hughes, B. O., 1992. Diurnal and individual variation in behaviour of restricted-fed broiler breeders. *Applied Animal Behaviour Science*, 32:361–374.

Leeson, S. and Summers, J. D., 1991. *Commercial Poultry Nutrition*. Guelph, Canada, University Books.

——. 2000. *Broiler Breeder Production*. Guelph, Canada, University Books.

Leeson, S., Diaz, G. and Summers, J. D., 1995. *Poultry Metabolic Disorders and Mycotoxins*. Guelph, Canada, University Books.

Lindberg, A. C. and Nicol, C. J., 1993. Group size preferences in laying hens. . In: *Proceedings of the Fourth European Symposium on Poultry Welfare* (Eds. Savory, C. J. and Hughes, B. O.), pp. 249–250. Potters Bar, U.K., Universities Federation for Animal Welfare.

——. 1996. Space and density effects on group size preferences in laying hens. *British Poultry Science*, 37: 709–721.

Malleau, A. E., Duncan, I. J. H. and Widowski, T. M., 1997. Effects of simulated brooding cycles on growth and behaviour of broiler and layer chicks. *Proceeding of the 31st International Congress of the International Society for Applied Ethology* (Eds. Hemsworth, P. H., Špinka, M. and Košt'àl, L.) p. 93. Prague, Czech Republic, Research Institute of Animal Production.

Mashaly, M. M., Webb, M. L., Youtz, S. L., Roush, W. B. and Graves, H. B., 1984. Changes in serum corticosterone concentration of laying hens as a response to increased population density. *Poultry Science*, 63: 2271–2274.

McLean, K. A., Baxter, M. R. and Michie, W., 1986. A comparison of the welfare of laying hens in battery cages and in a perchery. *Research and Development in Agriculture*, 3: 93–98.

McMillan, I., 2000. Selection for improved growth and reduced ascites syndrome incidence. *Proceedings of the 21st World's Poultry Congress*, Montreal, Canada, 20–24 August, 2000. Paper S2.4.05.

Mench, J. A., 1992. The welfare of poultry in modern production systems. *Poultry Science Review*, 4:107–128.

——. 1993. Problems associated with broiler breeder management. In: *Proceedings of the Fourth European Symposium on Poultry Welfare* (Eds. Savory, C. J. and Hughes, B. O.), pp. 195–207. Potters Bar, U.K., Universities Federation for Animal Welfare.

Mench, J. A. and Falcone, C., 2000. Welfare concerns in feed-restricted meat-type poultry parent stocks. In: *Proceedings of the 21st World's Poultry Congress*, Montreal, Canada, 20–24 August, 2000. Paper S3.3.03.

Millman, S. T. and Duncan, I. J. H., 2000a. Strain differences in aggressiveness of male domestic fowl in response to a male model. *Applied Animal Behaviour Science*, 66: 217–233.

——. 2000b. Effect of male-to-male aggressiveness and feed-restriction during rearing on sexual behaviour and aggressiveness toward females by male domestic fowl. *Applied Animal Behaviour Science*, 70: 63–82.

——. 2000c. Do female broiler breeder fowl display a preference for broiler breeder or laying strain males in a Y-maze test? *Applied Animal Behaviour Science*, 69: 275–290.

Millman, S. T., Duncan, I. J. H. and Widowski, T. M., 2000. Male broiler breeder fowl display high levels of aggression toward females. *Poultry Science*, 79: 1233–1241.

Mills, A. D., Duncan, I. J. H., Slee, G. S. and Clark, J. S. B., 1985a. Heart rate and laying behaviour in two strains of domestic chicken. *Physiology and Behaviour*, 35: 145–147.

Mills, A. D., Wood-Gush, D. G. M. and Hughes, B. O., 1985b. Genetic analysis of strain differences in pre-laying behaviour in battery cages. *British Poultry Science*, 26: 182–197.

Mitchell, M. A. and Kettlewell, P. J., 1993. Catching and transport of broiler chickens. In: *Proceedings of the Fourth European Symposium on Poultry Welfare* (Eds. Savory, C. J. and Hughes, B. O.), pp. 219–229. Potters Bar, U.K., Universities Federation for Animal Welfare.

Mitchell, M. A., Carlisle, A. J., Hunter, R. R., and Kettlewell, P. J., 2000. The responses of birds to transportation. In: *Proceedings of the 21st World's Poultry Congress*, Montreal, Canada, 20–24 August 2000. Paper S3.13.05.

Muir, W. M. and Craig, J. V., 1998. Improving animal well-being through genetic selection. *Poultry Science*, 77: 1781–1788.

Newberry, R. C., 1992. Influence of increasing photoperiod and toe-clipping on breast buttons of turkeys. *Poultry* Science, 71: 1471–1479.

Nicol, C. J., 1987a. Effect of cage height and area on the behaviour of hens housed in battery cages. *British Poultry Science*, 28: 327–335.

——. 1987b. Behavioural responses of laying hens following a period of spatial restriction. *Animal Behaviour*, 35: 1709–1719.

Norgaard-Nielsen, G., 1990. Bone strength of laying hens kept in an alternative housing system, compared with hens in cages and on deep litter. *British Poultry Science*, 31: 81–89.

North, M. O. and Bell, D. D., 1990. *Commercial Chicken Production Manual* (4th ed.). New York, Chapman and Hall.

Olsson, I. A. S. and Keeling, L. J., 2000. Night-time roosting in laying hens and the effect of thwarting access to perches. *Applied Animal Behaviour Science*, 68: 243–256.

Owings, W. J., Balloun, S. L., Marion, W. W. and Thomson, G. M., 1972. The effect of toe-clipping turkey poults on market grade, final weight and percent condemnation. *Poultry Science*, 51: 638–641.

Raj, A. B. M., 1993. Stunning procedures. In: *Proceedings of the Fourth European Symposium on Poultry Welfare* (Eds. Savory, C. J. and Hughes, B. O.), pp. 230–236. Potters Bar, U.K., Universities Federation for Animal Welfare.

——. 1996. Aversive reactions of turkeys to argon, carbon dioxide and a mixture of carbon dioxide and argon. *Veterinary Record*, 138: 592–593.

——. 1998. Welfare during stunning and slaughter of poultry. *Poultry Science*, 77: 1815–1819.

——. 2000. Recent developments in stunning of poultry. In: *Proceedings of the 21st World's Poultry Congress*, Montreal, Canada, 20–24 August 2000. Paper S3.13.03.

Renema, R. A. and Robinson, F. E., 2000. Reproductive implications of full–feeding female meat-type poultry parent stocks. In: *Proceedings of the 21st World's Poultry Congress*, Montreal, Canada, 20–24 August 2000. Paper S3.3.02.

Richter, F., 1954. Experiments to ascertain the causes of feather-eating in the domestic fowl. *Proceedings of the 10th World's Poultry Congress, Edinburgh*, 258–262.

Riddell, C., Helmboldt, C. F., Singson, E. P., and Matterson, L. D., 1968. Bone pathology of birds affected with cage layer fatigue. *Avian Diseases*, 12: 285–297.

Rowland, L. O., Fry, J. L., Christmas, R. B., O'Sheen, A. W. and Harris, R. H., 1972. Differences in tibia strength and bone ash among strains of layers. *Poultry Science*, 51: 1612–1615.

Savory, C. J., 1989. Stereotyped behavior as a coping strategy in restricted-fed broiler breeding stock. In: *Proceedings of the Third European Symposium on Poultry Welfare* (Eds. Faure, J. M. and Mills, A. D.). Tours, France, French Branch of the WPSA.

Savory, C. J. and Maros, K., 1993. Influence of degree of food restriction, age and time of day on behaviour of broiler breeder chickens. *Behavioural Processes*, 29:179–190.

Savory, C. J., Hocking, P. M., Mann, J. S. and Maxwell, M. H., 1996. Is broiler breeder welfare improved by using qualitative rather than quantitative food restriction to limit growth. *Animal Welfare*, 5: 105–127.

Savory, C. J., Wood-Gush, D. G. M. and Duncan, I. J. H., 1978. Feeding behaviour in a population of domestic fowl in the wild. *Applied Animal Ethology*, 4: 13–27.

Siegel, P. B. and Wisman, E. L., 1966. Selection for body weight at eight weeks of age. 6. Changes in appetite and feed utilization. *Poultry Science*, 45: 1391–1397.

Singer, P., 1990. *Animal Liberation* (2nd ed.). New York, Avon Books.

Tauson, R., 1980. Cages: how could they be improved? In: *The Laying Hen and its Environment* (Ed. R. Moss), pp. 269–299. Boston, Martinus Nijhoff.

——. 1989. Cages for laying hens: yesterday and today—tomorrow? *Proceedings of the Third European Symposium on Poultry Welfare*, (Eds. Faure, J. M. and Mills, A. D.), pp. 165–181. Tours, France, French Branch of the WPSA.

Vestergaard, K., Hogan, J. A. and Kruijt, J. P., 1990. The development of a behavior system: Dustbathing in the Burmese red junglefowl. I. The influence of the rearing environment on the organization of dustbathing. *Behaviour*, 112: 35–52.

Vince, M. A., 1974. Vocalization and communication in the natural situation. In: *Development of the Avian Embryo* (Eds. Freeman, B. M. and Vince, M. A.), pp. 38–42. London, Chapman and Hall.

Webster, A. B., 1995. Immediate and subsequent effects of a short fast on the behavior of laying hens. *Applied Animal Behaviour Science*, 45:255–266.

——. 2000. Behavior of White Leghorn laying hens after withdrawal of feed. *Poultry Science,* 79:192–200.

Webster, A. B., Fletcher, D. L. and Savage, S. I., 1996. Humane on-farm killing of spent hens. *Journal of Applied Poultry Research*, 5: 191–200.

Webster, A. J. F., 1995. *Animal Welfare—A Cool Eye Toward Eden*. Oxford, Blackwell.

Widowski, T. M. and Duncan, I. J. H., 2000. Working for a dustbath: Are hens increasing pleasure rather than reducing suffering? *Applied Animal Behaviour Science*, 68: 39–53.

Wood-Gush, D. G. M., 1956. The agonistic and courtship behaviour of the Brown Leghorn cock. *British Journal of Animal Behaviour*, 4: 133–142.

——. 1972. Strain differences in response to sub-optimal stimuli in the fowl. *Animal Behaviour*, 20: 72–76.

Wood-Gush, D. G. M. and Gilbert, A. B., 1975. The physiological basis of a behaviour pattern in the domestic hen. *Symposium of the Zoological Society of London*, 35: 261–276.

Woolley, S. C. and Gentle, M. J., 1988. Physiological and behavioural responses of the domestic hen to hypoxia. *Research in Veterinary Science*, 45: 377–382.

Zayan, R. and Doyen, J., 1985. Spacing patterns of laying hens kept at different densities in battery cages. In: *Social Space for Domestic Animals* (Ed. R. Zayan), pp. 37–70. The Hague, Martinus Nijhoff.

Zayan, R., Doyen, J. and Duncan, I. J. H., 1983. Social and space requirements for hens in battery cages. In: *Farm Animal Housing and Welfare* (Eds. Baxter, S. H., Baxter, M. R. and MacCormack, J. A. C.), pp. 67–90. The Hague, Martinus Nijhoff.

Zuidhof, M. J., Robinson, F. E., Feddes, J. J. R., Hardin, R. T., Wilson, J. L., McKay, R. I. and Newcombe, M., 1995. The effects of nutrient dilution on the well-being and performance of female broiler breeders. *Poultry Science*, 74: 441–456.

15

Rethinking Painful Management Practices

Daniel M. Weary and David Fraser

Introduction

Tail docking sheep, branding cattle, castrating pigs, dehorning calves—these are some of the common practices in animal agriculture that are widely acknowledged to cause pain to the animals. The procedures are also unpleasant chores for farmers and sources of concern to many consumers of animal products. Scientists and veterinarians have developed some practical alternatives that cause less pain, yet actual changes in this area remain slow. In some cases, painful procedures may be necessary to ensure human and animal health and safety, but in other cases, evidence of such benefits is lacking. In some cases, less-painful alternatives can be used to achieve the same aims, while in other cases available alternatives seem impractical for producers or no less painful for the animals.

In this chapter, we provide a framework for reconsidering the conventional methods of performing painful management practices on farm animals using examples from some of the most common procedures and promising alternatives.

What Are the Aims of the Procedure?

Practices in production agriculture often become routine, in part because this allows a complex series of tasks to be performed efficiently. Practicing dairy farmers, for example, may need to plant corn, harvest hay, buy grain, sell animals, spread manure, repair equipment, clean the barn, milk the cows, care for sick animals, and direct staff; little wonder that they may not have the time or inclination for critical reflection on whether it is really necessary to dehorn calves, or for research on which methods are most effective and least painful. The role of the academic (whose job *is* critical reflection and research) is therefore to begin with a simple question: why is this procedure performed? With a clear understanding of the aims of the procedure, livestock industries, with input from consumers and society at large, can then enter a meaningful conversation on whether these aims justify any suffering that is caused.

To start on relatively safe ground, let us consider a non-farm-animal example: cosmetic surgeries on companion animals, such as tail docking of dogs like the cocker spaniel, miniature pinscher, and Yorkshire terrier. These procedures are typically performed to meet specifications of breed associations like the American Kennel Club (The American Kennel Club, 1998), with little credible evidence of any benefit to the animal. Traditional reasons for docking (such as improved performance in fighting, ratting, and bearbaiting) no longer apply, and contemporary arguments (such as reduced injuries to the tail and improved hygiene) are not well supported by evidence (Wansbrough, 1996). The only benefit is that the dog will conform to the appearance standards of animal breeders.

Some practices performed on farm animals would seem to fall into a similar category. For example, horses of certain European breeds are branded as part of the breed specification, and, in other cases, cuts are sometimes made to the undersurface of the tail of horses to make them carry their tails at an angle that is aesthetically pleasing to the owner.

In other cases, however, painful procedures are used for important practical goals or, indeed, to prevent other significant animal welfare problems from developing. For cattle grazing unfenced rangeland in North America, branding is used to identify ownership and prevent theft. In the past, hot-iron branding has been the only feasible method of doing this in remote areas. Tail docking of pigs and beak trimming of chickens are done with the aim of preventing tail biting and feather pecking—two behavioral problems that can inflict significant injury and economic loss. Ideally, these behavioral problems would be solved by changing the animals' genetics or environment; but until that is achieved, the behavioral problems provide the main rationale for the painful procedures.

DOES THE PROCEDURE ACHIEVE ITS AIMS AND WHAT ARE THE NEGATIVE EFFECTS ON THE ANIMAL?

If some consensus can be achieved regarding the value of the aims, the next step is to determine if, in fact, these aims are met by the procedure. In some cases, the success of the procedure will seem obvious. For example, the horns of cattle cannot prove a threat to workers and other animals if the horns are removed. Hornless animals can still cause injuries, but the extent of these injuries is reduced (Meischke, Ramsay, and Shaw, 1974). However, even in this example, assessing the downside for the animal requires study; horns may function in dominance interactions, social signaling, and even grooming, and little is known about how loss of horns affects the cow. In many cases, research is also required to judge how successfully the procedure meets its aims. In this section we review two examples. In the first, we show that tail docking of dairy cows fails to provide an anticipated improvement in udder health. In the second, we show that clipping the needle teeth of piglets does succeed in reducing facial injuries caused by fighting.

Stalls for dairy cows are typically designed so that the rear end of the cow extends to or just beyond the end of the stall. This is done to prevent the cows from defecating on the lying surface; but with this design, tails can extend into the alley or gutter behind the stall, where they become soiled. The result, a feces-and-urine-soaked flyswatter, can then become something of a threat to milkers who must navigate themselves and their equipment around the tail. In addition, feces and the bacteria therein can be spread if the tail comes in contact with the cow's body, soiling the cow and her udder and potentially increasing the risk of mastitis.

Some dairy producers have begun tail docking their herds with the aims of increasing milker comfort and improving cow cleanliness and udder health (fig. 15.1). Adult dairy

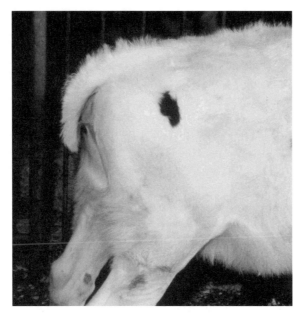

Figure 15.1.   Dairy calf with docked tail.   Recent results show that docked cows are no cleaner and no less likely to develop udder infections than cows with intact tails.

cows are normally docked by placing a tight elastic ring around the tail approximately 12 cm below the vulva. The elastic restricts blood flow killing the distal portion of the tail. Elastic rings are also used to dock calves, although some producers favor a docking iron that both cuts the tail and cauterizes the stump (see Tom et al., 2002, for a comparison of these two methods). There is also variation in the age of docking and the amount of tail removed (Stull et al., 2002).

Some studies have reported improved milker comfort when tails are docked (Matthews et al., 1995; Petrie et al., 1996a), but more modern milking parlors can prevent contact with the tail making this a less-important issue on many farms (Stull et al., 2002). Mastitis, however, remains one of the most important welfare problems for dairy cows, and procedures that could reduce the incidence of udder infections deserve consideration. To determine if tail docking really improves cow cleanliness and udder health, Tucker, Fraser, and Weary (2001) performed an experiment on a large commercial dairy farm. The farmer had decided to dock the five hundred cows in his herd, but agreed, for the purposes of this study, to begin by docking only half the cows. Over the following two months, Tucker et al. monitored cows but found no difference between docked and undocked cows in the amount of debris and feces on the backs, sides, and udders of animals, and no difference in somatic cell counts in the milk (SCC; an indication of udder infections) or in clinical cases of mastitis. A second study (Schreiner and Ruegg, 2002) compared cleanliness, SCC, and bacterial cultures of mastitis-causing pathogens from docked and undocked cattle on nine commercial farms and found no differences in these variables over the eight to nine months of the study. Eicher et al. (2001) also found no difference in udder cleanliness between docked and undocked animals. Thus, tail docking dairy cows does not seem to provide the intended benefits in terms of cow cleanliness and udder health.

Tail docking also has disadvantages to the cow, including possible pain from the procedure and the loss of functions normally served by the tail. For example, cows use their tails to control flies, and studies have shown that flies are more likely to disturb docked cows than cows with intact tails (e.g., Eicher et al., 2001). Given these disadvantages, and the lack of evidence for the purported benefits, dairy producers have little to gain from docking cows.

Piglets are born with eight fully erupted "needle teeth" (the deciduous canines and third incisors), which the animals use to deliver sideward bites to the faces of littermates when fighting at the udder. Producers often clip these teeth soon after birth using clippers or side-cutting pliers. Farmers perform the procedure with the intention of preventing injuries caused by the teeth to either the sow's udder or the faces of other piglets. The procedure actually seems to have little effect in reducing injuries to the udder, as these injuries are rare even when piglets have intact teeth (Robert, Thompson, and Fraser, 1995; Brown et al., 1996). In contrast, intact teeth are clearly associated with facial lesions on littermates (Fraser, 1975; Brown et al., 1996). In one experiment, we tested the effect of clipping by performing the procedure on just one side of the mouth, leaving some litters with intact teeth on the left side and others on the right. Due to the side-to-side biting typical of competition for teats, facial lesions were much more frequent on the left side of the face for those litters that had intact teeth on their right (fig. 15.2), and vice versa for those with intact teeth on the left (Weary and Fraser, 1999).

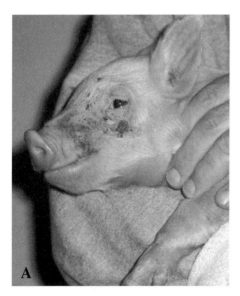 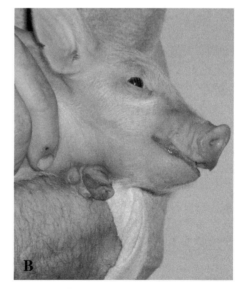

Figure 15.2.   The effect of teeth clipping on facial lacerations.   Piglets in this litter had clipped teeth on the left and intact teeth on the right. The side-to-side fighting for teats caused lesions on the left side of the faces of littermates (A), but not on the right side (B).

Unfortunately, teeth clipping also involves some negative consequences for the piglet. In addition to any pain and distress associated with the handling and operation, clipping exposes the pulp cavity and allows for pulpitis and gingivitis. Clipping can also damage the gums and cause splintering of the teeth and subsequent damage to the mucous membrane of the lips (Burger, 1983; Hutter et al., 1994).

CAN THE PROCEDURE BE MODIFIED TO REDUCE THE PAIN AND DISTRESS?

For procedures such as teeth clipping, which achieve important aims but have certain disadvantages to the animals' well-being, the challenge is to search for alternatives that address the disadvantages while meeting the aims and remaining feasible in practice.

Refining the Procedure

In some cases, relatively minor changes in how the procedure is performed can have important consequences in reducing pain and negative side effects. For example, removing just the tips of the needle teeth in piglets, as opposed to the conventional practice of clipping the teeth right to the gum line, has been shown to reduce damage to the teeth and gums (Hutter et al., 1994). In addition, we have found that partial clipping of teeth is as effective as full clipping in reducing facial lacerations to littermates (Weary and Fraser, 1999). In this case, we can recommend the alternative: removing just the tip of the tooth (with either clippers or a grinding tool) can be as effective in reducing lacerations to other piglets, while minimizing negative effects of the procedure such as damage to the teeth and gums.

There are several other good examples in the scientific literature showing how refinements to painful procedures can provide improvements for the animals. For instance, the use of freeze branding has been shown to cause less pain to cattle than does the more traditional hot-iron branding (Schwartzkopf-Genswein et al., 1998). Similarly, there is evidence that the use of tight elastics to castrate and tail dock lambs is less painful to the animals than the common alternative of cutting with a knife (Lestor et al., 1991).

Much work remains to be done to identify promising refinements. Fortunately, some painful procedures are done in a variety of ways on different farms. Hence, better procedures may already be in use and are now just waiting to be found and more widely adopted. Unfortunately, at least some of these alternatives appear to provide little or no advantage to the animal. For example, piglets are castrated in a bewildering variety of manners: in the way piglets are held, in the methods used to cut the scrotum, and in the way the spermatic cords are severed. In a series of experiments testing commonly used alternatives (Weary, Braithwaite, and Fraser, 1998; Taylor and Weary, 2000; Taylor et al., 2001), we found no evidence that any one method was less painful or distressing to piglets than others.

One important variable is the age at which the procedure is performed. Many procedures, such as piglet castration, are done at an early age in the belief that this reduces the pain and distress associated with the procedure. It has been a long-standing assumption among producers, veterinarians, and researchers that neonatal animals have a reduced ability to perceive pain. This assumption is reflected in husbandry recommendations to perform routine on-farm surgical procedures such as castration, tail docking, and dehorning within the first few weeks of life (e.g., Canadian Veterinary Medical Association, 1996, p. 8).

In some cases, an age effect will seem obvious. For example, much more tissue damage results from removing fully developed horns on adult cattle than from cauterizing the horn buds on week-old calves. Similarly, castrating a sexually mature boar is likely more damaging than castrating a week-old piglet. McGlone and Hellman (1988) compared the pain response to castration of weaned piglets (7 to 8 weeks old) versus preweaned piglets less than 20 days of age and found that the older piglets showed a stronger and longer lasting response to castration.

Unfortunately, this result does not mean that invasive procedures can be considered innocuous if performed at young ages, or that further improvements can be made by moving to progressively younger ages. In one experiment, Taylor et al. (2001) found that preweaned piglets responded strongly to castration regardless of whether the procedure was performed at 3, 10, or 17 days of age. The castrated piglets produced many more high-frequency calls (in excess of 1 kHz) during the procedure than did piglets that were sham castrated (i.e., handled identically) (fig. 15.3). Although there were differences between the age groups, these occurred for both the castrates and the shams, so that the effect of castration was similar at the three different ages.

The findings from this study, together with recent work in human pediatric medicine (Wolf, 1999), tends to undermine the idea that the newborn's perception of pain is limited. Of particular concern are results indicating that pain experienced early in life has long-term developmental effects that can actually accentuate later sensitivity to painful events (Ruda et al., 2000). Performing painful operations at younger ages may have some advantages, but there are no bases for complacency; neonates can be highly sensitive to pain and, like older animals, require procedures that cause less pain.

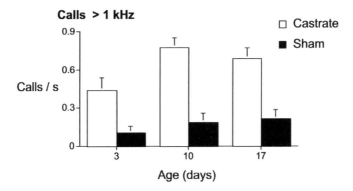

Figure 15.3.   Piglets vocalize during castration, especially producing calls greater than 1 kHz in frequency. The mean (+ S.E.) rates of these calls during the procedure are shown for piglets (*n* = 84) castrated or sham castrated at 3, 10, and 17 days of age. Piglets responded similarly to castration at all three ages (Adapted from Taylor et al., 2001).

In conclusion, there is often a range of alternative methods, and some provide real advantages to animals. In many cases, however, even the most humane of these alternatives will still result in significant pain. Thus, we also need to consider if analgesics, anesthetics, or other methods of managing the pain can be practically included as part of the procedure.

Anesthetics and Analgesics

If procedures like dehorning and castration cause pain, then surely we can improve the procedures simply by controlling the pain. Unfortunately, as we will show in the examples below, effective methods of pain control are not always available and some of these have other drawbacks. We review two examples. The first shows that a series of interventions can successfully reduce pain and distress associated with hot-iron dehorning in dairy calves. The second example reviews some less-successful attempts to mitigate pain due to castration in piglets. For further discussion on issues related to pain management, please see chapter 4.

Hot-iron dehorning of calves involves applying an iron, heated to about 600°C, to the area around the horn bud so as to cauterize the blood supply and other tissue feeding the developing horn. The procedure causes a pronounced pain response, as evidenced by behaviors during the procedure including tail wagging, head movements, tripping, and rearing (e.g., Graf and Senn, 1999); behaviors associated with postoperative pain such as head rubbing, head shaking, and ear flicking (e.g., McMeekan et al., 1999); and increased levels of circulating corticosteroids in the hours following the procedure (e.g., Petrie et al., 1996b). It has long been acknowledged that use of a local anesthetic can reduce the pain caused by the procedure and thus dampen cortisol and behavioral responses, but the use of local anesthetic alone is unsatisfactory for several reasons.

One reason is that local anesthetic does not provide adequate postoperative pain relief. The most popular local anesthetic, lidocaine, is effective for only two to three hours after administration (McMeekan et al., 1998). Indeed, some studies indicate that calves treated with local anesthetic actually have higher plasma cortisol levels than untreated animals after the local anesthetic loses its effectiveness (Graf and Senn, 1999; McMeekan et al., 1998; Petrie et al., 1996b). However, the use of nonsteroidal anti-inflammatory drugs (such as ketoprofen), in addition to a local anesthetic, can much reduce postoperative pain responses. One study (Faulkner and Weary, 2000) monitored how often calves shook their heads and flicked their ears during the 24 hours after hot-iron dehorning. As illustrated in figure 15.4, calves that received ketoprofen in their milk meal before dehorning showed far fewer of these behaviors in the hours after dehorning than did the control calves that did not receive ketoprofen.

The use of local anesthetic alone is not a perfect solution for other reasons as well. Calves respond to both the pain of the procedure and to the physical restraint required to perform it. Calves dehorned using a local anesthetic still require restraint, and they respond so strongly to restraint that it can be difficult for observers to be certain if adequate nerve blockage has been achieved. Calves must also be restrained while the local anesthetic is administered, as well as during the actual dehorning. Thus, calves experience the distress

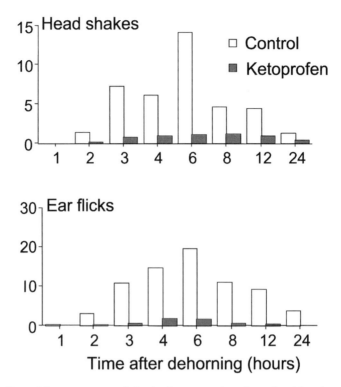

Figure 15.4. Two of the most common behavioral responses by calves after dehorning are head shakes and ear flicks. This figure shows the mean frequency of these behaviors during the 24 hours after hot-iron dehorning of dairy calves ($n = 20$) either with or without ketoprofen (Adapted from Faulkner and Weary, 2000).

associated with restraint on two occasions, and still may not receive an adequate nerve block. The use of a sedative (such as xylazine) can essentially eliminate calf response to the administration of the local anesthetic and the need for physical restraint during the administration of the local anesthetic and during dehorning (Grøndahl-Nielsen et al., 1999).

Thus, a combination of three treatments—a sedative, local anesthetic, and a nonsteroidal anti-inflammatory—provides effective pain management. The sedative allows for careful administration of the local anesthetic, with no response by the calf. The combination of sedative and local anesthetic allows for dehorning with no immediate pain response or other signs of distress. The combination of all three treatments reduces the pain responses both during dehorning and in the hours that follow.

However, such interventions may also have drawbacks for the animal. For example, the sedative xylazine can be dangerous; cattle are highly sensitive to this drug and mistakenly delivering a higher dose could kill the calf. In addition, the lack of behavioral response by sedated animals can be difficult to interpret—does this mean that the calf is oblivious to the handling, or is it simply difficult for the animal to move? Also, the recovery from the sedative may itself be distressing for the animal. In the dehorning example, other concerns are associated with both the local anesthetics (e.g., repeated injections necessary for the ring block) and the nonsteroidal anti-inflammatories (e.g., risk of gastric ulcers). Progress in this area will require collaboration with veterinary anesthesiologists to find a combination of procedures that works best for the animals.

Methods of pain mitigation must also be practical. The ideal alternatives are those that actually make the procedure easier or cheaper for producers to perform. In the dehorning example, the degree of physical restraint required to dehorn nonsedated calves often makes this a two-person job. A sedative makes the procedure easy to perform alone, and arguably makes the chore safer and less unpleasant for the farmer.

Castration typically involves two types of painful event: the incision of the scrotum, followed by pulling and severing the spermatic cord. Behavioral responses to these two aspects indicate that the latter is more painful (Taylor and Weary, 2000). A number of studies have shown that the immediate response to castration can be much reduced by infusing the scrotum with local anesthetic. For example, White et al. (1995) compared responses of piglets to castration, with and without local anesthetic delivered in this way, and found much reduced behavioral and physiological responses by piglets that had received the local anesthetic.

Unfortunately, it is not clear whether this treatment is ultimately beneficial to the piglet. Piglets show evidence of great distress when simply restrained, and delivery of the local anesthetic means that piglets have to be restrained twice—once to receive the injection and a few minutes later (after the local has taken effect) when they are castrated. Moreover, the injections themselves may be painful.

There have been attempts to use general anesthesia with piglets to control both the pain and distress due to restraint. Unfortunately, one of these attempts (McGlone and Hellman, 1988) had problems with either the dosage or the combination of drugs (an injection of xylazine, ketamine hydrochloride, and glyceryl guaiacolate) so that about 30 percent of the piglets died under anesthesia. In a more recent experiment, Kohler et al. (1998) found that piglets could be safely and effectively anesthetized for castration using carbon dioxide, but the piglets showed a strong behavioral and physiological response to the induction. Thus, at this stage, it seems that satisfactory methods of reducing the pain and distress due to castration are not readily available. In such cases, we need to reconsider whether the procedure needs to be done at all, or if the aims can be achieved in a much different manner.

Rethinking the Procedure

Meat from intact males can have an unpleasant flavor known as boar taint. The main compounds associated with boar taint are androstenone and skatole stored in the fat of sexually mature males. Male pigs that have been castrated produce little of these compounds, and are no more likely to have tainted meat than are female pigs. This is the primary reason why piglets in North America are castrated.

However, castration is a poor solution from the perspective of both the piglets and the producers. The piglets experience the pain and distress caused by castration. The farmers bear the costs of time taken to perform the chore combined with the reduced growth rate, poorer feed conversion, and poorer carcass quality typical of castrated piglets (e.g., Campbell and Taverner, 1988). In such cases, there is a role for more radical innovations, such as immunocastration. Gonadotropin releasing hormone (GnRH) is a naturally occurring hormone that initiates reproductive development by stimulating the release of other reproductive hormones and growth of the testicles. Immunologists have taken the creative approach of injecting animals with an altered form of GnRH. These injections act to immunize the pigs against the GnRH in their own bodies, much reducing testicular growth, production of other sex hormones, and the compounds responsible for boar taint. In one recent study, Dunshea et al. (2001) injected uncastrated pigs with a modified form of GnRH eight and four weeks before slaughter. They found that the carcasses from these immunocastrated pigs had very low levels of both androstenone and skatole, similar to those of castrated pigs, and much less than the levels found in boars (fig. 15.5). The immunocastrated pigs also had fewer skin lesions than did untreated boars, likely reflecting a lower level of fighting among these pigs. Thus, immunocastration avoids the pain and distress from castration and fighting, while allowing for the improved growth rate, feed conversion, and carcass quality typical of intact males.

Beak trimming of laying hens is another procedure that may be phased out in the future. Group-housed hens often peck at one another, and this pecking can result in feather and skin damage, and occasionally in death. To reduce the severity of injuries due to pecking, chicks typically have the distal portion of their beaks amputated, a procedure thought to cause both acute and chronic pain. Part of the problem of bird aggression may be due to genetic selection by poultry breeders. In selecting individual birds with the highest egg production in a group, geneticists may have been breeding inadvertently for aggressive, competitive behavior. In contrast, when geneticists keep related birds together, and select whole cages of birds that achieve high production on average, they breed for an ability to do well in a social setting. Given that laying hens are typically housed in groups on commercial farms, selecting productive groups would seem a better strategy than productive individuals. Indeed, experimental work has shown that such group-level selection can lead,

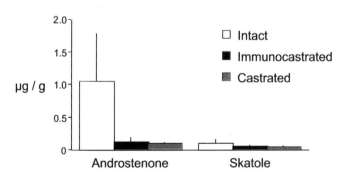

Figure 15.5.   Mean (+ S.E.) concentrations of androstenone and skatole in fat of carcasses of intact male pigs, immunocastrated males, and castrated males when slaughtered at 26 weeks of age. Immunocastration reduced the level of both compounds to that found in castrated males (Adapted from Dunshea et al., 2001).

in just a few generations, to birds that are both highly productive and relatively nonaggressive, to the extent that beak trimming may become unnecessary (Muir, 1995).

IMPLEMENTING CHANGE

Given our current knowledge about animal pain and methods to control it, how can we achieve implementation of better pain management in practical farm animal production?

The way animal industries are structured can either facilitate or discourage the replacement of painful procedures. In countries such as Australia and New Zealand, many pig producers avoid castration (and boar taint) by slaughtering pigs at lighter weights, well before the animals reach sexual maturity. In North America, meat processors, seeking to avoid the increased cost of slaughtering lighter animals, often refuse or discount pigs below a defined weight range. Thus, decisions by the slaughter industry limit the ability of North American producers to avoid castration of pigs. Similarly, companies that buy weaned pigs for further feeding may pay less for pigs with intact tails. Hence, even if the genetics and rearing environment are such that tail docking is unnecessary to prevent tail biting, docking may still be needed simply to ensure satisfactory prices for the animals.

In such cases, solutions may require cooperation between different parties in the animal industries. Elk ranchers in Alberta sell "velvet" antlers (partly grown antlers with active nerve and blood supply) for traditional oriental medicine. Presumably sawing the antlers at this stage is extremely painful for the animals. Effective anesthetic and analgesic drugs are available, but only veterinarians can buy the drugs, and it would be impractical to bring a veterinarian to the ranch every time the operation is done. To solve the problem, an agreement was reached between the elk ranchers and the Alberta Veterinary Medical Association whereby veterinarians train and certify ranchers to do the procedure themselves using local anesthetics obtained under the veterinarian's license. The agreement gives the animals the benefit of the anesthetics without being unduly onerous for the producer.

Economic incentives can sometimes help to reduce the use of painful procedures. For example, the Burger King Corporation has indicated that it will not buy beef from animals that have been subjected to wattling (cutting of the loose skin on the neck), severe ear notching, or repeated branding as means of animal identification. This provides an incentive for producers to stop these procedures.

The regulatory system sometimes promotes effective pain management and sometimes prevents it. In the United Kingdom, the law requires that anesthetic be used for dehorning or electrical disbudding of cattle. On the other hand, pain-management tools like ketoprofen, which are useful analgesics for such procedures, are not approved for this use in many countries; in this case, the regulatory controls over veterinary pharmaceuticals may stand in the way of improved pain management. Similarly, a procedure like immunocastration will require regulatory changes in various jurisdictions before it can be used to replace painful alternatives. In other cases, regulations actually require or encourage painful procedures to be carried out. In some states and provinces in North America, branding is the only legal means for identifying cattle grazing on publicly owned land; even if we had a workable alternative to branding for identifying free-ranging cattle, a regulatory change would still be required for the practice to end.

Simple traditions also play a role. As we have seen, ear cropping of dogs and branding of horses are done for reasons of tradition and appearance. Traditional attitudes among producers are also involved in decisions about painful procedures. For example, polled (i.e., genetically hornless) sires are readily available for many breeds of beef cattle, so producers can avoid both the cost and the pain of dehorning simply by mating cows to these sires. The range and quality of these sires is similar to that for horned animals, and many beef producers are now using polled genetics. However, some breeders remain opposed to the change. As one rancher was quoted as saying, the push toward the use of polled sires and away from dehorning "is scary and quite frankly, it's bullshit—it's like hot iron branding, there's really no effect on the cattle" (Thomas, 2000).

SUMMARY

In summary, we have provided a simple framework for addressing painful management practices. First, we considered the aims of the procedure. In some cases, such as the cosmetic branding of horses, a re-examination of the aims may suggest to the industry (or its critics) that these are too trivial to justify the resulting pain. Second, we asked whether the procedure actually meets these aims. As shown in the example of tail docking dairy cows, the aim of reducing the incidence of udder infections is commendable, but there is no evidence that tail docking achieves this end. Third, we asked whether the procedure can be modified to reduce the pain, while still meeting the aims and the practical constraints of the production system. In some cases, a refinement of the procedure can make an important difference, such as clipping just the distal third of the needle teeth in piglets as opposed to the conventional practice of clipping the teeth right to the gum line. In other cases, anesthetics and analgesics can be effective, as with dehorning of dairy calves. In yet other cases, such as castration of piglets, simple refinements and pain control methods seem inadequate or impractical, so that a major innovation (immunocastration) or changing the production constraints (reducing body weight at slaughter) is required. Ultimately, the best solutions need to be adopted by livestock producers; this may require incentives, regulatory changes, and altered attitudes of individuals who work with animals.

ACKNOWLEDGMENTS

We thank Sarah Murphy, Cassandra Tucker, and Cathy Schuppli for their contributions to this chapter. We are also grateful to our collaborators in the scientific work on these procedures including Allison Taylor, Leah Braithwaite, and Paul Faulkner. Our work is supported by the Natural Sciences and Engineering Research Council of Canada through the Industrial Research Chair in Animal Welfare, and by contributions from the Dairy Farmers of Canada, the Beef Cattle Industry Development Fund, the BC Dairy Foundation, the British Columbia SPCA, members of the BCVMA, and many other donors listed on our web site at www.agsci.ubc.ca/animalwelfare.

REFERENCES

American Kennel Club. 1998. The Complete Dog Book. 19th Edition. Howell Book House, New York.

Brown, J. M. E, Edwards, S. A., Smith, W. J., Thompson, E. and Duncan, J. 1996. Welfare and production implications of teeth clipping and iron injection of piglets in outdoor systems in Scotland. Prev. Vet. Med., 27: 95–r105.

Burger, A. 1983. Untersuchungen über die Folgen der Zahnresektion beim Ferkel. Inaugural Dissertation, Tierärztlichen Fakultät der Ludwig Maximilians-Universität, Munich.

Campbell, R. G. and Taverner, M. R. 1988. Genotype and sex effects on the relationship between energy intake and protein deposition in growing pigs. J. Anim. Sci. 66: 676–686.

Canadian Veterinary Medical Association. 1996. Animal welfare position statements. Canadian Veterinary Medical Association, Ottawa.

Dunshea, F. R., Colantoni, C., Howard, K., McCauley, I., Jackson, P., Long, K. A., Lopaticki, S., Nugent, E. A., Simons, J. A., Walker, J., and Hennessy, D. P. 2001. Vaccination of boars with a GnRH vaccine (Improvac) eliminates boar taint and increases growth performance. J. Anim. Sci. 79:2524–2535.

Eicher, S. D., Morrow-Tesch, J. L., Albright, J. L. and Williams, R. E. 2001. Tail-docking alters fly numbers, fly-avoidance behaviors, and cleanliness, but not physiological measures. J. Dairy Sci. 84: 1822–1828.

Faulkner, P. and Weary, D. M. 2000. Reducing pain after dehorning in dairy calves. J. Dairy Sci. 83: 2037–2041.

Fraser, D. 1975. The "teat order" of suckling pigs. II. Fighting during suckling and the effects of clipping the eye teeth. J. Agric. Sci., Camb. 84: 393–399.

Graf, B. and Senn, M. 1999. Behavioral and physiological responses of calves to dehorning by heat cauterisation with or without local anaesthesia. Appl. Anim. Behav. Sci. 62: 153–171.

Grøndahl-Nielsen, C., Simonsen, H. B., Lund, J. D. and Hesselholt, H. 1999. Behavioral, endocrine and cardiac responses in young calves undergoing dehorning without and with the use of sedation and analgesia. Vet. J. 158: 14–20.

Hutter, S., Heinritzi, K., Reich, E. and Ehret, W. 1994. Efficacitéde différentes méthodes de résection des dents chez le porcelet non sevré. Revue Med. Vet. 145: 205–213.

Kohler, I., Moens, Y., Busato, A., Blum, J. and Schatzmann, U. 1998. Inhalation anaesthesia for the castration of piglets: CO_2 compared to halothane. J. Vet. Med. A. 45: 625–633.

Lestor, S. J., Mellor, D. J., Ward, R. N. and Holmes, R. J. 1991. Cortisol responses of young lambs to castration and tailing using different methods. N.Z. Vet. J. 39: 134–138.

McGlone, J. J. and Hellman, J. M. 1988. Local and general anesthetic effects on behavior and performance of two- and seven-week-old castrated and uncastrated piglets. J. Anim. Sci. 66: 3049–3058.

McMeekan, C. M., Stafford, K. J., Mellor, D. J., Bruce, R. A., Ward, R. N. and Gregory, N. G. 1998. Effects of regional analgesia and/or non-steroidal anti-inflammatory analgesic on the acute cortisol response to dehorning calves. Res. Vet. Sci. 64: 147–150.

——. 1999. Effects of a local anaesthetic and a non-steroidal anti-inflammatory analgesic on the behavioral responses of calves to dehorning. N.Z. Vet. J. 47: 92–96.

Matthews, L.R., Phipps, A., Verkerk, G.A., Hart, D., Crockford, J.N., Carragher, J.F. and Harcourt, R.G. 1995. The effects of taildocking and trimming on milker comfort and dairy cattle health, welfare and production. Animal Behaviour and Welfare Research Centre, Hamilton, NZ.

Meischke, H. R. C., Ramsay, W. R. and Shaw, F. D. 1974. The effect of horns on bruising cattle. Aust. Vet. J. 50: 432–434.

Muir, W. M. 1995. Group selection for adaptation to multiple-hen cages: selection program and direct responses. Poult. Sci. 75: 447–458.

Petrie, N. J., Mellor, D. J., Stafford, K. J., Bruce, R. A., Ward, R. N. 1996a. Cortisol responses of calves to two methods of tail docking used with or without local anaesthetic. N.Z. Vet. J. 44: 4–8.

——. 1996b. Cortisol responses of calves to two methods of disbudding used with or without local anaesthetic. N.Z. Vet. J. 44: 9–14.

Robert, S., Thompson, B. K. and Fraser, D. 1995. Selective tooth clipping in the management of low-birth-weight piglets. Can. J. Anim. Sci. 75: 285–289.

Ruda, M. A., Ling, Q.-D., Hohmann, A. G., Peng, Y. B. and Tachibana, T. 2000. Altered nociceptive neuronal circuits after peripheral inflammation. Science 289:628–630.

Schreiner, D. A. and Ruegg, P. L. 2002. Tail docking and milk quality. J. Dairy Sci. 85: 2513–2521.

Schwartzkopf-Genswein, K. S., Stookey, J. M., Crowe, T. G. and Genswein, B. M. A. 1998. Comparison of image analysis, exertion force, and behavior measurements for use in the assessment of beef cattle responses to hot-iron and freeze branding. J. Anim. Sci. 76: 972–979.

Stull, C. L., Payne, M. A., Berry, S. L. and Hullinger, P. J. 2002. Evaluation of the scientific justification for tail docking dairy cattle. J. Am. Vet. Med. Assoc. 220: 1298–1303.

Taylor, A. A. and Weary, D. M. 2000. Vocal responses of piglets to castration: identifying procedural sources of pain. Appl. Anim. Behav. Sci. 70: 17–26.

Taylor, A. A., Weary, D. M., Lessard, M. and Braithwaite, L. A. 2001. Behavioral response of piglets to castration: the effect of piglet age. Appl. Anim. Behav. Sci. 73:35–43.

Thomas, L. 2000. Is it time to go polled? Canadian Cattlemen, December 20, 22–23.

Tom, E. M., Rushen, J., Duncan, I. J. H. and de Passillé, A. M. 2002. Behavioral, health and cortisol responses of young calves to tail docking using a rubber ring or docking iron. Can. J. Anim. Sci. 82: 1–9.

Tucker, C. B., Fraser, D. and Weary, D. M. 2001. Tail docking dairy cattle: effects on cow cleanliness and udder health. J. Dairy Sci. 84: 84–87.

Wansbrough, P. K. 1996. Cosmetic tail docking of dogs. Am. J. Vet. 74: 59–63.

Weary, D. M. and Fraser, D. 1999. Partial tooth-clipping of suckling pigs: effects on neonatal competition and facial injuries. Appl. Anim. Behav. Sci. 65: 21–27.

Weary, D. M., Braithwaite, L. A. and Fraser, D. 1998. Vocal response to pain in piglets. Appl. Anim. Behav. Sci. 56: 161–172.

White, R. G., DeShazer, J. A., Tressler, C. J., Borcher, G. M., Davey, S., Waninge, A., Parkhurst, A. M., Milanuk, M. J. and Clemens, E. T. 1995. Vocalization and physiological response of pigs during castration with or without a local anesthetic. J. Anim. Sci. 73: 381–386.

Wolf, A. R. 1999. Pain, nociception and the developing infant. Paediatr. Anaesth. 9: 7–17.

16

Alternatives to Conventional Livestock Production Methods

Michael C. Appleby

INTRODUCTION

Methods used in livestock production change frequently and vary between geographical areas, so one response to the title of this chapter might be that it is impossible to say what are conventional methods and what are alternatives. Tethering of dairy cows is usual in some countries and regions, rare in others.

However, a common tendency in developed countries over the last 50 years has been the drive for efficiency in agriculture, for cutting the cost of producing each egg or pound of meat or pint of milk. This was initiated by public policies—before, during, and after World War II—in favor of more abundant, cheaper food. It subsequently became market driven, with competition between producers and between retailers to sell food as cheaply as possible, and thereby acquired its own momentum. The specific methods that producers use to achieve efficiency vary with circumstances, but the general tendency of attempting to cut unit costs is defined here as the conventional approach to livestock production, and alternatives to that approach will be considered. Obviously, no producer ignores costs, so all producers will have some methodology in common that can be described as conventional by this definition. The point here is that "alternative livestock production methods" have some motivation in addition to cost cutting. "Livestock" is used here to include poultry.

In fact, the conventional approach, emphasizing efficiency, has not always identified the best methods even to achieve its own aims. It took an alternative approach, aimed at reducing problems for the animals concerned, to identify the fact that humane treatment of livestock by workers improves growth rate and reproduction (see chapter 2). A similar approach showed that understanding animal behavior can improve design of handling systems and, hence, efficient use of labor in handling livestock (see chapters 7 and 8). In both cases, the unit cost of producing or handling animals can be reduced, after an initial investment in worker training or facilities, while also improving animal welfare. There are doubtless many other aspects of livestock production where both cost efficiency and welfare can be increased, for example by reducing disease. Concern for animal welfare may be important in recognizing such opportunities, but clearly that concern, as expressed throughout this book, will not be satisfied by making only those improvements for welfare that also increase production efficiency. It is necessary to address alternative approaches to agriculture that do not only emphasize efficiency. In doing so, it becomes apparent that other alternative concerns, in addition to that for welfare, also have an impact on welfare.

SPECIAL CONCERNS AND NICHE MARKETS

For most people purchasing food, cheapness is attractive, and so, most of the animal products they buy have been produced by conventional production methods. However, in recent years many different concerns have been expressed over the impact of such methods on animal welfare, the environment, food safety and quality, food security, family farms, farmworkers, rural communities, and developing countries. Some people are willing to seek out and pay more for food produced by alternative methods that take these concerns into account. There have always been some producers who use such methods and obtain higher selling prices to offset their higher production costs—if, indeed, their production costs are really higher, which is often a matter of debate. They do this either because they share the concerns or for business reasons, or both.

The concerns listed are not mutually exclusive: they tend to overlap. Correspondingly, methods that diverge from the conventional emphasis on efficiency tend to address several concerns. This makes economic sense for the producers, as they may be able to sell their products to people with different concerns.

One of the most important of these alternative, specialty or niche markets is organic food. Sales have risen so fast in the last decade or so, that demand has often exceeded supply. The two main reasons why people buy organic food are probably health—people worry about hormones, pesticides, and other artificial chemicals in food—and a perception that organic production is less damaging to the environment.

But the meaning of "organic" is not self-evident, so many countries have drawn up specifications. And these specifications include husbandry methods for animals. For example, most require that livestock have access to the outdoors. This is true in the United States, for instance, which introduced its National Organic Plan in October 2002. Husbandry methods affect the impact of the operation on the environment: thus, allowing animals outdoors spreads their manure directly instead of by liquid slurry. They also affect the product: giving animals more space is essential if they are to be kept in good health without antibiotics or other chemicals.

Agencies drawing up the specifications, such as the Soil Association in the UK, have another reason for requiring special treatment of livestock. They say that consumers do not expect organic food to come from animals in conventional, close confinement. They expect animals kept for organic production to be looked after well, to be in "natural conditions." The end result is that the welfare of these animals is probably, on balance, better than in conventional production, because they have more space, more varied environment, and so on. Concern is sometimes expressed that there may be pest infestations and disease outbreaks on organic farms that are left untreated because chemical treatments would lead to loss of organic status, but this is probably rare. There are many successful organic farms where the animals are apparently healthier than in conventional conditions, without either such health problems or the need to treat them.

Another niche market that overlaps with organic food is that for "free-range" products. People's reasons for buying these are again diverse. In the case of free-range meat, the main factor is probably taste, which is affected by the animals' diet, their activity, and their rate of growth: in some cases slower growing breeds are used. This market has developed particularly strongly in France, where concern for food quality is high. Concern for welfare in France is not particularly strong, but the welfare of chickens and pigs reared for this production appears to be generally good: cost cutting is not a priority, and often animals are not just outdoors but in woodlands. In the case of free-range eggs, consumers' reasons for purchase often explicitly include the welfare of the hens themselves. Whether the welfare of free-range hens is better than that of hens in houses will be discussed below, but people certainly perceive it to be so. Criteria for free-range egg production will also be covered below.

The theme of freedom has also been emphasized in niche markets that specifically address concern for animal welfare. The leader in this field is the UK's Royal Society for Prevention of Cruelty to Animals, which launched its Freedom Food program in 1994. There are detailed criteria that must be met by producers who want to join the program. They can then use the Freedom Food label. This includes the name "RSPCA," which has widespread recognition and confidence from the British public. The RSPCA also helps with marketing. The program has grown steadily, helped by the overlap in criteria between this and other schemes. If producers are already certified organic or for producing free-range eggs, they do not usually have to make many additional changes to be able to use the Freedom Food label, which is therefore well worthwhile.

Similar programs have begun in North America. The American Humane Association started its Free Farmed scheme in 2000; Certified Humane was launched by Humane Farm Animal Care in 2003; and in Canada, SPCA Certified food was launched in British Columbia in 2002. The first and third of those programs have a label with a red barn that conveys other messages as well as that about welfare standards—for example, that the farming methods used are traditional. Another welfare organization involved in a similar way is the United States' Animal Welfare Institute, which has humane husbandry criteria for pigs. One large cooperative of family pig farmers has adopted these criteria and uses this fact as part of its marketing strategy.

Other concerns, and labels and niche markets that address those concerns, may also have an impact on welfare. Examples include concerns about use of genetic engineering in farm animals and injection of dairy cows with bovine growth hormone. Another example with a less obvious connection is the increasing interest shown in buying locally produced food. The motivation for this is probably mainly related to the environment (cutting "food miles" uses less fuel and produces less pollution) and to considerations of community. However, farms advertising to local consumers also use their own image as part of the sales pitch, and often welcome visitors, and are therefore much more likely to treat their animals well than to use close confinement and other "industrial" animal production methods.

The fact that all these niche markets, and the methods used to supply them, address overlapping concerns is not coincidental. They all place a much greater emphasis on the animals themselves than do conventional methods. These alternative methods can be said to be animal centered, to recall that animal production is first and foremost a biological process rather than taking the technological approach that has become conventional. This can be contrasted with one other, narrower feature often used in marketing food: its freshness. The freshness of milk, eggs, or meat says nothing about how the animals that produced it were treated.

Most of these niche markets could, in theory, expand until they include all food produced, with all producers meeting the relevant criteria. However, most will in practice continue to take a relatively small proportion of the total market for the foreseeable future. Nevertheless, these alternatives have had a disproportionately large influence on how farm animals are treated, by leading the way to wider changes. This topic will recur later in this chapter, under Mechanisms for Change.

How are animals actually treated, under alternative approaches to livestock production, and what effects does this have on welfare? In the next section, specific methods will be considered briefly: those intended to tackle a specific problem or promote a specific advantage. One important area will then be covered separately, namely, methods of feeding. After this, whole environments will be addressed: first the special case of environments for handling and transport—because during these procedures the environment is new to the animals and all-important—and then general approaches to environmental design.

SPECIFIC METHODS

This section will be brief, for two related reasons. First, the fact that alternatives to conventional livestock production methods address diverse, overlapping concerns means that producers rarely use one specific alternative method in isolation. When they do, it is likely to be for a special marketing pitch, for example for grain-fed beef or the "five grain eggs" that were sold in the UK for some years. These examples are similar to the marketing of freshness already mentioned, in not being animal centered. That is because—and this is the second reason for the section's brevity—in a complex environment, few specific changes will have restricted effects. For example, a controversial aspect of conventional livestock housing is use of bare concrete or wire for flooring. This can cause injury, particularly in large animals that have high weight to area ratio for parts of the body in contact with the floor. One response is use of bedding for dairy cows. Nilsson (1992, p. 100) has emphasized that in prevention of injury, softness of the floor is important: "Lying areas for dairy cows must have a certain degree of softness to lessen the incidence of injuries and to provide comfort. Studies of this problem showed that the incidence of injuries decreases with an increase in the softness of the floor in standings used for tied dairy cows." However, floors must not be too soft because "animals experience a very soft underlay as being unstable for standing on. They must have a firm footing for the hooves." Indeed, different characteristics and effects of floors interact (pp. 94, 107):

> The most important physical properties of the walking and lying surfaces in livestock buildings are: thermal comfort, softness, friction, abrasiveness. . . . It is obvious that the

> optimal values of all the floor properties are difficult if not impossible to fulfil simulta-
> neously. Instead the aim must be to work out a compromise which as much as possible
> fulfils the different demands. . . . Other important properties of the floors in livestock
> houses are mechanical strength, cleaning ability, toxicity, pathogenicity, etc.

Furthermore, changing animals' flooring influences not just their standing and lying, but
other behavior such as exploration, nesting, aggression, and often feeding.

To express the same issue in a different way, a producer who makes one change in rearing methods—such as stopping use of antibiotics, or tail docking, or early weaning—will
certainly have to be vigilant in subsequent husbandry and will probably have to make other
changes in routine practices, to cope with the varied effects of that change. So no attempt
will be made here to draw up a comprehensive "wish list" of alternative practices that
would improve animal welfare, although such a list could readily be compiled from the
other chapters of this book.

FEEDING METHODS

Feeding is often very closely controlled in animal agriculture, for obvious reasons: feed is
one of the most costly inputs, and growth and production are the main outputs. There are
benefits to the animals of such control, but also clear disadvantages when animals have difficulties adapting to environments different from those in which their behavior evolved.
So, although in production terms the effectiveness of an environment can be judged in
terms of efficiency of food intake, the design of the environment often leads to problems
in which individuals within the system are compromised in some way. For example, pregnant sows are usually fed well below voluntary intake, in one or two small concentrate
meals per day. When they are kept in stable groups, most aggression is related to feeding
(Martin and Edwards, 1994). Attempts to solve such problems are most likely to be successful if the causes of the problems are understood. Thus,

> feed related aggression depends on both the accessibility of the feed and the space
> around the feeding area. Outdoor sows have more space available than housed animals,
> and their food is typically distributed over a greater area. It is possible that the prob-
> lems [of aggression] experienced by low-ranking sows may be less pronounced. (Mar-
> tin and Edwards, 1994, p. 64)

In fact, such modification of the environment not only may lead to reduction in undesirable food related behavior such as high levels of aggression, but also may increase food
conversion efficiency.

Modifications can range from a total change in environment, as in the example above,
to small changes in the way food is offered. For example, the diet itself can be modified to
make it more palatable using flavorings or more bulky to increase gut fill. Thus, sugar beet
or chopped straw added to concentrate feeds can lead to a decrease in vulva biting in sows
(van Putten and van de Burgwal, 1990).

There has been considerable research on feeding methods, and sometimes on their implications for welfare, but few methods studied experimentally have been widely adopted because of economic constraints. A notable exception is electronic feeders for sows, and this is a good illustration of the importance of understanding animal behavior—of designing animal-centered methods.

The main impetus for development of electronic sow feeders was not improvement of welfare but reduction of labor, and this may account for the fact that little attention was initially given to the behavior of the animals who would actually be using them. The first models launched commercially had a single rear opening for both entry and exit, with no gate. Sows waiting to eat, hungry because of restricted rations, often directed severe aggression against the sow currently using or leaving the feeder. Another problem was that high-ranking sows sometimes lay down inside, blocking access for others. These problems were so significant that it was apparent these models had not been properly tested with groups of sows. Addition of an automatic gate prevented aggression while a sow was inside but not while she was leaving. The problem was finally solved by addition of a front exit. This also reduced the incidence of blocking—because a sow pushing in at the rear entrance can usually persuade the incumbent to leave rather than to lie down—and allowed animals that have eaten to be shed into a separate pen, preventing them from attempting reentry. The method is now common in some countries. This is doubtless mainly because its labor requirements are lower than hand-feeding, but it has also facilitated the introduction of group housing. Further, it can be argued that the availability of this method was an important factor in the European Union's decision to phase out stalls and tethers for pregnant sows.

Feeding methods do vary fairly widely; for example, they obviously differ for animals kept housed or on pasture. However, the example of electronic feeders demonstrates that, as with other specific methods discussed in the previous section, changes to feeding methods cannot be made in isolation but must be considered in the context of whole systems.

Handling and Transport

It is important to mention the handling and transporting of animals, because these procedures involve changes to their whole environment, or at least to many of its most important aspects, to the extent that it is common for welfare to be compromised in all the areas indicated by the Five Freedoms. These are promulgated by the UK's Farm Animal Welfare Council (FAWC) and comprise (1) freedom from hunger and thirst, (2) freedom from discomfort, (3) freedom from pain, injury, and disease, (4) freedom from fear and distress, and (5) freedom to express normal behavior (FAWC, 1997).

Considerable progress has been made in handling methods (see chapters 7 and 8), for the reason, mentioned above, that here improvements in welfare are also economic. With transport, as with feeding, research has elucidated many implications for welfare. For example, Stephens and Perry (1990, p. 50) used the operant approach to test response of pigs to vibration and noise in a transport simulator:

All the pigs learned to press the switch panel which turned the transport simulator off. The animals usually began to make responses during the first training session of 30 min and by the fourth session they kept the apparatus switched off for about 75% of the time. . . . These experiments clearly demonstrate that young growing pigs find the vibration to be aversive and that the pigs responded behaviourally to terminate the vibration of their pen.

This sort of work is being used to identify methods of transport that have less impact on welfare than those currently in use. However, also as with feeding, implementation has been limited, affected by practicality, expense, and the relative priority given to welfare. This whole area of management requires more thought than it has previously been given: for example, such issues as whether preslaughter transport is necessary at all or whether animals could be slaughtered on the farm deserve much more attention. A promising advance in this respect is a mobile unit for slaughtering and processing meat on-farm, currently being developed for use in the San Juan Islands of Washington State, USA, where otherwise animals have a long boat journey to slaughter (Lopez Community Land Trust, undated).

GENERAL METHODS

The clearest example of alternatives to conventional methods in environmental design for farm animals is that of systems for laying hens in Europe. This probably stems from the fact that the demand for eggs is inelastic: eggs are not readily interchangeable with other items in the diet, and people tend to buy a set number whatever the price. And there have always been some consumers who prefer to pay more for eggs, apparently with the feeling that by doing so they are getting a better quality product. This background may explain why, almost uniquely among animal production sectors, the system in which eggs were produced became a selling point. A niche market began to develop, particularly in northern Europe, for eggs that did not come from cages: free-range eggs in some countries, deep litter or "scratching" eggs in others. Initially, this was mostly roadside sales in the country from farmyard flocks, but in the 1980s such eggs also began to be produced by larger companies and sold in shops. Some people bought them—at a higher price—because they perceived them to be more nutritious, tastier, or healthier. Some were also concerned about the welfare of the hens, and this concern led to the development of other noncage systems in the 1970s and 1980s. A problem was that eggs sold as free range might come from hens allowed to range only inside a house, or allowed outside only if they could find one small exit from a large building, and other terms were similarly ill defined.

The European Community acted in 1985 by imposing legislation on its member countries, defining four labels that can be put on eggs and the corresponding conditions in which hens must be kept (table 16.1). Absence of any of these labels implies that eggs come from battery cages. The latter are generally called conventional laying cages in the industry, and battery cages are also conventional in the sense used in this chapter: designed

Table 16.1. Criteria Defined by the European Community for Labeling of Eggs

Label	Criteria
Free range	Continuous daytime access to ground mainly covered with vegetation Maximum stocking density 1,000 hens/hectare
Semi-intensive	Continuous daytime access to ground mainly covered with vegetation Maximum stocking density 4,000 hens/hectare
Deep litter	Maximum stocking density 7 hens/m^2 A third of floor covered with litter Part floor for droppings collection
Perchery or barn	Maximum stocking density 25 hens/m^2 Perches, 15 cm for each hen

Source: CEC (1985).

to maximize economic efficiency. The European Union is currently revising the categories in table 16.1. From 2004, all eggs must be labeled and only three descriptions will be allowed: free range (a compromise between the current free range and semi-intensive criteria), barn (with changed criteria), and caged.

A similar trend for marketing of eggs from alternative systems began in North America in the 1990s, but is still small to date. Terminology varies and eggs are sold with descriptions such as "cage free." In the United States, use of the term *free range* is regulated, but only minimally: it requires that birds should be given *some* outdoor access, not how much or for how long.

By the 1990s, about 20 percent of eggs sold in the UK were free range, and an additional proportion of barn eggs. In the late 1990s, some supermarket chains actively promoted this trend. Some sold barn eggs at the same price as cage eggs, while one chain stopped stocking cage eggs altogether. In other countries, such as Denmark and Germany, deep litter eggs are more popular. It should be noted, though, that these sales are mostly of eggs sold whole. Few ready-made meals or other products containing eggs indicate how the hens were kept, and few customers think to ask—although commercial purchasers may do so, as discussed in the next section.

Battery cages compromise most or all of FAWC's (1997) Five Freedoms, and even contravene the very limited freedoms recommended in the Brambell Report (1965), which said that farm animals should have freedom "to stand up, lie down, turn around, groom themselves and stretch their limbs." Noncage systems alleviate these problems. However, there is one major welfare problem that is generally worse in all these systems than in battery cages. If birds are not beak trimmed, cannibalism is likely, often affecting a high proportion of birds. Beak trimming is practiced as a preventative measure, but this mutilation has become increasingly controversial. Promise that this problem is soluble is offered by developments in Switzerland, which banned both laying cages and beak trimming in 1992.

Various systems based on the Dutch tiered-wire floor designs are used (Matter and Oester, 1989). It seems that performance of these, and welfare of the birds, was relatively poor at first but improved with experience (Fröhlich and Oester, 2001). Their farms are small compared to other countries, though, and their success has yet to be replicated elsewhere. Cannibalism is rare in battery cages, even among birds with untrimmed beaks, but beak trimming is nevertheless common in pullets intended for cages, partly to reduce feather pecking. A possible causal factor for cannibalism in noncage systems is their larger group size, although this is not proven. This led to development of another alternative, modified or enriched cages for small groups, providing increased area and height compared to conventional cages, and also a perch, a nest box, and a litter area (Sherwin, 1994; Appleby et al., 2002).

In 1996, the Scientific Veterinary Committee of the European Community produced a report on welfare in different housing systems. It noted that all systems have welfare benefits and deficiencies. For example (p. 109):

> [In c]urrent battery cage systems . . . the risk of cannibalism is low and there is no necessity for beak trimming. . . . [However,] because of its small size and its barrenness, the battery cage as used at present has inherent severe disadvantages for the welfare of hens.
>
> To retain the advantages of cages and overcome most of the behavioural deficiencies, modified enriched cages are showing good potential in relation to both welfare and production.
>
> Housing systems such as aviaries, percheries, deep litter or free range provide . . . improved possibility for the birds to express a wider range of behaviour patterns. . . . [However,] mainly because of the risk of feather pecking and cannibalism, these systems have severe disadvantages for the welfare of laying hens.

Consequently, the European Union passed a Directive (CEC, 1999) that will phase out battery cages (conventional cages) by 2012 but still allow enriched cages.

However, there is no complete consensus on the merits of different systems. Germany decided in 2001 that, in the context of a Europewide phasing out of conventional battery cages, it will also disallow enriched cages within its own borders, producing a situation similar to that in Switzerland. A similar response is being considered by The Netherlands and the UK. This must depend partly on the weighting by these countries of the welfare advantages of noncage systems—primarily freedom of movement and increased variety of behavior—against the disadvantages—primarily the need for beak trimming. There are thus some elements of science in the decision, and some elements of general attitudes to welfare. It is recognized that people vary in their attitude to welfare, emphasizing either animal feelings, functioning, or naturalness (Fraser et al., 1997). This decision may reflect an increased emphasis on naturalness in Germany, sometimes expressed in the criticism "an enriched cage is still a cage."

This variety in approaches to welfare offers a useful explication of the idea expressed earlier, that many alternatives to conventional livestock production methods can be said to be animal centered. In general, such alternative methods will take account of all these approaches: feelings, functioning, and naturalness. The three approaches can also be identified in the Five Freedoms (FAWC, 1997), which include freedom from mental problems such as hunger and physical problems such as disease, as well as freedom to perform normal or natural behavior.

As one example of a housing system that fits such a model, an alternative to crates for veal calves was developed by Webster (1995) and colleagues. The following passage considers the interaction between different aspects of welfare—nutrition, health, and behavior—and while mental aspects are not mentioned explicitly, it is clear that feelings, functioning, and naturalness are all involved here.

> We called our approach the Access system. Calves wearing transponders were reared in groups of 14 to 20 in straw yards and given access to a computer-controlled feeding station which dispensed rationed amounts of milk replacer and a small amount of solid feed containing sufficient digestible fibre to stimulate rumen development. All the calves had to learn was that a teat would appear in one station if they were due for a milk feed but would not appear if they had already had enough; similarly for the solid ration. All calves acquired these basic computer skills within two days. The Access system has, to date, only been used on an experimental scale but it did show that when calves are given just enough of the sort of solid food necessary to normalize rumen development, enteric diseases can be reduced to the low level considered acceptable in normal calf rearing units. Furthermore, since enteritis triples the risk that calves will subsequently contract pneumonia, respiratory infections were normalized as well. Simply put, the calves were now healthy because their development was normal and because they were healthy they could be run in groups. (p. 188)

MECHANISMS FOR CHANGE

The increasing numbers of people, throughout the developed world, who are concerned about farm animal welfare, do not want improvements in the welfare of just the animals that supply them personally with food, but of all farm animals. As such, the developments in the egg market described in the previous section are particularly important: the fact that a significant proportion of people—albeit still a minority—were willing to pay to support their principles was taken as grounds for politicians to introduce more widespread improvements, not only to poultry welfare but also to welfare of other farm animals. This is reasonable. Surveys have shown that more people say they want welfare of farm animals to be improved, even if this increases food prices, than actually buy higher-priced welfare-friendly products such as free-range eggs in the shops (Bennett, 1997). In other words, they are behaving as citizens when they answer the questionnaire, as consumers juggling varied priorities when they do the shopping. The only case where people have actually been asked to vote on legislation to improve animal welfare, with associated higher costs, was in Switzerland, and they did approve that legislation: the ban on battery cages was the result of a referendum.

The introduction to this chapter mentioned the pressure for cheap food production that has been widespread over the last 50 years or so. This pressure is sometimes described—including by the animal production industry—as a consumer demand for cheap food, but this is an oversimplification implying that people want cheapness at the expense of all other considerations and that cutting prices is an end that justifies all possible means. It is not surprising, indeed it is reasonable, that offered two otherwise similar products most shoppers will buy the cheaper. In fact, it is not reasonable to expect shoppers to take day-by-day responsibility for animal welfare at the point of sale, any more than they are expected to do so for other issues that are of concern to society such as pollution. It is increasingly apparent that people who do not look after farm animals themselves expect those who do to take responsibility for doing so properly—either voluntarily or involuntarily.

This expectation is being realized in both Europe and the United States, but by different mechanisms. In the United States, the lead is now being taken by the retail sector. A senior executive of one of the major fast food chains has commented that their customers expect them—the restaurant company—to ensure that the animals supplying them with food are properly looked after (England, 2002). That company is following the lead of the McDonalds Corporation, which in 2000 started requiring its suppliers to provide laying hens with the same space allowance as in Europe, and not to practice forced molting. McDonalds buys 2.5 percent of U.S. eggs. Subsequently, the National Council of Chain Restaurants and the Food Marketing Institute (which represents the major supermarket chains) developed a collaborative program, producing Husbandry Guidelines for their suppliers of animal products in 2002. These do not go as far as European legislation, but they are significant in acknowledging the importance of animal welfare and in forming a basis for possible future raising of welfare standards.

Both legislation and retail pressure avoid the limitations inherent in "purchasing power," for example the tendency of the latter to apply to whole eggs but not to egg products. This is important because an increasing proportion of food is sold in processed form.

In fact, the shift toward sale of preprocessed food in developed countries offers hope for widespread improvement of farm animal welfare. If a meal containing animal products is bought in a supermarket or restaurant, those products account for only about 5 percent of the price. So an increase in cost of animal production by, say, 10 percent would only increase the cost of such meals by 0.5 percent. Most customers would not notice such a change and would approve it, if asked, to benefit animal welfare or the environment. McInerney (1998) has analyzed this approach for real examples such as the banning of battery cages and sow gestation crates and shown that there is little financial impact on either consumers, or on farmers—who can offset increased costs with increased income as discussed above.

Finding mechanisms for change is difficult in an industry largely driven by competition, especially as that competition is intensifying with the burgeoning international trade in agricultural produce. Alternative livestock production methods, benefiting animal welfare, can and should replace those based solely on narrow, short-term financial criteria that have become conventional over the last few decades. Achieving such a change will, however, be a slow process.

REFERENCES

Appleby, M.C., Walker, A.W., Nicol, C.J., Lindberg, A.C., Freire, R., Hughes, B.O., and Elson, H.A., Development of furnished cages for laying hens, *British Poultry Science,* 43 (2002), 489–500.

Bennett, R.M., Economics, in M.C. Appleby, and B.O. Hughes (eds.), *Animal Welfare.* Wallingford, UK: CAB International, 1997, pp. 235–48.

Brambell, F.W.R., *Command Paper 2836.* London, UK: Her Majesty's Stationery Office, 1965.

CEC (Commission of the European Communities), Amendment 1943/85 to Regulation 95/69, also amended by 927/69 and 2502171, *Official Journal of the European Communities, 13 July 1985.*

——. Council Directive 1999/74/EC laying down minimum standards for the protection of laying hens, *Official Journal of the European Communities 3rd August 1999,* L 203, 53–57.

England, C., Burger King and animal welfare: Why did this company get involved? *Proceedings, Canadian Association for Laboratory Animal Science & Alberta Farm Animal Care Conference.* Edmonton, Canada: CALAS, 2002, p. 13.

FAWC (Farm Animal Welfare Council), *Report on the Welfare of Laying Hens.* Tolworth, UK: FAWC, 1997.

Fraser, D., Weary, D.M., Pajor, E.A., and Milligan, B.N., A scientific conception of animal welfare that reflects ethical concerns, *Animal Welfare,* 6 (1997), 187–205.

Fröhlich, E.K.F., and Oester, H., From battery cages to aviaries: 20 years of Swiss experience, in H. Oester and C. Wyss (eds.), *Proceedings, 6th European Symposium on Poultry Welfare.* Zollikofen, Switzerland: World's Poultry Science Association, 2001, pp. 51–59.

Lopez Community Land Trust, San Juan County Food Processing Center. Lopez, WA, USA: Lopez Community Land Trust, undated.

Martin, J.E., and Edwards, S.A., Feeding behaviour of outdoor sows: the effects of diet quantity and type. *Applied Animal Behaviour Science,* 41 (1994), 63–74.

Matter, F., and Oester, H., Hygiene and welfare implications of alternative husbandry systems for laying hens, in J.M. Faure and A.D. Mills (eds.), *Proceedings, Third European Symposium on Poultry Welfare.* Tours, France: World's Poultry Science Association, 1989, pp. 201–12.

McInerney, J.P., The economics of welfare, in A.R. Michell, and R. Ewbank (eds.), *Ethics, Welfare, Law and Market Forces: The Veterinary Interface.* Wheathampstead, UK: Universities Federation for Animal Welfare, 1998, pp. 115–132.

Nilsson, C., Walking and lying surfaces in livestock houses, in C.J.C. Phillips and D. Piggins (eds.), *Farm Animals and the Environment.* Wallingford, UK: CAB International, 1992, pp. 93–110.

Scientific Veterinary Committee, *Report on the Welfare of Laying Hens.* Brussels, Belgium: Commission of the European Communities Directorate-General for Agriculture VI/B/II.2, 1996.

Sherwin, C.M. (ed.), *Modified Cages for Laying Hens.* Potters Bar, UK: Universities Federation for Animal Welfare, 1994.

Stephens, D.B., and Perry, G.C., The effects of restraint, handling, simulated and real transport in the pig (with reference to man and other species). *Applied Animal Behaviour Science,* 28 (1990), 41–55.

Van Putten, G., and van de Burgwal, J.A., Vulva biting in group-housed sows: preliminary report, *Applied Animal Behaviour Science,* 26 (1990), 180–86.

Webster, A.J.F., *Animal Welfare: A Cool Eye Towards Eden.* Oxford, UK: Blackwell, 1995.

17

Euthanasia

Robert E. Meyer and W. E. Morgan Morrow

INTRODUCTION

While the public accepts and demands animal products, it also wants assurances that the animals are not miserable (Rollin, 1995). Despite the best efforts of managers to provide for animals under their care, we often see animals on the farm that have failed to respond to treatment, are suffering from conditions for which there are no treatments, or suffer conditions that have effective but prohibitively expensive treatments. Euthanasia (derived from the Greek as "good death") is the humane and responsible management solution for these animals. Euthanasia is not, and should never be considered as, the "easy way out" for poor managers. Rather, euthanasia should be considered a tool for managers: a means to alleviate the suffering of individual animals and protect the health of all animals under their care.

By definition, euthanasia should be timely and humane; in practice, however, achieving both goals on the farm is difficult. Most managers intuitively understand that euthanasia is an important part of good husbandry, but that doesn't necessarily make the actual process any easier to carry out for an individual affected animal. Also, the rapid industrialization of production agriculture, as exemplified in the swine industry, has brought about many changes, most notably fewer individuals with a farming background looking after the animals. Publicity following recent prosecutions of people mistreating animals during the euthanasia process has resulted in industrywide concern with the issue of on-farm euthanasia.

Because the euthanasia process combines physical restraint of an animal with a lethal action or chemical agent, animal handlers are at risk for physical injury or even death. Moreover, some farmworkers suffer psychological distress when asked to euthanatize animals in their care. We know this is a problem because farm managers tell us it is and researchers have documented the problem for companion animal handlers involved in the euthanasia process. Worker distress associated with on-farm euthanasia is a poorly understood area in production agriculture; who is most affected, how can their concerns be addressed, how can their distress be alleviated? An especially vexing industry problem is that of euthanatizing the well, but uneconomic, farm animal. Providing clear criteria for treatment or euthanasia of farm animals seems likely to provide at least some psychological relief.

In this chapter, we address what we believe to be some of the major challenges to animal welfare facing the animal production industry: (1) defining criteria for on-farm euthanasia during normal steady-state production, (2) the impact of on-farm euthanasia practices on farmworkers, and (3) euthanasia during an emergency such as a foreign animal disease (FAD) outbreak.

THE EUTHANASIA PROCESS

Guidelines for euthanasia methods have been established by the American Veterinary Medical Association (AVMA) (Beaver et al., 2001). These guidelines discuss relevant physiology, animal and human behavioral considerations, modes of action, and the relative merits of the available methods. Industry-specific guidelines for euthanasia, such as the National Pork Producers Council guide *On Farm Euthanasia of Swine* (NPPC, 1997) and university-produced extension training materials such as *On-Farm Euthanasia: Better Ways* (Morrow and Meyer, 2001), agree with AVMA-accepted methods and processes. When questions arise as to acceptable euthanasia methods and processes, the AVMA guidelines should be considered the final arbiter.

The euthanasia process should be painless and distress free. Pain is the sensation that results when nerve impulses from peripheral nociceptors reach a functioning cerebral cortex and associated subcortical brain structures. Anesthetized animals and properly euthanatized animals do not feel pain because the necessary sensory processing within the cerebral cortex is blocked or disrupted. Reflex motor activity and movement, such as limb withdrawal or generalized seizures, may still occur, however pain is not consciously perceived by the animal in the absence of a functioning cerebral cortex. When evaluating euthanasia methods, it is important to remember that loss of consciousness should precede loss of muscle movement activity. Agents and methods that prevent movement through muscle paralysis but do not block or disrupt the cerebral cortex are not acceptable as the sole agent for euthanasia because they result in conscious perception of pain and distress.

All euthanatizing agents cause death by three basic mechanisms: direct depression of neurons necessary for life function, hypoxia, and physical disruption of brain activity (Beaver et al., 2001). Direct depression of neurons necessary for life function can be achieved through overdose of inhaled anesthetics, such as halothane or isoflurane, or through overdose of injectable barbiturate anesthetics, such as Beuthanasia-D. Consciousness is usually lost quickly, movement and motor activity are minimal, especially with the barbiturates, and death occurs from cardiac and respiratory arrest. These agents are not routinely used to euthanatize farm animals for several reasons, including, in the case of the barbiturates, the need for prescribed use and strict inventory controls and tracking, as well as the potential to poison animals or people ingesting the carcass. From a worker safety perspective, these drugs should not be available to farmworkers (Morrow, 1999).

Hypoxia is commonly achieved by exposing animals to high concentrations of gasses that displace oxygen, such as carbon dioxide, nitrogen, or argon, or by exposure to carbon monoxide to block uptake of oxygen by red blood cells. Preslaughter carbon dioxide stunning of swine is currently used in parts of Europe (Troeger and Waltersdorf, 1991). Exsanguination is another method of inducing hypoxia, albeit indirectly, and is often recommended as a way to ensure death in an unconscious or moribund animal.

Physical disruption of brain activity is the most commonly used method of euthanasia for on-farm euthanasia. This can be produced through a blow to the skull resulting in concussive stunning, through direct destruction of the brain with a captive bolt or bullet, or through depolarization of brain neurons following electrocution. Death follows when the midbrain centers controlling respiration and cardiac activity fail. Physical disruption methods are often followed by exsanguination. These methods are inexpensive, humane, and painless if performed properly, and leave no drug residues in the carcass. Furthermore, animals presumably experience less fear and anxiety with methods that require little preparatory handling. However, physical methods usually require a more direct association of the operator with the animals to be euthanatized, which can be offensive to, and upsetting for, the operator. Reflex movement following the onset of unconsciousness can be particularly unsettling.

EUTHANASIA AND THE FARMWORKER

The physical and potential psychological hazards of euthanasia methods to animal workers have been reviewed (Morrow, 1999). While the specific dangers of the various agents and methods are well documented, information on the risks farmworkers face when euthanatizing animals are often only intuitively understood or recognized from anecdotal reports of injury.

Adverse psychological reactions are reported in shelter animal handlers and laboratory technicians having to perform euthanasia (Rollin, 1986). Shelter workers are particularly at risk because they have to euthanatize so many animals. Estimates for the number of animals euthanatized annually in the United States vary from 8 million (HSUS, 1992) to 14 million (MSPCA, 1987). Depression, unresolved grief, anger, and nightmares have been reported by shelter workers following euthanasia of animals under their care (Ellis, 1993). Other shelter workers reported anger, guilt, frustration, and sadness or suffered sleepless nights, bouts of crying, and severe depression (White and Shawhan, 1996). In contrast, others reported that they had little or no emotional feelings about euthanasia. Laboratory technicians report it is very stressful for them when they are asked to euthanatize a group of animals they have been tending for months or years (Arluke, 1999). Another dissatisfied group is veterinarians who are asked to euthanatize healthy pets. The unpleasantness of the task is exacerbated when the reason has little to do with the welfare of the animal but more for the convenience of the owner. An interesting finding is that cultural differences do exist among veterinarians in their acceptance of euthanasia. In two studies reported in 1990, 74 percent of 167 veterinarians in England reported that, if requested by the owner, they would euthanatize a healthy animal (Fogle and Abrahamson, 1990) whereas in Japan only 44 percent of 2,500 veterinarians would do likewise (Kogure and Yamazaki, 1990).

Although peer-reviewed studies on the attitudes of farm-animal workers toward the task of euthanasia are scarce, most farming people we ask state that they do not enjoy it. In a survey of job satisfaction, farrowing managers reported the most dissatisfaction with their job (31.3 percent reporting their job satisfaction as "needs changes" or "poor") compared with managers (17.2 percent), assistant managers (26.9 percent), and herdsmen (24.4 percent) (Kliebenstein, Hurley, and Orazem, 1996). We surmise that at least a part of their dissatisfaction is associated with their job requirement of having to euthanatize many compromised piglets (Matthis, 2002). For business in general, and for the agricultural animal industry in particular, hiring and retaining quality employees is a major responsibility of management and an increasingly difficult task. To help decrease labor turnover, management must be sensitive to factors contributing to employee unease; and if it is related to euthanasia, a special effort will be needed to resolve these issues.

We suspect farmworkers' attitudes to euthanasia vary according to their prior experience. For example, people raised on farms who have euthanatized animals before, or seen others do it, may be less likely to find it objectionable. Increasingly, the people working on farms do not have a farming background and have no prior experience of euthanasia. Part of the reason people dislike euthanatizing animals is that they transfer their fear and the unpleasantness they feel to the animal and assume it is experiencing the same feelings. This is normal, we all do it, but each of us does it to varying degrees. Farm managers must recognize differences among people in their aversion to euthanasia and delegate the responsibilities accordingly. If people are constantly and reluctantly exposed to euthanasia, they can experience and/or exhibit dissatisfaction with their work, absenteeism, belligerence, or careless and callous handling of animals. To ease the stress, managers should discuss the euthanasia protocol in detail, including the necessity for euthanasia, and encourage the handlers to participate in supportive discussion groups (Wolfe, 1985).

As discussed previously, we are "limited" to methods of euthanasia that act through the mechanisms of direct neuronal depression, disruption of brain activity, and hypoxia. Regardless of the method, however, people are disturbed less by the euthanasia process when they feel distanced from the physical act of euthanasia or when animals exhibit little or no movement. For example, laboratory technicians reported they felt more comfortable gassing animals, where they were more dissociated from the animals' death, than directly killing the animal with cervical dislocation (Arluke, 1999). Focus groups of North Carolina swine farm managers have told us they would prefer euthanasia methods "where you give a shot and the animal goes to sleep" over the physical methods currently in use.

The challenge with regard to euthanasia and the farmworker will be twofold: to determine how the euthanasia process impacts farmworkers, and then to use that information to refine existing euthanasia methods to be more acceptable to the individuals charged with performing the task.

EUTHANASIA IN STEADY-STATE PRODUCTION OPERATIONS

Generally, an animal should be culled when it is no longer profitable or euthanatized when it is inhumane to let it live. The difficulty all managers encounter is defining when animals become uneconomic and whether to treat or euthanatize the challenged animal. While simply stated, both "uneconomic" and "inhumane" are enormously difficult to quantify. Individual managers usually resort to a very subjective assessment often heavily weighted by the perceived economic value of the animal (its ability to return a profit). Practically, both criteria should be considered to create better guidelines for farm managers. Again, focus groups of North Carolina farm managers have told us that having clear criteria for when to euthanatize an animal would help reduce some of the job stress they feel.

Economic Perspective: Market Pigs

Market pigs have no individual performance records and the decision to treat or euthanatize is usually based on a subjective, often cursory, usually superficial, clinical examination. Implementing a program that consistently addresses the care and treatment of the compromised market pig has never been easy.

When pigs are moved into the next stage of production (e.g., weaner pigs to a nursery and then into a grow-finish barn), management usually weight-sorts the pigs and places compromised pigs into special (hospital) pens. Pigs are added to these special pens throughout the production cycle as they fall behind their pen-mates or develop conditions requiring special care and attention. Unfortunately, this does not solve the problem, because on many farms there are still too many gaunt, rough-coated, compromised pigs that will never make it to market let alone return a profit.

Economic Perspective: Sows

Deciding when to cull sows is easier because over successive parities managers have accumulated some information on their individual performance. Economically, a sow should stay in the herd as long as the expected profit from her next litter is higher than the lifetime average of a replacement gilt. The exception is when she needs to be euthanatized to ease her suffering. Managers can determine from the herd records what she is likely to do in her next parity based on performance of other similar sows, and they can use that information to help them make a more informed decision based on the economic value of the sow.

DETERMINING PAIN AND SUFFERING

Assessment of animal pain is difficult. Physical suffering can be conceptualized as the product of pain and its duration. Managers can usually identify those animals suffering the most because, for example, they exhibit aberrant behavior or have visible lesions (e.g., burns, lacerations, compound fractures) making their condition obvious. However, the issue is clouded because a condition may be visually striking but less painful (e.g., prolapses) or inconspicuous but more painful (e.g., arthritis). Pain may reduce normal pig social behaviors and vocalization, while vocalization in response to handling may be more pronounced. Changes in gait, reluctance to move, and hiding in bedding may also be observed (Hardie, 2000; Dobromylskyj et al., 2000).

By daily monitoring, farm managers can usually estimate pain duration but the difficulty of estimating pain intensity remains. Objective measures, such as blood pressure, temperature, and heart rate, are considered unreliable guides to the presence of pain (Conzemius et al., 1997) and are difficult to determine in the pig. Clinicopathological measurements of humoral factors, such as epinephrine, norepinephrine, and cortisol, are also unreliable estimators of pain (Dobromylskyj et al., 2000).

Behavior-based pain scoring systems, scored by an experienced observer, have been developed to assess pain in nonverbal human infants (McGrath and Unruh, 1989). Behavior-based pain scales use a variety of methods to quantify pain (Hardie, 2000; Dobromylskyj et al., 2000). The *simple descriptive scale* consists of three to five expressions describing various levels of pain intensity (e.g., "no pain" through "severe pain"). Each expression is assigned an index value, and the sum of the index values becomes the pain score. The *visual analog scale* is generally a 100 mm line with "no pain" at one end and "severe pain" at the other. A mark is made on the line to indicate the amount of pain being suffered; the distance from the "no pain" end to the mark becomes the pain score. The *numerical rating scale* is similar, in that the observer picks a number between 0 and 10 or 0 and 100. The *multifactorial pain scale* is usually a composite of many simple descriptive scale values that relate behavior to pain. When the multifactorial pain scale also includes physiologic variables, it is sometimes confusingly called a *numerical rating scale* or a *variable rating scale*. These scales have all been adapted for use in companion and farm animals; however, studies suggest that behavioral monitoring may be difficult unless animals are in moderate-to-severe pain (Flecknell, 1996). Further, the ability of human observers to discriminate between levels of pain based on behavioral clues appears to be limited to between three and six levels of pain (Hardie, 2000).

Thus, in deciding how to dispose of a sick animal, the farm manager needs to consider not only the economic implications but also the animal's welfare. Too often, particularly in the past, economics and the person's aversion to perform euthanasia have been the primary deciding factors, to the detriment of the animal's welfare. Animals that are unable to walk or fend for themselves, or that are sick, have not responded to treatment, and are unlikely to recover, should be euthanatized on the farm rather than sent to slaughter or market. Compromised animals should not be penned in trucks or vehicles with normal animals and their individual needs for transport should be addressed. The positions of the American Veterinary Medical Association and the Canadian Veterinary Medical Association on disabled farm animals are detailed in the appendix.

THE NEED FOR SPECIFIC CRITERIA FOR EUTHANASIA

Unlike the companion animal literature, which contains much discussion and many suggested guidelines on the appropriateness and timing for euthanasia, farm animal literature holds little discussion and few guidelines for when a farm animal should be euthanatized. Many of the companion animal guidelines are very subjective (e.g., ability to enjoy food, ability to breathe freely and without difficulty, ability to eat and drink without pain, ability to respond to owner and family), but when taken together are helpful in creating a euthanasia profile. Other guidelines are more objective. Duncan (1988) recommends that companion animals should be euthanatized if they have:

- *Weight loss:* 20–25 percent of total body weight, characterized by muscle wasting
- *Extreme weakness/inability:* no desire to eat or drink, persisting for 24 hours or more
- *Moribund state:* depression and body temperature below 99°F (37°C)
- *Infection:* involving one or more organ systems, which fails to respond to treatment within an appropriate amount of time
- *Respiratory/cardiovascular:* failure of these systems, including blood loss or anemia resulting in a hematocrit below 20 percent
- *Nervous/musculoskeletal:* injuries that cannot be healed, resulting in uncontrolled seizures or the loss of a limb

These guidelines could be adapted for farm animals. For example, the following general guidelines could apply to pigs of any weight or age:

- Weight loss of 20–25 percent of total body weight, characterized by muscle wasting
- Extreme weakness or inability with a lack of desire to eat or drink, persisting for 24 hours or more
- Suffering from any infection/disease that fails to respond to treatment

Adhering to these guidelines would ensure that pigs with broken legs, unresolved prolapses, or lameness that prevents the animal from walking unassisted would be promptly euthanatized.

In addition, some farming systems have adopted specific protocols to help managers cope with the difficult decision on what to euthanatize and what to keep. For example, the "two-strike" system (Roberts, 2002) has two criteria that must be fulfilled before a weaner pig is euthanatized:

- Underweight (e.g., less that 8 lb on a farm with 18-day weaning)

and

- Has a disability such as a rupture, or navel ill, or lameness, or poor body condition

This introduces a special category of concern for pork producers, the lightweight pig. Since the work of England (England, 1974), it has been long accepted that lightweight piglets at birth are lightweight at weaning. Lightweight pigs at weaning remain small and are a significant contributor to the variation in slaughter weight and, as such, a major problem in assembling slaughter loads. In three-site production where the system rewards nursery managers for dispatching more pigs, there tends to be more pigs shipped than there should be. Consequently, finishing managers struggle with the issue of how to handle the underweight/disadvantaged pigs they are shipped.

Given the economic incentives to produce and deliver similarly sized "cookie-cutter" type pigs to slaughter, various techniques have been pursued to improve the profitability of lightweight pigs. Some have concluded that it is cheaper to euthanatize them as soon as they are identified; others have advocated special treatment including penning by size, special accommodations, and special diets including liquid diets (Azain, Jones, and Glaze, 1998; Azain et al., 1994).

Additional benefits from euthanatizing lightweight pigs may arise if they are, in fact, asymptomatic carriers of disease. While this hypothesis is difficult to prove, some researchers are reporting extra mortality that cannot be explained simply by the fact that the mortality of light pigs is greater (Deen, 2002). A much higher mortality in nurseries is being observed as the proportion of weaned lightweight pigs increases. This has major implications if it is true because it is a further economic incentive to euthanatize the lightweight pigs. Euthanatizing the lightweight pigs could decrease the risk of infecting other members of their cohort, and, more important from the public health perspective, may decrease the risk of infecting those who care and work with them or consume them from possible zoonotic diseases they may carry (e.g., salmonellosis).

The advantages of culling the lightweights include:

* Increased floor space for the remaining pigs
* A market for the lightweights, such as the barbecue market in the Southeast
* An increase in the throughput (turns) for the building
* A decrease in the risk of disease transmission

The additional advantages for euthanatizing the lightweights include

* Avoidance of the antibiotic residue problem
* No need for special housing or handling
* No mixing problems post accumulation
* No marketing issues
* No biosecurity risk from cull trucks picking up lightweights from multiple farms

The challenge with regard to euthanasia in the steady-state production operation will be to better understand the relative painfulness and discomfort associated with the range of common conditions; to define and validate specific criteria for when to treat, cull, or euthanatize individual animals; and to effectively communicate this information to managers so they can better care for their animals. Development of a pain rating scale, validated for species-specific behaviors, which forces treatment when a certain score is reached (Hardie, 2000), may be the most accurate method of assuring prompt treatment in the production farm setting.

EUTHANASIA IN THE FACE OF A FOREIGN ANIMAL DISEASE OUTBREAK

The outbreak of foot-and-mouth disease (FMD) in the United Kingdom (UK) and Europe in 2001 illustrates the distinction between euthanasia as performed under the steady-state conditions of normal farming and the conditions that would prevail under an emergency such as the outbreak of a foreign animal disease.

The 2000 report of the AVMA panel on euthanasia states that "under unusual conditions, such as disease eradication and natural disasters, euthanasia options may be limited. In these situations, the most appropriate technique that minimizes human and animal health concerns must be used. These options include, but are not limited to, carbon dioxide and physical methods such as gunshot, penetrating captive bolt, and cervical dislocation" (Beaver et al., 2001).

In the case of FMD, infected animals are to be humanely killed and disposed of within 24 hours of diagnosis to limit viral replication and subsequent disease spread, and all susceptible animals on adjacent farms within a specified radius are to be humanely killed and disposed of within 48 hours (Ferguson, Donnelly, and Anderson, 2001). Animals identified for slaughter during the FMD outbreak in the UK were euthanatized by government-licensed slaughter teams, each of which included at least one veterinarian, using a combination of accepted humane methods, including captive bolt, gunshot to the brain, and lethal injection.

The Department for the Environment, Food, and Rural Affairs (DEFRA) failed to achieve the recommended goals for timely euthanasia of infected and susceptible animals. If there had been no delays (within 24 hours) in slaughter of animals on infected premises, the epidemic could have been reduced by 40 percent (Ferguson et al., 2001). Further, if animals on contiguous farms had been euthanatized within 48 hours, then the epidemic could have been reduced by 66 percent (Ferguson et al., 2001). Clearly, timely euthanasia would likely have greatly limited the spread of the disease and the period the country was designated as non-FMD disease free.

According to DEFRA, 4,189,000 animals were killed during the 2001–2002 UK foot-and-mouth outbreak (DEFRA, 2002), with an average of 10,000–12,000 animals being euthanatized each day of the outbreak. As sobering as these numbers are, the potential situation for the United States in the event of an outbreak of a foreign animal disease is much, much worse due to greater numbers of animals and extensive interstate animal movement. North Carolina alone has nearly 9,000,000 pigs in production. At a slaughter rate of 12,000 animals per day, it would take nearly two years just to depopulate the pigs currently in production, without taking into account infected ruminants or wildlife. The economic effect of a FAD outbreak in the United States would be devastating. Economists have estimated that the direct costs of an FMD outbreak could reach $10 billion in the first year with indirect costs ten times that amount (Morrow, 2001).

The methods of euthanasia used in the UK FMD outbreak would be difficult to apply in the United States, especially to large numbers of swine. Captive bolt, gunshot, and lethal injection each require that each animal be handled and restrained, and that operators are properly trained in the correct application of each technique. Given that large swine operations commonly have a thousand or more animals in each building and very few animal workers, handling individual animals would greatly slow the euthanasia process and increase the potential for viral replication and spread. Worker safety, as well as emotional trauma, would be significant issues. Clearly, faster, less labor intensive, but equally humane euthanasia methods would be required if the goals of humane slaughter and timely disposal were to be met in the event of an FMD or other foreign animal disease outbreak in the United States. Preliminary studies conducted by the authors in collaboration with the North Carolina swine industry have demonstrated the feasibility of applying the current AVMA guidelines for carbon dioxide euthanasia to adult pigs contained within a dump truck; much work, however, remains to validate and develop this method for widespread on-farm use in an FAD outbreak.

The challenge with regard to euthanasia for an FAD outbreak will be for the agricultural animal industry, USDA, and the individual states to proactively develop suitable guidelines and strategies for rapid and humane euthanasia of unprecedented numbers of animals. Taking a page from the UK experience, veterinarians should be involved in all stages of the planning and implementation process. Without such planning, it would be all too easy for those more concerned with expediency to apply inhumane killing techniques at the expense of animal welfare (e.g., suffocation of confined animals by closing up buildings; pumping carbon monoxide into buildings directly from the exhaust pipes of gasoline engines; indiscriminate mass shootings rather than precisely placed single gunshot to the brain). It is unrealistic in this day and age to expect the slaughter of vast numbers of animals during an FAD action to occur without public awareness of the processes involved. By employing the most humane euthanasia methods possible under the circumstances, the agricultural animal industry can publicly demonstrate its commitment to animal welfare.

SUMMARY OF CHALLENGES

A significant challenge for improving farm animal welfare will be for agricultural researchers and the animal production industry to develop humane euthanasia methods that are more acceptable to the individuals charged with performing the euthanasia task. To this end, more research will be required on the effect of the euthanasia process on the farmworker as well as toward the implementation of novel humane methods. Given that we are limited to direct neuronal depression, disruption of brain activity, and hypoxia to produce humane death, it is unrealistic to think that substantially different euthanasia methods are forthcoming. Rather, the task will be to refine existing euthanasia methods in more acceptable ways such that farmworker stress and discomfort are reduced. An example of this is the substitution of carbon dioxide hypoxia for a blow to the head for euthanasia of lightweight or compromised weanling pigs (Morrow and Meyer, 2001). Other challenges will be in educating farmworkers in the role euthanasia plays in good husbandry practice and in validating behavioral assessment scales for farm managers to determine when to treat, cull, or euthanatize the compromised animal. Development of humane methods suitable for timely euthanasia of unprecedented numbers of animals in the face of an FAD outbreak is urgently needed, both to limit spread of disease as well as to proactively address the public's concern for the humane treatment of farm animals.

REFERENCES

Arluke A. 1999. Uneasiness among laboratory technicians. *Occupational Medicine* 14:305–316.
Azain MJ, Arentson RA, Tomkins T, Sowinski JS. 1994. The effect of pelleted or liquid diets on performance of pigs weaned at 7 to 10 days of age. *Journal of Animal Science* 72(Suppl 1):215.

Azain MJ, Jones R, Glaze T. 1998. Management of lightweight pigs. Annual report, pp. 164–167, University of Georgia, Athens.

Beaver BV, Reed W, Leary S, et al. 2001. 2000 Report of the AVMA Panel on Euthanasia. *Journal of the American Veterinary Medical Association* 218:669–696.

Conzemius MG, Hill CM, Sammarco JL, Perowski SZ. 1997. Correlation between subjective and objective measures to determine severity of postoperative pain in dogs. *Journal of the American Veterinary Medical Association* 210:210–222.

Deen J. 2002. *International Pigletter,* March 22(1).

Department for Environment, Food, and Rural Affairs (DEFRA). 2002. Statistics on Foot and Mouth Disease. http://www.defra.gov.uk/animalh/diseases/fmd/cases/statistics/generalstats.asp. Accessed 5/8/2002.

Dobromylskyj P, Flecknell PA, Lascelles BD, et al. 2000. Pain assessment. In *Pain Management in Animals*, edited by PA Flecknell and A Waterman-Pearson. London: W.B. Saunders.

Duncan JC. 1988. *Careers in Veterinary Medicine*. New York: Rosen Publishing Group.

Ellis BJ. 1993. *Paws for Thought: A Look at the Conflicts, Questions, and Challenges of Animal Euthanasia*. Columbia, SC: Pawprint Press.

England DC. 1974. Husbandry components in prenatal and perinatal development in swine. *Journal of Animal Science* 38:1045–1049.

Ferguson NM, Donnelly CA, Anderson RM. 2001. Transmission intensity and impact of control policies on the foot and mouth epidemic in Great Britain. *Nature* Oct 4; 413(6855):542–548.

Flecknell PA. 1996. *Laboratory Animal Anaesthesia*, 2nd ed. London: Academic Press.

Fogle B, Abrahamson D. 1990. Pet loss: A survey of the attitudes and feelings of practicing veterinarians. *Anthrozoos* 3:143–150.

Hardie EM. 2000. Recognition of pain behaviour in animals. In *Animal Pain. A Practice-oriented Approach to an Effective Pain Control in Animals*, edited by LJ Hellebrekers. Utrecht: Van der Wees Uitgeverij.

Humane Society of the United States (HSUS). 1992. Pet Overpopulation Fact Sheet. Washington, DC: The Humane Society of the United States.

Kliebenstein J, Hurley T, Orazem P. 1996. Personnel Management Issues and Job Satisfaction in Pork Production. Swine Extension Educators Conference, Des Moines, IA.

Kogure N, Yamazaki K. 1990. Attitudes to animal euthanasia in Japan: A brief review of cultural influences. *Anthrozoos* 3:151–154.

Massachusetts Society for the Prevention of Cruelty to Animals (MSPCA). 1987. *Stop Pet Overpopulation*. Boston: Massachusetts Society for the Prevention of Cruelty to Animals.

Matthis S. 2002. Unpublished research, personal communication to the authors. North Carolina State University, Raleigh.

McGrath PJ, Unruh AM. 1989. *Pain in Children and Adolescents*. Amsterdam: Elsevier.

Morrow WEM. 1999. Euthanasia hazards. *Occupational Medicine* 14:235–246.

——. 2001. Foot-and-Mouth Disease Facts. http://mark.asci.ncsu.edu/Swine_News/2001/sn_v2403.htm. Accessed 5/8/2002.

Morrow WEM, Meyer RE. 2001. *On-Farm Euthanasia: Better Ways*. Raleigh: North Carolina State University College of Veterinary Medicine Biomedical Communications.

National Pork Producers Council (NPPC). 1997. *On Farm Euthanasia of Swine—Options for the Producer*. Publication #04259–4/97. Des Moines, IA: National Pork Producers Council.

Roberts J. 2002. Personal communication to the authors. North Carolina State University, Raleigh.

Rollin B. 1986. Euthanasia and moral stress. In: *Loss, Grief and Care*, R. DeBellis, ed. Binghamton, NY: Haworth Press.

Rollin BE. 1995. *Farm Animal Welfare: Social, Bioethical, and Research Issues*. Ames: Iowa State University Press.

Troeger K, Waltersdorf W. 1991. Gas anaesthesia of slaughter pigs. *Fleischwirtsch Int.* 4:43–49.

White DJ, Shawhan R. 1996. Emotional responses of animal shelter workers to euthanasia. *Journal of the American Veterinary Medical Association* 208:846–849.

Wolfe T. 1985. Laboratory animal technicians: Their role in stress reduction and human companion animal bonding. *Veterinary Clinics of North America Small Animal Practitioner* 15:449–454.

Appendix

U.S. and Canadian Veterinary Medical Associations' Positions on Food Animals

AMERICAN VETERINARY MEDICAL ASSOCIATION
GENERAL POSITION ON FOOD ANIMALS

Disabled Livestock: The AVMA recommends that disabled livestock be handled humanely in all situations.

If an animal is down on the farm:

- If the animal is in extreme distress or the condition is obviously irreversible, the animal should be moved humanely and directly to a state or federally inspected slaughter plant, slaughtered on the farm if possible (with appropriate precautions taken to maintain the safety of the food product), or immediately and humanely euthanatized.
- If the animal is not in extreme distress and continues to eat and drink, the producer should contact a veterinarian for assistance and provide food, water, and appropriate shelter and nursing care to keep the animal comfortable.
- If the condition involves a recent injury to a healthy animal, the animal should be shipped directly to a state or federally inspected slaughter plant or slaughtered on the farm (where state laws permit).
- Nonambulatory animals should never be sent through intermediate marketing channels. They should be euthanatized or shipped directly to a state or federally inspected slaughter plant.

If an animal is down at the market:

- If the animal is in extreme distress or the condition is obviously irreversible, the animal should be moved humanely and directly to a state or federally inspected slaughter plant or immediately and humanely euthanatized. If immediate euthanasia is not possible, pain relief should be provided in the interim before euthanasia.

See: http://www.avma.org/care4pets/polfood.htm(accessed 5/08/2002).

CANADIAN VETERINARY MEDICAL ASSOCIATION POSITION ON DISABLED LIVESTOCK

Animal Welfare Position Statements: Nonambulatory Animals

Definition: A nonambulatory animal is defined as an animal that is unable to stand and walk without assistance.

Position: The Canadian Veterinary Medical Association (CVMA) recommends that nonambulatory livestock only be transported to a processing facility if the following criteria are met:

1. A veterinary inspection of the nonambulatory animal has been performed on the premises of origin, and this inspection certifies that the animal has passed an ante mortem, preslaughter inspection;

2. the loading and transportation of the nonambulatory animal is performed in a manner to avoid pain, suffering, and distress to the animal; and

3. upon arrival at the processing facility, the animal is humanely stunned or euthanized on the vehicle prior to unloading. The processing facility must be properly equipped to perform these procedures.

Background: The humane handling of the nonambulatory animal is a major concern for all parties involved. A number of factors will influence the decision as to the proper and humane handling of the nonambulatory animal. These factors include the size and weight of the animal, its condition, the reason for its nonambulant state, the animal's location, proximity to destination, and the availability of proper loading and conveying equipment, along with qualified attending personnel.

A nonambulatory animal must not be moved prior to a veterinary inspection on the premises of origin. A diagnosis and prognosis are a prerequisite for making a decision regarding the further handling of the animal. If the animal/carcass is to be moved to a processing facility, it must be accompanied by an ante-mortem veterinary certificate. This certificate must state the diagnosis; a statement that the animal can or cannot be humanely loaded; a statement that the animal is fit for slaughter; and a statement that the owner has observed all applicable withdrawal times for drugs used.

Nonambulatory animals that are deemed unfit for slaughter should be humanely euthanized on location and the carcass disposed of in accordance with local regulations.

In those situations where the nonambulatory animal is deemed to be fit for slaughter, but where the veterinarian's opinion is that loading and transportation is deemed to be inhumane, on-farm slaughter is recommended. The carcass may be used for private consumption, or, in jurisdictions where permissible, the carcass can be taken to a processing facility for dressing and postmortem inspection.

Education of the producer in the prevention, proper care and handling, and the humane disposition of the nonambulatory animal is a major responsibility for the veterinarian. (November 2000)

See: http://www.cvma-acmv.org/welfare1.asp?subcat=Priorities&num=18(accessed 5/08/2002).

Index